# Aspects of
# Neuroendocrinology

*V. International*
*Symposium on Neurosecretion*

August 20th — 23rd, 1969, Kiel

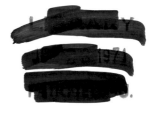

Edited by

## W. Bargmann and B. Scharrer

With 145 Figures

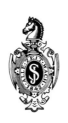

Springer-Verlag Berlin · Heidelberg · New York 1970

© by Springer-Verlag Berlin · Heidelberg 1970
Printed in Germany
Library of Congress Catalogue Card Number 76–135967
Universitätsdruckerei H. Stürtz AG, Würzburg

Title-No. 1698

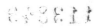

# Vorwort

Der hiermit vorgelegte Band enthält die Mehrzahl der Vorträge, die im August 1969 auf dem V. Internationalen Symposium über Neurosekretion im Anatomischen Institut der Universität Kiel unter reger internationaler Beteiligung gehalten wurden. Folgende Hauptthemen wurden behandelt:

1. Neurosecretion in invertebrates,
2. Adrenergic neurons,
3. Mechanisms of release of neurohypophyseal materials,
4. Hypothalamic control of anterior pituitary.

Weitere Kurzvorträge waren verschiedenen Problemen der Neurosekretion gewidmet.

Das Internationale Komitee für die Vorbereitung des Symposiums, dem außer den Unterzeichneten die Herren Professoren H. S. HELLER (Bristol), G. STERBA (Leipzig) und FR. STUTINSKY (Strasbourg) angehörten, dankt dem Springer-Verlag für die Sorgfalt, die er dieser Publikation wiederum angedeihen ließ, dem Kultusministerium des Landes Schleswig-Holstein für materielle Förderung des Symposiums und Fräulein Dr. B. VON GAUDECKER (Kiel) für redaktionelle Unterstützung.

W. BARGMANN (Kiel)                    B. SCHARRER (New York)

# Contents

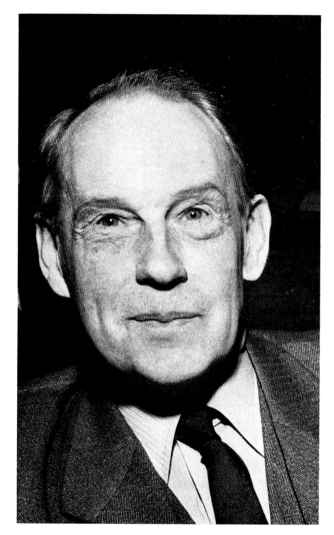

BERTIL HANSTRÖM 1891—1969

# Opening Remarks

W. Bargmann

Anatomisches Institut der Neuen Universität Kiel

Meine Damen und Herren!

Im Namen des Internationalen Komitees, das die Vorbereitung dieses 5. Symposions über Neurosekretion übernommen hat, und zugleich als Hausherr begrüße ich Sie alle sehr herzlich im Kieler Anatomischen Institut. Zugleich danke ich Ihnen im Namen des Rektors unserer mehr als dreihundert Jahre alten Christiana Albertina, daß Sie die nördlichste deutsche Universität mit Ihrem Besuch beehren, im besonderen das Anatomische Institut, an dem einst die Anatomen FLEMMING, Graf SPEE, v. MÖLLENDORFF und BENNINGHOFF lehrten. Am Rande sei zu Ihrer Information bemerkt, daß dieses Gebäude, in dem wir uns befinden, ursprünglich kein Anatomisches Institut war, sondern eines der wenigen Fabrikgebäude in Kiel, die der Zerstörung im 2. Weltkrieg entkamen und daher in ein Universitätsinstitut umgewandelt werden konnten. Professor HELLER, der unsere Universität als einer der ersten Kollegen aus dem Ausland nach dem Krieg besuchte, war ein hilfreicher Zeuge unserer damaligen Bemühungen um den Wiederaufbau der Kieler Universität. Ich freue mich daher auch aus diesem Grunde, ihn heute in diesem Hörsaal begrüßen zu können.

Eine Reihe von Kollegen hat zu unserem Bedauern aus schwerwiegenden persönlichen oder aus organisatorischen Gründen von einer Teilnahme an diesem Symposion absehen müssen und mich gebeten, Ihnen Grüße zu übermitteln, nämlich Dr. ANNICA DAHLSTRÖM (Göteborg), Mme. HERLANT-MEEWIS und Professor MARC HERLANT (Brüssel), Professor LEGAIT (Nancy), Dr. STETSON (Seattle) und aus den sozialistischen Ländern die Kollegen Prof. AKMAYEV (Moskau), die Prof. GERSCH (Jena), JASINSKI (Krakau) und POLENOV (Leningrad).

Unter denen, die unserer Tagung noch vor wenigen Wochen einen guten Verlauf gewünscht haben, befindet sich auch ein alter Freund, der inzwischen Abschied von dieser Welt genommen hat. BERTIL HANSTRÖM, einer der Pioniere auf dem Gebiete der Neurosekretionsforschung, verstarb am 17. Juli 1969 im Alter von 77 Jahren. Die Neuroendokrinologie verdankt ihm u.a. einen großen Überblick über die hormonal aktiven Elemente im Nervensystem von Invertebraten und Vertebraten und ihm wie ERNST und BERTA SCHARRER die fruchtbare Konzeption, wonach neurohormonale Systeme verschiedener funktioneller Bedeutung bei nicht miteinander verwandten Tierformen nach dem gleichen Prinzip organisiert sind, d.h. sich in Produktionsstätten von Wirkstoffen, Transportwege und Organe der Stapelung und Ausschüttung gliedern. Ein Thema, dessen Bedeutung BERTIL HANSTRÖM in der ,,Introduction'' unterstrich, mit der er als charmanter Gastgeber das 2. Internationale Symposion über Neurosekretion in Lund 1957 eröffnete.

Die Themen der Vorträge unseres Kieler Symposions, deren Veröffentlichung
dem Andenken BERTIL HANSTRÖMs gewidmet sein wird, gruppieren sich um *main
topics*, deren Bedeutung bereits auf dem Strasbourger Symposion des Jahres 1966
hervorgehoben wurde, das unter der Leitung unseres verdienten Kollegen FRED
STUTINSKY einen so harmonischen Verlauf nahm. Zunächst ein Wort über das
Thema „Current problems in invertebrate neurosecretion", das Professor BERTA
SCHARRER und Dr. MARY WEITZMAN in einem Überblick behandeln werden. Von
ihrer Erforschung sind nicht nur wichtige Einblicke in die Regulation biologischer
Prozesse bei Wirbellosen zu erwarten, die den Untersucher als solche faszinieren.
Die Aufdeckung neuroendokriner Mechanismen und ihrer morphologischen Grundlagen bei Wirbellosen kann den Blick für gleichartige bzw. ähnliche Phänomene
bei Vertebraten schärfen und unter Umständen dazu beitragen, biologische Grund-
fragen zu beantworten, wenn man sich der geeigneten Species bedient. So sei, um
ein Beispiel zu nennen, in einem Intermezzo an die Diskussion über die submikroskopischen Grundlagen der Speicherung und des Transportes von Neurohormonen
erinnert:

Sir FRANCIS KNOWLES in his studies on the crustacean *Squilla mantis* (1960)
has found neurosecretory vesicles of varying submicroscopical structure, one of
which displays crystalline order, while I and B. v. GAUDECKER (1969) described
neurosecretory elementary granules with crystalloid ultrastructure in mammals.
These granules are related to other more conventional forms by transitional structures so that it is impossible to separate two distinct classes of granules.

We interpret the crystalline pattern as attributable to carrier protein, namely
neurophysin. Further analysis of the data of KNOWLES in comparison with our
own promise to contribute to the understanding of neurosecretory granules in
invertebrates especially in reference to the question if the latter contain carrier
protein of the neurophysin type.

In Strasbourg wurde auch die Frage erörtert, ob die Neurosekretionisten noch
immer auf dem rechten Wege sind, wenn sie die adrenergen Neurone nicht in die
Gruppe der neurosekretorischen Zellen einbeziehen. Wir bedauern außerordentlich,
daß Dr. ANNICA DAHLSTRÖM wegen Erkrankung nicht imstande ist, ihr Referat
über „Adrenergic neurons" zu halten und uns so erneut Gelegenheit zu geben, die
Gültigkeit klassischer Vorstellungen anhand neuer Befunde zu prüfen. Dieses
Thema steht in innerem Zusammenhang mit dem aktuellen, auch klinisch wich-
tigen Problem der hypothalamischen Kontrolle des Hypophysenvorderlappens,
über die Dr. SCHNEIDER (Dallas) und Dr. FUXE und Dr. HÖKFELT (Stockholm)
berichten werden.

Eine Fortsetzung der Strasbourger Diskussion stellen auch die Vorträge über
den — oder die ? — Mechanismen des release neurohypophysärer Hormone dar,
über die Dr. THORN (Kopenhagen) in einem einleitenden Referat sprechen wird.
Auch und gerade dieses Thema zeigt, daß sich die Forscher, die sich mit den Fragen
der Neurosekretion befassen, auf einem Grenzgebiet zwischen Endokrinologie,
Neurophysiologie und Pharmakologie befinden.

I should like to take this opportunity to say a word of thanks to Dr. MARY
WEITZMAN for making it easier for all of us to keep up with the increasing amounts
of literature in neurosecretion and related subjects by her painstaking and excellent efforts in preparing „Bibliographia Neuroendocrinologica". Dieser Titel

unterstreicht die Tatsache, daß die Probleme der Neurosekretionsforschung, denen unser schon zur Tradition gewordenes Symposium sich seit der Neapler Tagung widmet, nicht isoliert gesehen und untersucht werden können, sie sind in der Tat Probleme der *Neuroendokrinologie*.

Es entspräche den internationalen Gepflogenheiten, wenn ich diese kurzen Bemerkungen nun auch in anderen Sprachen vortragen würde. Der Reichtum unseres Programms veranlaßt mich jedoch zu der Bitte, mit diesen kurzen Ausführungen vorlieb zu nehmen und mich das 5. Internationale Symposion über Neurosekretion mit den Worten eröffnen zu lassen: Thanks for coming, Welcome in the Kiel Department of Anatomy, Soyez les bienvenues — Herzlich willkommen!

# Neurosecretion in Invertebrates

## Current Problems in Invertebrate Neurosecretion*

Berta Scharrer and Mary Weitzman

Department of Anatomy, Albert Einstein College of Medicine, Bronx, N.Y. 10461 (USA)

### Introduction

In the course of years, a broad comparative approach to the study of neuro-secretory phenomena has proved not only rewarding but mandatory. Much insight continues to be gained from the analysis of relatively simple systems. A valid definition of the very concept of neurosecretion requires a comprehensive spectrum of information, including that on the phylogenetic origin of neuroglandular activity. Ideally, therefore, progress in this field should be viewed along its entire front. The line drawn between invertebrates and vertebrates for purposes of the present survey must not be interpreted as an indication of fundamental disparities between the two groups. In fact, an outline of current problems in invertebrate neurosecretion might well serve as a general introduction to this Symposium. As will become apparent, these problems include the elucidation of the neuronal and glandular attributes of neurosecretory neurons, properties of afferent control mechanisms, the chemical nature and mode of release of neurosecretory mediators, the extraneuronal pathways by which they reach their sites of operation, and the manner in which these messengers control their effector cells.

In terms of sheer quantity, the reports on invertebrate neurosecretion available in the current literature exceed by far the framework of this survey. A cursory look at the material published since the last Symposium indicates that much of it serves to substantiate previously existing information. Valuable as they are, such studies need not be given primary consideration here. Rather, our selection will focus on those recent contributions that represent new approaches to the analysis of the phenomenon of neurosecretion in general, and that will set the course for future investigation.

If the list of references selected is by necessity incomplete, it is hoped that it may nevertheless serve as a guideline to topics of major current interest. It should be understood that a publication cited in the text does not necessarily represent the only documentation of a given statement, and often not the first that appeared in print. (For general orientation the following references may be useful: Bern and Hagadorn, 1965; Bern and Knowles, 1966; Gabe, 1966; Hagadorn, 1967a, b.)

### Methodology

The analysis of neurosecretory centers in invertebrates, as in higher forms, depends on the combined application and evaluation of morphological, physiological, and biochemical methods.

A recent addition in light microscopy is the bulk staining technique which, especially among small invertebrates, permits the visualization of entire neurosecretory systems in whole

* Supported by grant NB-00840 from the U.S.P.H.S.

mounts rather than serial sections. The use of mixtures that demonstrate the cysteine and/or cystine components of neurosecretory material reveals certain details; for example, its presence in dendritic branches arising from initial processes of neurosecretory perikarya in the pars intercerebralis of insects (Adiyodi and Bern, 1968; Dogra, 1968).

The histochemical approach has proved especially successful in the application of highly specific fluorescence methods, in particular the pseudoisocyanine method of Schiebler and Sterba (Sakharov et al., 1965; Gaude and Weber, 1966; Bassurmanova and Panov, 1967), and the formaldehyde condensation reaction for biogenic amines developed by Hillarp and his coworkers (Frontali, 1968; Chanussot et al., 1969; and others). The characterization of various types of neurosecretory neurons by other (e.g. enzyme-histochemical) methods is being carried out in various invertebrate species (Schreiner, 1966; Vigh-Teichmann and Goslar, 1968; Tewari and Awasthi, 1968).

At the electron microscopic level, attention is being paid to the conditions of tissue preparation and their relative value for obtaining reproducible results. A pertinent example are the guidelines contributed by Hökfelt (1968) and others for the identification of aminergic neurosecretory elements (B fibers of Knowles, 1965). These seem to apply also to invertebrate material, but studies in this direction have only barely begun (Mancini and Frontali, 1970).

Measurements of nucleolar, nuclear, and cellular diameters, and estimations of the amounts of stainable material in perikarya and axons of neurosecretory neurons are useful in establishing morphological criteria for "active" versus "inactive" states (Rensing, 1964; Bloch et al., 1966; Panov, 1967; Vitz, 1967; E. Thomsen and Lea, 1969).

Classical physiological methods, such as extirpation and reimplantation of tissues, preparation of active extracts, organ culture, etc. (Schaller and Meunier, 1967; Gianfelici, 1968), are still in use in the investigation of neurohormones. Among recent additions are attempts to effect the release of neurosecretory substances from neurohemal storage centers, *in vivo* or *in vitro*, by electrical stimulation of nerves known to control such release (Bunt and Ashby, 1968; Gosbee et al., 1968; Kater, 1968; Normann, 1969).

Increasingly sophisticated biochemical methods have been adapted for the determination of the chemical constitution of the active principles furnished by neurosecretory centers of invertebrates, a task that is rather tedious because of the smallness of the source. Among those used with success are gel-filtration on Sephadex (Ishizaki and Ichikawa, 1967; Gersch and Stürzebecher, 1968); density gradient centrifugation (Bartell et al., 1968); enzymatic digestion (Brown, 1965), and incorporation studies by means of administration of radioactive precursors such as $^{35}$S-cysteine (Mordue and Goldsworthy, 1969) or $^3$H-uridine (Nolte and Kuhlmann, 1966).

## Occurrence and Characterization of Neurosecretory Neurons

Many detailed and comprehensive studies in recent years have strengthened the thesis that neurosecretory neurons and organ systems occur in all multicellular animals including coelenterates (Hanström, 1965; Davey, 1966; Gabe, 1966; Simpson et al., 1966; Davey and Breckenridge, 1967; Davis et al., 1968; Lentz, 1968; Joly and Descamps, 1968; Heurtault, 1969; M. Thomsen, 1969) (see Figs. 1—4). New and varied information has modulated our views on what features all neurosecretory neurons have in common, in contradistinction to those of conventional neurons. Some of the criteria once thought to be essential have to be abandoned or modified, since they no longer generally apply, whereas other features emerge into sharper focus than before.

The most pertinent characteristic is that neurosecretory neurons engage in the production of specific neurochemical mediators to such a degree that here, and here alone, glandular activity outweighs all other neuronal attributes. Another point, likewise supported by recent invertebrate data, is that not all of the existing neurosecretory messengers act in a neurohormonal capacity, but instead may be

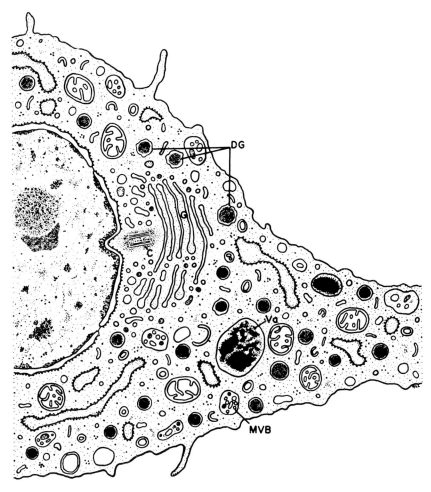

Fig. 1. Large granule-containing cell with processes in mesenchyme of the sponge *Sycon*. The membrane-bounded granular material is of medium electron-density (*DG*); the diameters range from 1,100 to 1,700 Å. *G* Golgi apparatus; *MVB* multivesicular bodies; *Va* phagocytic vacuole; *C* centriole. (From LENTZ, 1968)

effective over very short distances. In brief, such versatility seems plausible in a group of animals so much more varied than the vertebrates. In contrast to the latter, the more primitive forms also show a relatively larger proportion of their nervous systems to be taken up by neurosecretory cells. New sites of neurosecretory activity are being added to the roster of known centers at several levels of invertebrate organization. Examples are the perisympathetic organs (RAABE, 1965, 1967; DE BESSÉ, 1967; GRILLOT, 1968; PROVANSAL, 1968), and the peripheral neurosecretory cell groups in insects (FINLAYSON and OSBORNE, 1968). Furthermore, possible neuroendocrine organ systems analogous to those in arthropods, have recently been discovered among polychetes (BASKIN and GOLDING, 1968; GOLDING et al., 1968).

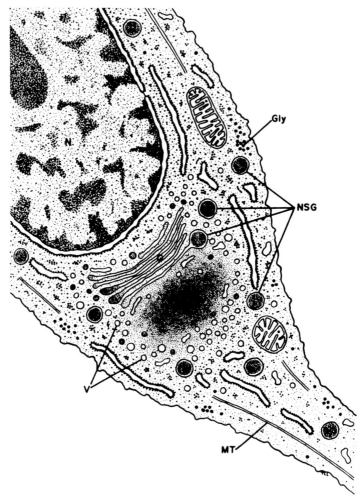

Fig. 2. Neurosecretory cell of *Hydra*. Membrane-bounded granules of moderate density (*NSG*) seem to originate within Golgi cisternae (*G*). *V* small vesicles; *MT* microtubules; *Gly* glycogen; *N* nucleus. (From Lentz, 1968)

## Types of Neurosecretory Cells

Morphological, biochemical, and functional criteria are combined in distinguishing several classes of neurosecretory neurons. Our knowledge about them is still too incomplete for the determination of homologous cell types among various species. Therefore, more or less temporary and neutral designations, such as by capital letters (A, B, C . . ., P, Q, etc.), or Roman numerals (I—XIII) are currently in use. More or less detailed surveys are available for individual representatives of insects (Raabe, 1965, 1967; Girardie, 1967; Fletcher, 1969), crustaceans (Szudarski, 1963), annelids (Gersch and Wohlrabe, 1965; Herlant-Meewis, 1966), nemerteans (Bianchi, 1969), and molluscs (Wautier *et al.*, 1961; Simpson *et al.*, 1966; Schmekel and Wechsler, 1968).

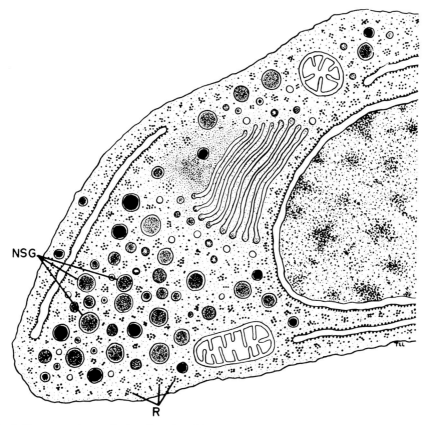

Fig. 3. Neurosecretory cell of a planarian. Note numerous large membrane-bounded granules of varying electron density (*NSG*). The Golgi cisternae contain electron-dense material in peripheral location from which small vesicles with comparable content seem to be derived. *R* free ribosomes. (From LENTZ, 1968)

It is also often difficult to identify in the electron microscope a cell type known by its light microscopic properties. An exceptionally favorable material in this regard is the oligochete *Enchytraeus albidus* with its paired Q cells, whose secretory cycle can be manipulated and correlated with changes in their ultrastructural appearance (UDE and GERSCH, 1968). Similar studies along these lines in insects were made by BASSURMANOVA and PANOV (1967), and RAMADE (1969), and in molluscs by SAKHAROV et al. (1965).

Whereas the ultrastructural appearance of classical neurosecretory granules and their mode of formation are well established (see, for example, GIRARDIE and GIRARDIE, 1967; BOER et al., 1968; DHAINAUT-COURTOIS, 1968; NEWMAN et al., 1968; SCHMEKEL and WECHSLER, 1968), those of aminergic neurosecretory elements are only beginning to be recognized. In current efforts to correlate subcellular appearance with cytochemical and neuropharmacological information, the wide variety of available invertebrate material may provide favorable model systems.

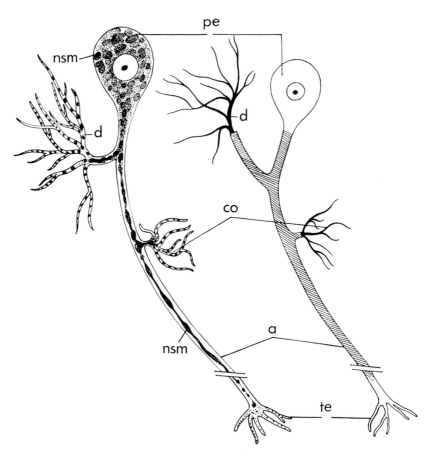

Fig. 4. Diagram of a neurosecretory neuron in the pars intercerebralis of the insect *Periplaneta* (left) and a typical invertebrate neuron of the conventional type (right). *a* axons; *co* collaterals; *d* dendrites; *nsm* neurosecretory material; *pe* perikarya; *te* terminals. (From Adiyodi and Bern, 1968)

## Chemical Properties

Histochemically, the proteinaceous nature of most neurosecretory products of invertebrates seems beyond doubt. Aside from carrier proteins (neurophysins), classical ("peptidergic", aldehyde fuchsin-positive, A-type) neurosecretory neurons elaborate active polypeptides that are rich in cysteine or cystine (Schreiner, 1966; Dogra, 1968; Adiyodi and Bern, 1968). The presence of disulfide and sulfhydryl groupings is responsible for several histochemical reactions used for the demonstration of this material (Busselet, 1968; Zimmermann, 1968).

However, the demonstration of cysteine in itself does not permit conclusions as to whether or not this substance or at least part of it may be a component of the carrier protein. For example, in experiments by Mordue and Goldsworthy (1969) the injection of $^{35}$S-cysteine in insects yielded little radioactivity in the physiologically active fractions and most of it appeared in the protein presumed to be neurophysin. Current studies are aimed at a more precise characterization of the active principles in contrast to the carrier substance, and of the manner in which these components of the neurosecretory material are bound to each other. A closely related question concerns the possible modification of this arrangement while the material is in the process of being transported along the axon (GABE, 1967; LAKE, 1970).

The second class of active neurosecretory products (present in aminergic, aldehyde fuchsin-negative, B-type neurons) seems to contain little or no cystine (LAKE, 1970), but instead a large amount of biogenic amines (noradrenaline, 5-hydroxytryptamine; BIANCHI, 1967; COGGESHALL et al., 1968; EHINGER et al., 1968; FRONTALI, 1968; KLEMM, 1968; NEWMAN et al., 1968; CHANUSSOT et al., 1969; REUTTER, 1969). For the identification of this material fluorescence-histochemical and ultrastructural characteristics are equally important. Both are currently being used in efforts to learn more about B-type neurosecretory neurons in various classes of invertebrates.

The histochemical approach has yielded at least strong circumstantial evidence in support of the concept that the majority of active neurosecretory mediators in invertebrates, as well as vertebrates, are peptides. Attempts to substantiate these data by the application of biochemical methods such as those developed for the purification and isolation of neurosecretory principles from vertebrates to analogous systems in invertebrates are handicapped by the much smaller yields of the latter. The results of numerous painstaking studies in this direction are still difficult to interpret. On the one hand, several facts point to a proteinaceous character of purified materials with neurohormonal activities obtained from insect brains known to contain peptidergic neurons (ISHIZAKI and ICHIKAWA, 1967; NATALIZI and FRONTALI, 1967; GERSCH and STÜRZEBECHER, 1968; MORDUE and GOLDSWORTHY, 1969; SCHUETZ, 1969; SMITH and RALPH, 1970; TOEVS and BRACKENBURY, 1969). On the other hand, heat stability and resistance to certain peptidases, observed in some of these preparations call for caution (see also SCHREINER, 1966). According to WILLIAMS (1967), there is at least a possibility that the "brain hormone" of insects, for example, might turn out to be a mucopolysaccharide instead of a protein or a complex containing protein.

A class of non-proteinaceous mediators on which more attention began to be focused lately are the biogenic amines (COLHOUN, 1967; BAUCHAU, 1968; QUAY, 1968). In the present context, the relevance of biochemical studies on these compounds depends on whether or not the one or the other among them functions as a neurohormone rather than a neurotransmitter in any of the invertebrates investigated thus far. Physiological indications for a neurohormonal role will be discussed in another section (p. 14). Suffice it to say here that catecholamines have been demonstrated in the nervous systems of a variety of invertebrates in amounts suggestive of "neurosecretory" proportions. The same holds for serotonin whose presence has been reported, for example, in annelids, crustaceans and insects.

## Neuronal Properties

A problem approached with renewed interest in recent years concerns the neuronal properties of neurosecretory cells. Aside from close similarities in morphology, as shown for example in insects by ADIYODI and BERN (1968), there are physiological parallelisms. An important feature is the capacity for generating and conducting impulses. Action potentials with characteristic slow conduction velocity have been demonstrated in neurosecretory neurons of several invertebrates, in part by intracellular recordings (Cooke, 1967; Frazier et al., 1967; Gosbee et al., 1968; Strumwasser, 1968).

Various experimental methods were used to determine the nature and degree of afferent stimulation received by these cells as well as the kinds of response of which they are capable. An interesting system, recently analyzed with electro-physiological methods by Jahan-Parwar et al. (1969) in the aquatic gastropod *Aplysia*, consists of a group of large neurosecretory neurons in the abdominal ganglion. These elements behave like pacemaker cells, i.e., they are relatively unaffected by afferent synaptic input. Yet, their autogenic activity is stepped up by special sensory, particularly chemical, stimuli that are conveyed to the neuro-secretory neurons by way of the branchial nerve from the osphradium, a receptor organ in the mantle cavity. The transmission of this sensory information occurs by means of antidromic conduction. Such activation does not result in efferent synaptic transmission, and there is no significant production of acetylcholine in these neurosecretory neurons (Giller and Schwartz, 1968). Instead, the response may be release of the secretory product (see below).

More frequent than chemical or mechanical sensory input are photic stimuli whose influence on the activity of neurosecretory centers is documented by numerous studies (Claret, 1966; Fingerman et al., 1967; Bohm and Parker, 1968). Such photo-neuro-endocrine pathways were traced in insects (Brousse-Gaury, 1968a, b, 1969). Here, fibers of ocellar nerves synapse with neuro-secretory neurons of the cerebral ganglion. The amounts of stainable secretory products stored in their perikarya can be experimentally manipulated by selectively abolishing the photic input. Thus, changes in the axonal membrane effecting the release of secretory material may be restrained under the conditions of illumination.

## Discharge, Extracellular Pathways, and Mode of Action of Neurosecretory Material

Recent observations in invertebrates have substantially contributed to the important insight that the circulatory system is not the only vehicle for the extracellular transport of neurosecretory messengers. Animals whose organ systems lack a capillary blood supply clearly demonstrate that acellular stromal channels may serve as connecting links between sources of neurosecretory material and the general circulation, or effector cells nearby. In some instances, the distance that this material has to traverse may be no greater than the space between two con-tiguous cells.

Physiological evidence that release into the extracellular compartment occurs (assay of incubation medium, etc.; Cooke, 1967; Kater, 1968; Normann and Duve, 1969) is available. The active material manufactured by neurosecretory neurons is discharged in morphologically distinctive areas of the axons that are not restricted to the terminal region (Figs. 5, 6). Such sites of release ("synaptoids") are not equivalent to standard presynaptic specializations even though

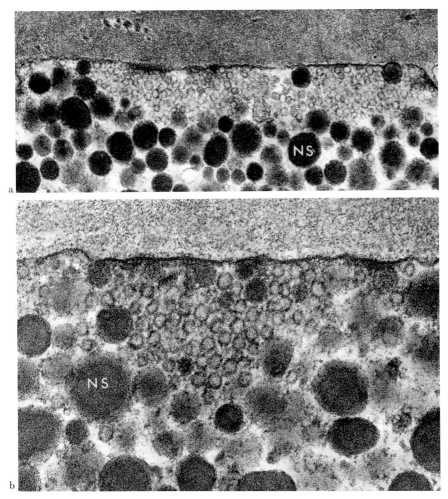

Fig. 5a and b. Sites of release of neurosecretory material facing extracellular stroma in corpus cardiacum of the insect *Leucophaea*. Note A-type neurosecretory granules (*NS*), numerous small "clear", and few dense-core vesicles, plus diffuse, opaque material pressing against axolemma. a ×48,000; b ×74,000. (From SCHARRER, 1968)

they resemble them morphologically. They are more or less transient structures that appear and disappear according to demand, as evidenced by the fact that their numbers were increased in the corpus cardiacum of insects following electrical stimulation of the nervi corporis cardiaci (SCHARRER and KATER, 1969).

Synaptoids of this kind have been studied in a variety of arthropods. The conclusion reached is that the steps leading to the discharge of neurosecretory material are not precisely the same in every species. In some arthropods examined (SMITH and SMITH, 1966; NORMANN, 1969; WEITZMAN, 1969), exocytosis seems to be the predominant mechanism (Fig. 6); in others more or less intact neurosecretory granules outside of the confines of axons are seen rarely or not at all (SCHARRER, 1968). The same may hold for gastropods (NOLTE, 1967).

An interesting ultrastructural feature in the neurosecretory terminals of the crayfish, *Procambarus clarkii*, are coated pits and vesicles which, like the adjacent "synaptic" vesicles, incorporate tracer particles. Their functional role is still unclear (Bunt, 1969).

The elucidation of ultrastructural details in reference to the mode of discharge of neurosecretory material is perhaps less pertinent for functional interpretations than the fact that synaptoids may be located close to the circulatory system as

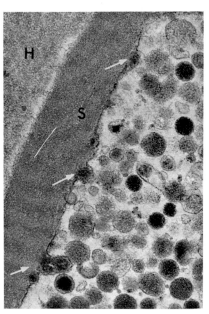

Fig. 6. Part of neurosecretory axon facing stromal sheath (*S*) in sinus gland of land crab, *Gecarcinus*. Arrows point to intermediate stages in the release of granules by the process of exocytosis. *H* hemocoele. ×35,200. (From Weitzman, 1969)

well as contiguous cellular structures. The latter arrangement suggests that release of neurosecretory material may take place in direct apposition to effector sites, even though this seems relatively rare. Examples among insects are muscles, pericardial cells, salivary gland cells (Bowers and Johnson, 1966; Maddrell, 1967), corpus allatum cells (Scharrer, 1964), and neurosecretory axons (Scharrer, 1963); among annelids, the putative endocrine cells of the infracerebral gland of nereids (Golding *et al.*, 1968). More often the active principles have to traverse at least small spaces filled with acellular stroma unless they reach their "targets" by way of the hemolymph.

In the case of contiguous cells, submicroscopic specializations at the "postsynaptic" side are more often than not missing. The crucial question still remaining to be answered is whether there actually exists a direct cell-to-cell interaction comparable to, if not identical with, neurohumoral events in regular synaptic transmission. The proposal that such cases be interpreted as examples of neurotransmitter action on the part of neurosecretory messenger substances (Maddrell, 1967) seems to be at least premature. An alternative interpretation that cannot be entirely excluded would be that neurosecretory material released in close proximity to a cell has nothing to do with the latter's control but merely gains access to an extracellular pathway in a circuitous fashion.

Equally incomplete is our knowledge of what causes the discharge of neurosecretory material from its intraneuronal storage sites. There are reasons to believe that this process is correlated with action potentials conducted by neurosecretory axons (COOKE, 1967; GOSBEE et al., 1968). Visibly demonstrable reduction or depletion of neurosecretory material can be accomplished in some neurohemal organs by appropriate physiological intervention, but the interpretation of these results requires caution. For example, not all attempts at manipulating the release of neurosecretory material by electrical stimulation have avoided changes in ultrastructure that can be attributed to direct stimulation of the gland (see SCHARRER and KATER, 1969). There is some evidence that the release of neurosecretory material in invertebrates, like that in vertebrates, is a calcium-dependent process (BERLIND and COOKE, 1968).

The manner in which neurosecretory substances exert their influence on the various "target" cells of invertebrates is almost entirely unexplored. A move in this direction was made by FINGERMAN and his coworkers (FINGERMAN, 1969; FREEMAN et al., 1968) who focused their attention on the elucidation of possible hormone-membrane interactions in the control of crustacean chromatophores. Different chromatophorotropins controlling certain pigment cells are singularly influenced in their activities by specific cations. For example, in the prawn Palaemonetes vulgaris, the sodium ion favors the response to the red pigment-concentrating hormone. The application of drugs, known to affect the transport of sodium across the axonal membrane, showed that the effect of the red pigment-concentrating hormone was inhibited by ouabain and enhanced by tetrodotoxin.

Furthermore, this hormone causes membrane hyperpolarization whose magnitude parallels the degree of pigment concentration in the effector cell, but no major change in ion permeability. Therefore, the hormonal signal to the erythrophores may require interaction with some membrane component that does not involve ion permeability but results in changes of intra- and extracellular sodium concentration. The administration of cyclic AMP (adenosine monophosphate), a known mediator of hormone actions at the level of the effector cells, had no influence on the concentration of red pigment. However, this compound seems to participate in the response of the same pigment to a second chromatophorotropin, the red pigment-dispersing hormone.

Many more studies of this and a similar kind will have to be carried out before a more general idea of the possible modes of interaction with the target cell can be formulated.

## Functional Significance of Neurosecretory Substances

There is hardly a physiological process in existence for which control by neurosecretory mediators cannot be claimed in at least one or another invertebrate animal (Table). In some of these control mechanisms the signal reaches the terminal target directly, in others it does so by involving at least one endocrine way station. There is a division of labor in that the products of certain groups of neurosecretory

Table. *Functional roles of neurosecretory substances in invertebrates*

| | | |
|---|---|---|
| Growth and development | Crustaceans | Matsumoto (1962), Aiken (1969) |
| | Insects | Fraenkel and Hsiao (1965), Claret (1966), Rinterknecht (1966), Fukuda and Takeuchi (1967), Girardie (1967), Hasegawa and Yamashita (1967), Hintze (1968), Morohoshi and Oshiki (1969), Pipa (1969), Seligmann *et al.* (1969) |
| | Chilopoda | Scheffel (1965a, b) |
| Regeneration | Annelids | Gersch and Wohlrabe (1965), Juberthie and Meštrov (1965), Gallisian (1968), Porchet and Durchon (1968) |
| | Crustaceans | Bauchau (1966) |
| | Insects | Joly (1968) |
| **Reproduction** | | |
|   Asexual | Planarians | Lender and Zghal (1968) |
|   Gonads | Worms | Bierne (1964, 1966), Hauenschild (1966), Hagadorn (1968) |
| | Echinoderms | Kanatani (1967), Kanatani *et al.* (1969), Schuetz (1969) |
| | Molluscs | Strumwasser *et al.* (1969), Toevs and Brackenbury (1969) |
| | Crustaceans | Aiken (1968), Berreur-Bonnenfant (1968) |
| | Insects | Adiyodi and Nayar (1966), Girardie (1966), Girardie and Joly (1967), Davey (1967), De Bessé (1967), Geldiay (1967), Barth (1968), Engelmann (1968), Thomas (1968), Naisse (1969), Wilkens (1969) |
|   Accessory organs | Crustaceans | Juchault and Legrand (1968), Meusy (1968) |
| | Insects | Naisse (1969) |
| **Metabolism** | | |
|   Protein | Molluscs | Meenakshi and Scheer (1969) |
| | Crustaceans | Bauchau and Hontoy (1968), Puyear (1969) |
| | Insects | E. Thomsen (1966), Wyss-Huber and Lüscher (1966), Clarke and Gillott (1967a, b), Osborne *et al.* (1968), Mordue and Goldsworthy (1969) |
|   Carbohydrate | Crustaceans | Ramamurthi *et al.* (1968) |
| | Insects | Kobayashi *et al.* (1967), Natalizi and Frontali (1967), Mordue and Goldsworthy (1969), Normann and Duve (1969) |
|   Lipid | Crustaceans | O'Connor and Gilbert (1968) |
| | Insects | Mayer and Candy (1969) |
|   Water | Molluscs | Chaisemartin (1968), Jahan-Parwar *et al.* (1969) |
| | Crustaceans | Bauchau and Hontoy (1968), Bliss (1968), Mantel (1968), Kamemoto and Ono (1969) |
| | Insects | Unger (1965a), Cazal and Girardie (1968), De Bessé and Cazal (1968), Smalley and Brown (1968), Maddrell *et al.* (1969), Mordue and Goldsworthy (1969) |
| | Spiders | Kühne (1959) |

Table (continued)

| | | |
|---|---|---|
| Electrolyte | Lineidae | LECHENAULT (1965) |
| | Molluscs | CHAISEMARTIN (1968) |
| | Crustaceans | RAMAMURTHI and SCHEER (1967), KALBER and COSTLOW (1968), KAMEMOTO and ONO (1969), KATO and KAMEMOTO (1969) |
| Respiratory | | WYSS-HUBER and LÜSCHER (1966), MÜLLER and ENGELMANN (1968), KEELEY and FRIEDMAN (1969) |
| Nucleic acids | | MIYAWAKI (1966), CLARKE and GILLOTT (1967a, b), FINGERMAN et al. (1967) |
| Color change | Crustaceans | BAUCHAU (1966), FINGERMAN (1966, 1969) |
| | Insects | RAABE (1965), GIRARDIE (1967) |
| Glandulotropic effects | Crustaceans | BAUCHAU (1966) |
| | Insects | GIRARDIE (1966), LOHER and HUBER (1966), CASSIER (1967), SCHARRER (1964, 1967), L. JOLY et al. (1968), SRIVASTAVA and SINGH (1968) |
| Neurotropic effects and behavior | | UNGER (1965b), LOHER and HUBER (1966), BARTH (1968) |
| Non-neural, non-glandular effectors | | BAUCHAU (1966), BOWERS and JOHNSON (1966), NAYLOR and WILLIAMS (1968) |
| Cardiac rhythmicity | | RAABE et al. (1966), NATALIZI and FRONTALI (1967), KATER (1968), MORDUE and GOLDSWORTHY (1969), SMITH and RALPH (1969) |
| Circadian rhythmicity | Crustaceans | BAUCHAU (1966), NAYLOR and WILLIAMS (1968) |
| | Insects | RENSING (1964), BRADY (1967a, b), HINKS (1967), NISHIISUTSUJI-UWO and PITTENDRIGH (1968), RAO (1968) |
| Neuroendocrine integration | | SCHARRER and SCHARRER (1963), B. SCHARRER (1967) |

cells are concerned with functions not carried out by those of other groups. Moreover, a given effect (e.g., cardiac acceleration) may result from the activity of more than one hormone principle. On the other hand, a given cardioaccelerator, such as that present in the corpus cardiacum of insects, also fulfills additional hormonal functions.

The concept that most of these substances reach their effector sites by way of the circulatory system, and therefore qualify as neurohormones, still holds for invertebrates as much as for vertebrates. Current interest concerns not only the further elucidation of these endocrine activities, but also the exploration of the non-hormonal roles of neurosecretory messengers about which our knowledge is still very fragmentary (see B. SCHARRER, 1969). It is not intended here to discuss in any detail the present status of neurohormonal activities in invertebrates. Hardly any comment is needed about the blood-borne peptides and their great versatility in the roles of metabolic regulators, morphogenetic hormones, etc. A number of comprehensive texts are available in which this subject is properly surveyed (see, for example, Bauchau, 1966; Joly, 1968).

The endocrine roles played by biogenic amines of neural origin are more difficult to assess, since this class of chemical mediators also furnishes neurotransmitter substances. Nevertheless, there are various indications that some invertebrate hormones belong to this class. An example is serotonin, furnished by a distinctive type of neurosecretory cell in the pars intercerebralis of the nocturnal moth *Noctua* where it seems to act as a hormone controlling the circadian rhythm of this insect (Hinks, 1967). Serotonin also proved to be a potent stimulator of fluid excretion by the Malpighian tubules, even though it does not seem to be identical with the known diuretic hormone (Maddrell *et al.*, 1969). Much more additional work will be required before the neurohormonal role of biogenic amines can be fully appreciated.

## Phylogeny of Neurosecretory Neurons

Two schemes have been proposed for the phylogenetic derivation of neurosecretory neurons (see Gabe, 1966; Lentz, 1968). One view maintains that conventional neurons were the first on the scene and, by a gradual process of differentiation, gave rise to highly specialized elements in which secretory activity became the dominant feature. A second proposition stresses that glandular elements, originally located in the epidermis, developed additional neuronal characteristics when they became secondarily incorporated into nervous centers.

Even though the first scheme seems to be supported by better evidence, a final solution of this problem requires much additional study of neurosecretory phenomena, especially among the most primitive metazoans in existence. For this reason, the discovery of neurosecretory cells in coelenterates (Lentz, 1968) is a welcome recent addition to our knowledge in that it provides possible early links in the phylogenetic sequence (compare Figs. 1—3).

What may perhaps be underlined at present is that the various views mentioned are not as far apart as it would appear at first sight. Since undifferentiated cells possess the basic properties of excitability, conductivity, and elaboration of physiologically active substances, they may give rise to glandular as well as neural elements. In both these derivatives the capacity for secretory activity is retained but, in the course of structural and functional specialization, differences in degree become increasingly pronounced. It is obvious that neurosecretory cells do not digress quite as much from the ancestral pattern as do conventional neurons. The questions to be considered then are merely how far back the dichotomy occurred, and where the dividing line between neurosecretory and conventional neurons should be drawn.

## Conclusions

What are the take-home lessons of our present survey ? An overall view of the current status of invertebrate neurosecretion indicates that it remains a vigorous field of investigation. Its major contribution consists in the substantiation of concepts that apply to the interpretation of the phenomenon of neurosecretion in general. Among these concepts, the central position of the neurosecretory neuron as a link between the neural and the endocrine systems of integration remains unchallenged (see SCHARRER and SCHARRER, 1963; B. SCHARRER, 1969). But only within recent years has it been generally appreciated that not all of the signals between nerve centers and glands of internal secretion need to be conveyed by means of neurohormones. This insight is based largely on ultrastructural evidence. In certain instances, a short extracellular pathway consisting of stromal elements replaces the circulatory system. In others, endocrine cells seem to be supplied with secretomotor junctions. These would appear to provide the machinery for "private" communication comparable to that in regular neuron-to-neuron contacts. But even though electron microscopy has become a major factor in the search for mechanisms of neuroendocrine mediation, the present data should be considered as highly suggestive and in need of physiological confirmation.

Moreover, the line of demarcation between neurohumoral and neurohormonal activities is somewhat blurred by the following points:

a) Instead of conventional transmitters, axonal contacts with endocrine cells may contain peptidergic principles.

b) Aminergic neurochemical mediators, in addition to their well established role in synaptic transmission, can also function as neurohormones. Therefore, the kind of interaction that occurs at sites of more or less close contact between neural and endocrine elements is probably akin to, but not identical with, conventional synaptic transmission.

The functional characteristics of neurochemical mediators operating in these special situations may turn out to be distinctive enough to require their classification as a separate type, somewhat intermediate between neurotransmitters and neurohormones.

Finally, outside of the realm of neuroendocrine communication, products of neurosecretory neurons are capable of affecting non-glandular "terminal targets" directly, and here again the extracellular pathway may consist in the vascular system or merely in a small space between adjacent cells.

Evidently, the spectrum of possibilities by which neurons fulfill their integrative functions is becoming increasingly enlarged. A major share of this versatility is based on the need for various forms of communication between neural centers and glands of internal secretion. The most impressive result of the development of appropriate mechanisms throughout the animal kingdom is the neurosecretory neuron, a cell which is highly specialized and at the same time capable of performing multiple tasks. It is safe to predict that further progress in this area will occur on many fronts, and that the invertebrates with their wealth of neurosecretory systems will continue to make substantial contributions to the advance of neuroendocrinology.

## References

ADIYODI, K. G., BERN, H. A.: Neuronal appearance of neurosecretory cells in the pars inter-cerebralis of *Periplaneta americana* (L.). Gen. comp. Endocr. **11**, 88—91 (1968).
—, NAYAR, K. K.: Some neuroendocrine aspects of reproductions in the viviparous cockroach, *Trichoblatta sericea* (Saussure). Zool. Jb., Abt. Physiol. **72**, 453—462 (1966).

16          B. Scharrer and M. Weitzman:

Aiken, D. E.: Environmental regulation of ovarian maturation and egg laying in the crayfish *Orconectes virilis*. Amer. Zool. **8**, 754 (1968).
— Photoperiod, endocrinology and the crustacean molt cycle. Science **164**, 149—155 (1969).
Bartell, C. K., May, K., Fingerman, M.: Electron microscopic examination of subcellular components containing melanophorotropic activity, separated by density gradient centrifugation, from neurosecretory cells in the eyestalks of the fiddler crab, *Uca pugilator*. Biol. Bull. **135**, 414 (1968).
Barth, R. H.: The comparative physiology of reproductive processes in cockroaches. Part I. Mating behaviour and its endocrine control. In: Advances in reproductive physiology, ed.: A. McLaren, vol. 3, p. 167—207. New York and London: Academic Press 1968.
Baskin, D. G., Golding, D. W.: Morphological evidence for a presumptive neuroendocrine complex in polynoids (Polychaeta). Amer. Zool. **8**, 756 (1968).
Bassurmanova, O. K., Panov, A. A.: Structure of the neurosecretory system in Lepidoptera. Light and electron microscopy of type A′-neurosecretory cells in the brain of normal and starved larvae of the silkworm *Bombyx mori*. Gen. comp. Endocr. **9**, 245—262 (1967).
Bauchau, A.: La Vie des Crabes. Paris: Paul Lechevalier 1966.
— La sérotonine dans le règne animal. Rev. Quest. sci. **139**, 379—399 (1968).
— Hontoy, J.: Métabolisme de l'azote et hormones pédonculaires chez *Eriocheir sinensis* H. Milne Edwards. Crustaceana **14**, 67—75 (1968).
Berlind, A., Cooke, I. M.: Effect of calcium omission on neurosecretion and electrical activity of crab pericardial organs. Gen. comp. Endocr. **11**, 458—463 (1968).
Bern, H. A., Hagadorn, I. R.: Neurosecretion. In: T. H. Bullock and G. A. Horridge, Structure and function in the nervous systems of invertebrates, vol. I, p. 353—429. San Francisco and London: W. H. Freeman & Co. 1965.
— Knowles, F. G. W.: Neurosecretion. In: Neuroendocrinology, ed.: L. Martini and W. F. Ganong, vol. I, p. 139—186. New York and London: Academic Press, 1966.
Berreur-Bonnenfant, J.: Action de la glande androgène et du cerveau sur la gamétogenèse de Crustacés Péracarides. Arch. Zool. exp. gén. **108**, 521—558 (1968).
De Bessé, N.: Neurosécrétion dans la chaîne nerveuse ventrale de deux blattes, *Leucophaea maderae* (F.) et *Periplaneta americana* (L.). Bull. Soc. Zool. Fr. **92**, 73—86 (1967).
— Cazal, M.: Action des extraits d'organes périsympathiques et de corpora cardiaca sur la diurèse de quelques Insectes. C. R. Acad. Sci. (Paris) **266**, Sér. D, 615—618 (1968).
Bianchi, S.: The amine secreting neurons in the central nervous system of the earthworm (*Octolasium complanatum*) and their possible neurosecretory role. Gen. comp. Endocr. **9**, 343—348 (1967).
— On the neurosecretory system of *Cerebratulus marginatus* (Heteronemertini). Gen. comp. Endocr. **12**, 541—548 (1969).
Bierne, J.: Maturation sexuelle anticipée par décapitation de la femelle chez l'Hétéronémerte *Lineus ruber* Müller. C. R. Acad. Sci. (Paris) **259**, 4841—4843 (1964).
— Localisation dans les ganglions cérébroïdes du centre régulateur de la maturation sexuelle chez la femelle de *Lineus ruber* Müller (Hétéronémertes). C. R. Acad. Sci. (Paris) **262**, Sér. D, 1572—1575 (1966).
Bliss, D. E.: Transition from water to land in decapod crustaceans. Amer. Zool. **8**, 355—392 (1968).
Bloch, B., Thomsen, E., Thomsen, M.: The neurosecretory system of the adult *Calliphora erythrocephala*. III. Electron microscopy of the medial neurosecretory cells of the brain and some adjacent cells. Z. Zellforsch. **70**, 185—208 (1966).
Boer, H. H., Slot, J. W., Andel, J. van: Electron microscopical and histochemical observations on the relation between medio-dorsal bodies and neurosecretory cells in the basommatophoran snails *Lymnaea stagnalis*, *Ancylus fluviatilis*, *Australorbis glabratus* and *Planorbarius corneus*. Z. Zellforsch. **87**, 435—450 (1968).
Bohm, M. K., Parker, R. A.: The fine structure of daphnid supraesophageal and optic ganglia, and its possible functional significance. J. Morph. **126**, 373—393 (1968).
Bowers, B., Johnson, B.: An electron microscope study of the corpora cardiaca and secretory neurons in the aphid, *Myzus persicae* (Sulz.). Gen. comp. Endocr. **6**, 213—230 (1966).

BRADY, J.: Control of the circadian rhythm of activity in the cockroach. I. The role of the corpora cardiaca, brain and stress. J. exp. Biol. **47**, 153—163 (1967a).

— Control of the circadian rhythm of activity in the cockroach. II. The role of the suboesophageal ganglion and ventral nerve cord. J. exp. Biol. **47**, 165—178 (1967b).

BROUSSE-GAURY, P.: Chez les Dictyoptères Mantidae, description d'arcs réflexes neuro-endocriniens depuis les ocelles. C. R. Acad. Sci. (Paris) **267**, Sér. D, 1468—1470 (1968a).

— Modification de la neurosécrétion au niveau de la pars intercerebralis de *Periplaneta americana* L. en l'absence de stimuli ocellaires. Bull. biol. Fr. Belg. **102**, 481—490 (1968b).

— Des stimulus photiques transmis par des nerfs tégumentaires contrôlent des cellules neurosécrétrices chez les Dictyoptères Blaberidae et Blattidae. C. R. Acad. Sci. (Paris) **268**, Sér. D, 383—386 (1969).

BROWN, B. E.: Pharmacologically active constituents of the cockroach corpus cardiacum: Resolution and some characteristics. Gen. comp. Endocr. **5**, 387—401 (1965).

BUNT, A. H.: Formation of coated and "synaptic" vesicles within neurosecretory axon terminals of the crustacean sinus gland. J. Ultrastruct. Res. **28**, 411—421 (1969).

— ASHBY, E. A.: Ultrastructural changes in the crayfish sinus gland following electrical stimulation. Gen. comp. Endocr. **10**, 376—382 (1968).

BUSSELET, M.: Données histochimiques sur les corps cardiaques d'*Antheraea pernyi* Guer. (Lepidoptera, Attacidae) et de *Rhodnius prolixus* Stal. (Hemiptera, Reduvidae). C. R. Acad. Sci. (Paris) **266**, Sér. D, 2280—2282 (1968).

CASSIER, P.: La reproduction des insectes et la régulation de l'activité des corps allates. Ann. Biol. **6**, 595—670 (1967).

CAZAL, M., GIRARDIE, A.: Contrôle humoral de l'équilibre hydrique chez *Locusta migratoria migratorioides*. J. Insect Physiol. **14**, 655—668 (1968).

CHAISEMARTIN, C.: Contrôle neuroendocrinien du renouvellement hydro-sodique chez *Lymnaea limosa* L. C. R. Soc. Biol. (Paris) **162**, 1994—1998 (1968).

CHANUSSOT, B., DANDO, J., MOULINS, M., LAVERACK, M. S.: Mise en évidence d'une amine biogène dans le système nerveux stomatogastrique des Insectes: Etude histochimique et ultrastructurale. C. R. Acad. Sci. (Paris) **268**, Sér. D, 2101—2104 (1969).

CLARET, J.: Mise en évidence du rôle photorécepteur du cerveau dans l'induction de la diapause, chez *Pieris brassicae* (Lepido.). Ann. Endocr. (Paris) **27**, 311—320 (1966).

CLARKE, K. U., GILLOTT, C.: Studies on the effects of the removal of the frontal ganglion in *Locusta migratoria* L. I. The effect on protein metabolism. J. exp. Biol. **46**, 13—25 (1967a).

— — Studies on the effects of the removal of the frontal ganglion in *Locusta migratoria* L. II. Ribonucleic acid synthesis. J. exp. Biol. **46**, 27—34 (1967b).

COGGESHALL, R. E., RUDE, S., ORDEN, L. S. VAN: A correlated electron microscopic and fluorescence study on two identified, 5-hydroxytryptamine containing, cells in the leech. Anat. Rec. **160**, 333 (1968).

COLHOUN, E. H.: Pharmacological tantalizers. In: Insects and physiology, ed.: J. W. L. BEAMENT and J. E. TREHERNE, p. 201—213. Edinburgh and London: Oliver & Boyd 1967.

COOKE, I. M.: Correlation of propagated action potentials and release of neurosecretory material in a neurohemal organ. In: Invertebrate nervous systems, ed.: C. A. G. WIERSMA, p. 125–130. Chicago and London: Chicago Univ. Press 1967.

DAVEY, K. G.: Neurosecretion and molting in some parasitic nematodes. Amer. Zool. **6**, 243—249 (1966).

— Some consequences of copulation in *Rhodnius prolixus*. J. Insect Physiol. **13**, 1629—1636 (1967).

— BRECKENRIDGE, W. R.: Neurosecretory cells in a cestode, *Hymenolepis diminuta*. Science **158**, 931—932 (1967).

DAVIS, L. E., BURNETT, A. L., HAYNES, J. F.: Histological and ultrastructural study of the muscular and nervous systems in *Hydra*. II. Nervous system. J. exp. Zool. **167**, 295—332 (1968).

DHAINAUT-COURTOIS, N.: Étude histologique et ultrastructurale des cellules nerveuses du ganglion cérébral de *Nereis pelagica* L. (Annélide Polychète). Comparaison entre les types cellulaires I–VI et ceux décrits antérieurement chez les Nereidae. Gen. comp. Endocr. **11**, 414—443 (1968).

Dogra, G. S.: The study of the neurosecretory system of *Periplaneta americana* (L.) *in situ* using a technique specific for cystine and/or cysteine. Acta anat. (Basel) **70**, 288—303 (1968).

Ehinger, B., Falck, B., Myhrberg, H. E.: Biogenic monoamines in *Hirudo medicinalis*. Histochemie **15**, 140—149 (1968).

Engelmann, F.: Endocrine control of reproduction in insects. Ann. Rev. Entomol. **13**, 1—26 (1968).

Fingerman, M.: Neurosecretory control of pigmentary effectors in crustaceans. Amer. Zool. **6**, 169—179 (1966).

— Cellular aspects of the control of physiological color changes in crustaceans. Amer. Zool. **9**, 443—452 (1969).

— Dominiczak, T., Miyawaki, M., Oguro, C., Yamamoto, Y.: Neuroendocrine control of the hepatopancreas in the crayfish *Procambarus clarki*. Physiol. Zool. **40**, 23—30 (1967).

Finlayson, L. H., Osborne, M. P.: Peripheral neurosecretory cells in the stick insect (*Carausius morosus*) and the blowfly larva (*Phormia terrae-novae*). J. Insect Physiol. **14**, 1793—1801 (1968).

Fletcher, B. S.: The diversity of cell types in the neurosecretory system of the beetle *Blaps mucronata*. J. Insect Physiol. **15**, 119—134 (1969).

Fraenkel, G., Hsiao, C.: Bursicon, a hormone which mediates tanning of the cuticle in the adult fly and other insects. J. Insect Physiol. **11**, 513—556 (1965).

Frazier, W. T., Kandel, E. R., Kupfermann, I., Waziri, R., Coggeshall, R. E.: Morphological and functional properties of identified neurons in the abdominal ganglion of *Aplysia californica*. J. Neurophysiol. **30**, 1288—1351 (1967).

Freeman, A. R., Connell, P. M., Fingerman, M.: An electrophysiological study of the red chromatophore of the prawn, *Palaemonetes:* Observations on the action of red pigment-concentrating hormone. Comp. Biochem. Physiol. **26**, 1015—1029 (1968).

Frontali, N.: Histochemical localization of catecholamines in the brain of normal and drug-treated cockroaches. J. Insect Physiol. **14**, 881—886 (1968).

Fukuda, S., Takeuchi, S.: Studies on the diapause factor-producing cells in the suboesophageal ganglion of the silkworm, *Bombyx mori* L. Embryologia **9**, 333—353 (1967).

Gabe, M.: Neurosecretion. Oxford-London: Pergamon Press 1966.

— Évolution du produit de neurosécrétion protocéphalique des Insectes Ptérygotes au cours du cheminement axonal. C. R. Acad. Sci. (Paris) **264**, Sér. D, 943—945 (1967).

Gallissian, A.: Greffe des ganglions cérébroïdes chez le Lumbricide *Eophila dollfusi* Tétry. Influence sur la diapause et la régénération. C. R. Acad. Sci. (Paris) **267**, Sér. D, 657—658 (1968).

Gaude, H., Weber, W.: Untersuchungen zur Neurosekretion bei *Acheta domesticus* L. Experientia (Basel) **22**, 396—397 (1966).

Geldiay, S.: Hormonal control of adult reproductive diapause in the Egyptian grasshopper *Anacridium aegyptium*, L. J. Endocr. **37**, 63—71 (1967).

Gersch, M., Stürzebecher, J.: Weitere Untersuchungen zur Kennzeichnung des Aktivationshormons der Insektenhäutung. J. Insect Physiol. **14**, 87—96 (1968).

— Wohlrabe, K.: Experimentelle Untersuchungen über die Beziehungen zwischen Neurosekretion und Regeneration bei *Enchytraeus*. Zool. Jb., Abt. Physiol. **71**, 393—413 (1965).

Gianfelici, E.: Différenciation *in vitro* du complexe cérébro-endocrinien chez *Calliphora erythrocephala*. Ann. Endocr. (Paris) **29**, 496—500 (1968).

Giller, E., Jr., Schwartz, J. H.: Choline acetyltransferase: Regional distribution in the abdominal ganglion of *Aplysia*. Science **161**, 908—911 (1968).

Girardie, A.: Contrôle de l'activité génitale chez *Locusta migratoria*. Mise en évidence d'un facteur gonadotrope et d'un facteur allatotrope dans la *pars intercerebralis*. Bull. Soc. Zool. Fr. **91**, 423—439 (1966).

— Contrôle neuro-hormonal de la métamorphose et de la pigmentation chez *Locusta migratoria cinerascens* (Orthoptère). Bull. Biol. Fr. Belg. **101**, 79—114 (1967).

— Girardie, J.: Etude histologique, histochimique et ultrastructurale de la pars intercerebralis chez *Locusta migratoria* L. (Orthoptère). Z. Zellforsch. **78**, 54—75 (1967).

— Joly, P.: Mécanisme physiologique de l'effet de groupe chez les acridiens. Coll. Int. C.N.R.S. Paris **173**, 127—145 (1967).

Golding, D. W., Baskin, D. G., Bern, H. A.: The infracerebral gland—a possible neuroendocrine complex in *Nereis*. J. Morph. **124**, 187—216 (1968).

GOSBEE, J. L., MILLIGAN, J. V., SMALLMAN, B. N.: Neural properties of the protocerebral neurosecretory cells of the adult cockroach *Periplaneta americana*. J. Insect Physiol. **14**, 1785—1792 (1968).

GRILLOT, J. P.: Description d'organes neurohémaux métamériques associés à la chaîne nerveuse ventrale chez deux coléoptères: *Chrysocarabus auronitens* Fabr. (Carabidae) et *Oryctes rhinoceros* L. (Scarabaeidae). C. R. Acad. Sci. (Paris) **267**, Sér. D, 772—775 (1968).

HAGADORN, I. R.: Neuroendocrine mechanisms in invertebrates. In: Neuroendocrinology, ed.: L. MARTINI and W. F. GANONG, vol. 2, p. 439—484. New York and London: Academic Press 1967a.

— Neurosecretory mechanisms. In: Invertebrate nervous systems—their significance for mammalian neurophysiology, ed.: C. A. G. WIERSMA, p. 115—124. Chicago and London: Chicago Univ. Press 1967b.

— The effect of gonadotropin lack upon the testes of *Hirudo*. Amer. Zool. **8**, 754 (1968).

HANSTRÖM, B.: Indications of neurosecretion and the structure of the Sokolow's organ in pycnogonids. Sarsia **18**, 25—36 (1965).

HASEGAWA, K., YAMASHITA, O.: Control of metabolism in the silkworm pupal ovary by the diapause hormone. J. sericult. Sci. Japan **36**, 297—300 (1967).

HAUENSCHILD, C.: Der hormonale Einfluß des Gehirns auf die sexuelle Entwicklung bei dem Polychaeten *Platynereis dumerilii*. Gen. comp. Endocr. **6**, 26—73 (1966).

HERLANT-MEEWIS, H.: Les cellules neurosécrétrices de la chaîne nerveuse d'*Eisenia foetida*. Z. Zellforsch. **69**, 319—325 (1966).

HEURTAULT, J.: Neurosécrétion et glandes endocrines chez *Neobisium caporiaccoi* (Arachnides, Pseudoscorpions). C. R. Acad. Sci. (Paris) **268**, Sér. D, 1105—1108 (1969).

HINKS, C. F.: Relationship between serotonin and the circadian rhythm in some nocturnal moths. Nature (Lond.) **214**, 386—387 (1967).

HINTZE, C.: Histologische Untersuchungen über die Aktivität der inkretorischen Organe von *Cerura vinula* L. (Lepidoptera) während der Verpuppung. Wilhelm Roux' Arch. Entwickl.-Mech. Org. **160**, 313—343 (1968).

HÖKFELT, T.: *In vitro* studies on central and peripheral monoamine neurons at the ultra-structural level. Z. Zellforsch. **91**, 1—74 (1968).

ISHIZAKI, H., ICHIKAWA, M.: Purification of the brain hormone of the silkworm *Bombyx mori*. Biol. Bull. **133**, 355—368 (1967).

JAHAN-PARWAR, B., SMITH, M., BAUMGARTEN, R. VON: Activation of neurosecretory cells in *Aplysia* by osphradial stimulation. Amer. J. Physiol. **216**, 1246—1257 (1969).

JOLY, L., JOLY, P., PORTE, A., GIRARDIE, A.: Étude physiologique et ultrastructurale des corpora allata de *Locusta migratoria* L. (Orthoptère) en phase grégaire. Arch. Zool. exp. gén. **109**, 703—727 (1968).

JOLY, P.: Endocrinologie des Insectes. Paris: Masson, Collection les Grands Problèmes de la Biologie, Monographie 7, 1968.

JOLY, R., DESCAMPS, M.: Étude comparative du complexe endocrine céphalique chez les Myriapodes Chilopodes. Gen. comp. Endocr. **10**, 364—375 (1968).

JUBERTHIE, C., MEŠTROV, M.: Régénération postérieure en milieu humide et activité neuro-sécrétrice de la chaîne nerveuse chez *Eophila pyrenaica* (Oligochètes Lumbricidae). C. R. Acad. Sci. (Paris) **260**, 991—994 (1965).

JUCHAULT, P., LEGRAND, J. J.: Rôle des hormones sexuelles, des neurohormones et d'un facteur épigénétique dans la physiologie sexuelle d'individus intersexués d'*Armadillidium vulgare* Latr. (Isopode Oniscoïde). C. R. Acad. Sci. (Paris) **267**, Sér. D, 2014—2016 (1968).

KALBER, F. A., COSTLOW, J. D.: Osmoregulation in larvae of the land-crab, *Cardisoma guanhumi* Latreille. Amer. Zool. **8**, 411—416 (1968).

KAMEMOTO, F. I., ONO, J. K.: Neuroendocrine regulation of salt and water balance in the crayfish *Procambarus clarkii*. Comp. Biochem. Physiol. **29**, 393—401 (1969).

KANATANI, H.: Neural substance responsible for maturation of oocytes and shedding of gametes in starfish. In: Gunma Symposia on Endocrinology, vol. 4, Sex and Reproduction, ed.: K. I. HANAOKA, p. 65—78. Maebashi, Japan: Gunma Univ. 1967.

— SHIRAI, H., NAKANISHI, K., KUROKAWA, T.: Isolation and identification of meiosis inducing substance in starfish *Asterias amurensis*. Nature (Lond.) **221**, 273—274 (1969).

KATER, S. B.: Cardioaccelerator release in *Periplaneta americana* (L.). Science **160**, 765—767 (1968).

Kato, K. N., Kamemoto, F. I.: Neuroendocrine involvement in osmoregulation in the grapsid crab *Metopograpsus messor*. Comp. Biochem. Physiol. **28**, 665—674 (1969).

Keeley, L. L., Friedman, S.: Effects of long-term cardiatectomy-allatectomy on mitochondrial respiration in the cockroach, *Blaberus discoidalis*. J. Insect Physiol. **15**, 509—518 (1969).

Klemm, N.: Monoaminhaltige Strukturen im Zentralnervensystem der Trichoptera (Insecta). Teil I. Z. Zellforsch. **92**, 487—502 (1968).

Knowles, F.: Neuroendocrine correlations at the level of ultrastructure. Arch. Anat. micr. Morph. exp. **54**, 343—357 (1965).

Kobayashi, M., Kimura, S., Yamazaki, M.: Action of insect hormones on the fate of $^{14}$C-glucose in the diapausing, brainless pupa of *Samia cynthia pryeri* (Lepidoptera: Saturniidae). Appl. Ent. Zool. **2**, 79—84 (1967).

Kühne, H.: Die neurosekretorischen Zellen und der retrozerebrale neuroendokrine Komplex von Spinnen (Araneae, Labidognatha) unter Berücksichtigung einiger histologisch erkennbarer Veränderungen während des postembryonalen Lebenslaufes. Zool. Jb., Abt. Anat. **77**, 527—600 (1959).

Lake, P. S.: Histochemical studies of the neurosecretory system of *Chirocephalus diaphanus* Prévost (Crustacea: Anostraca). Gen. comp. Endocr. **14**, 1—14 (1970).

Lechenault, H.: Neurosécrétion et osmorégulation chez les Lineidae (Hétéronémertes). C. R. Acad. Sci. (Paris) **261**, 4868—4871 (1965).

Lender, T., Zghal, F.: Influence du cerveau et de la neurosécrétion sur la scissiparité de la Planaire *Dugesia gonocephala*. C. R. Acad. Sci. (Paris) **267**, Sér. D, 2008—2009 (1968).

Lentz, T. L.: Primitive Nervous Systems. New Haven and London: Yale University Press 1968.

Loher, W., Huber, F.: Nervous and endocrine control of sexual behaviour in a grasshopper (*Gomphocerus rufus* L., Acridinae). Symp. Soc. exp. Biol. **20**, 381—400 (1966).

Maddrell, S. H. P.: Neurosecretion in insects. In: Insects and physiology, ed.: J. W. L. Beament and J. E. Treherne, p. 103—118. Edinburgh and London: Oliver & Boyd 1967.

— Pilcher, D. E. M., Gardiner, B. O. C.: Stimulatory effect of 5-hydroxytryptamine (serotonin) on secretion by Malpighian tubules of insects. Nature (Lond.) **222**, 784—785 (1969).

Mancini, G., Frontali, N.: On the ultrastructural localization of catecholamines in the beta lobes (corpora pedunculata) of *Periplaneta americana*. Z. Zellforsch. **103**, 341—350 (1970).

Mantel, L. H.: The foregut of *Gecarcinus lateralis* as an organ of salt and water balance. Amer. Zool. **8**, 433—442 (1968).

Matsumoto, K.: Experimental studies of the neurosecretory activities of the thoracic ganglion of a crab, *Hemigrapsus*. Gen. comp. Endocr. **2**, 4—11 (1962).

Mayer, R. J., Candy, D. J.: Control of haemolymph lipid concentration during locust flight: An adipokinetic hormone from the corpora cardiaca. J. Insect Physiol. **15**, 611—620 (1969).

Meenakshi, V. R., Scheer, B. T.: Regulation of galactogen synthesis in the slug *Ariolimax columbianus*. Comp. Biochem. Physiol. **29**, 841—845 (1969).

Meusy, J. J.: Effets de l'ablation des pédoncules oculaires et des organes Y sur les glandes androgènes et sur l'appareil génital chez le crabe mâle *Carcinus maenas* L. (Crustacé, Décapode) pubère. C. R. Acad. Sci. (Paris) **267**, Sér. D, 1861—1863 (1968).

Miyawaki, M.: Eyestalk hormones and $P^{32}$ incorporation of the hepatopancreas cells in the crayfish, *Procambarus clarkii*. Annot. zool. jap. **39**, 137—141 (1966).

Mordue, W., Goldsworthy, G. J.: The physiological effects of corpus cardiacum extracts in locusts. Gen. comp. Endocr. **12**, 360—369 (1969).

Morohoshi, S., Oshiki, T.: Effect of the brain on the suboesophageal ganglion and determination of voltinism in *Bombyx mori*. J. Insect Physiol. **15**, 167—175 (1969).

Müller, H. P., Engelmann, F.: Studies on the endocrine control of metabolism in *Leucophaea maderae* (Blattaria). II. Effect of the corpora cardiaca on fat-body respiration. Gen. comp. Endocr. **11**, 43—50 (1968).

Naisse, J.: Rôle des neurohormones dans la différenciation sexuelle de *Lampyris noctiluca*. J. Insect Physiol. **15**, 877—892 (1969).

Natalizi, G. M., Frontali, N.: Purification of insect hyperglycaemic and heart accelerating hormones. J. Insect Physiol. **12**, 1279—1287 (1967).

NAYLOR, E., WILLIAMS, B. G.: Effects of eyestalk removal on rhythmic locomotor activity in *Carcinus*. J. exp. Biol. **49**, 107—116 (1968).

NEWMAN, G., KERKUT, G. A., WALKER, R. J.: The structure of the brain of *Helix aspersa*. Electron microscope localization of cholinesterase and amines. In: Studies in the structure, physiology and ecology of molluscs, ed.: V. FRETTER, p. 1—17. London: Academic Press 1968.

NISHIITSUTSUJI-UWO, J., PITTENDRIGH, C. S.: Central nervous system control of circadian rhythmicity in the cockroach. III. The optic lobes, locus of the driving oscillation ? Z. vergl. Physiol. **58**, 14—46 (1968).

NOLTE, A.: The mode of release of neurosecretory material in the freshwater pulmonate *Lymnaea stagnalis* L. (Gastropoda). Symposium on Neurobiology of Invertebrates, p. 123—133. Budapest: Hungarian Acad. Sci. Publ. 1967.

— KUHLMANN, D.: Einbau von $^3$H-Uridin in den Schlundring von *Helix pomatia* L. Naturwissenschaften **53**, 281—282 (1966).

NORMANN, T. C.: Experimentally induced exocytosis of neurosecretory granules. Exp. Cell Res. **55**, 285—287 (1969).

— DUVE, H.: Experimentally induced release of a neurohormone influencing hemolymph trehalose level in *Calliphora erythrocephala* (Diptera). Gen. comp. Endocr. **12**, 449—459 (1969).

O'CONNOR, J. D., GILBERT, L. I.: Aspects of lipid metabolism in crustaceans. Amer. Zool. **8**, 529—539 (1968).

OSBORNE, D. J., CARLISLE, D. B., ELLIS, P. E.: Protein synthesis in the fat body of the female desert locust, *Schistocerca gregaria* Forsk., in relation to maturation. Gen. comp. Endocr. **11**, 347—354 (1968).

PANOV, A. A.: Reaction of A'-neurosecretory cells of the silkworm larvae to starvation during the period of facultative feeding. Dokl. Akad. Nauk SSSR, Otd. Biol. **176**, 543—546 (1967).

PIPA, R. L.: Insect neurometamorphosis. IV. Effects of the brain and synthetic α-ecdysone upon interganglionic connective shortening in *Galleria mellonella* (L.) (Lepidoptera). J. exp. Zool. **170**, 181—192 (1969).

PORCHET, M., DURCHON, M.: Influence de la maturité génitale sur la régénération postérieure, chez *Perinereis cultrifera* Grube (Annélide Polychète). C. R. Acad. Sci. (Paris) **267**, Sér. D, 194—196 (1968).

PROVANSAL, A.: Mise en évidence d'organes neurohémaux métamériques associés à la chaîne nerveuse ventrale chez *Vespa crabro* L. et *Vespula germanica* Fabr. (Hyménoptères Vespidae). C. R. Acad. Sci. (Paris) **267**, Sér. D, 864—867 (1968).

PUYEAR, R. L.: Molt cycle regulation of nucleotide pyrophosphatase in the hepatopancreas of the blue crab, *Callinectes sapidus* Rathbun. Comp. Biochem. Physiol. **28**, 159—168 (1969).

QUAY, W. B.: Comparative physiology of serotonin and melatonin. Advanc. Pharmacol. **6**, Part A, 283—297 (1968).

RAABE, M.: Etude des phénomènes de neurosécrétion au niveau de la chaîne nerveuse ventrale des phasmides. Bull. Soc. zool. Fr. **90**, 631—654 (1965).

— Recherches récentes sur la neurosécrétion dans la chaîne nerveuse ventrale des insectes. Bull. Soc. zool. Fr. **92**, 67—71 (1967).

— CAZAL, M., CHALAYE, D., BESSÉ, N. DE: Action cardioaccélératrice des organes neurohémaux périsympathiques ventraux de quelques Insectes. C. R. Acad. Sci. (Paris) **263**, Sér. D, 2002—2005 (1966).

RAMADE, F.: Mise en évidence de cellules neurosécrétrices Gomori négatives dans la Pars intercerebralis de *Musca domestica* L. par une étude comparative en microscopie ordinaire et électronique. C. R. Acad. Sci. (Paris) **268**, Sér. D, 1945—1947 (1969).

RAMAMURTHI, R., MUMBACH, M. W., SCHEER, B. T.: Endocrine control of glycogen synthesis in crabs. Comp. Biochem. Physiol. **26**, 311—319 (1968).

— SCHEER, B. T.: A factor influencing sodium regulation in crustaceans. Life Sci., Part II, **6**, 2171—2175 (1967).

RAO, K. P.: Circadian activity rhythm in the CNS and its control. In: Quantitative biology of metabolism. Ed.: A. LOCKER, p. 258—261. New York: Springer 1968.

RENSING, L.: Daily rhythmicity of corpus allatum and neurosecretory cells in *Drosophila melanogaster* (Meig). Science **144**, 1586—1587 (1964).

Reutter, K.: Das Verhalten des aminergen Nervensystems während der Regeneration des Vorderdarms von *Lineus sanguineus* Rathke (Nemertini). Z. Zellforsch. **102**, 283—292 (1969).

Rinterknecht, E.: Contrôle hormonal de la cicatrisation chez *Locusta migratoria*. Rôle de la pars intercerebralis chez les sujets larvaires. Bull. Soc. Zool. **91**, 789—802 (1966).

Sakharov, D. A., Borovyagin, V. L., Zs.-Nagy, I.: Light, fluorescence and electron microscopic studies on "neurosecretion" in *Tritonia diomedia* Bergh (Mollusca, Nudibranchia). Z. Zellforsch. **68**, 660—673 (1965).

Schaller, F., Meunier, J.: Résultats de cultures organotypiques du cerveau et du ganglion sous-oesophagien d'*Aeschna cyanea* Müll. (Insecte Odonate). Survie des organes et évolution des éléments neurosécréteurs. C. R. Acad. Sci. (Paris) **264**, Sér. D, 1441—1444 (1967).

Scharrer, B.: Neurosecretion. XIII. The ultrastructure of the corpus cardiacum of the insect *Leucophaea maderae*. Z. Zellforsch. **60**, 761—796 (1963).

— Histophysiological studies on the corpus allatum of *Leucophaea maderae*. IV. Ultrastructure during normal activity cycle. Z. Zellforsch. **62**, 125—148 (1964).

— The neurosecretory neuron in neuroendocrine regulatory mechanisms. Amer. Zool. **7**, 161—169 (1967).

— Neurosecretion. XIV. Ultrastructural study of sites of release of neurosecretory material in blattarian insects. Z. Zellforsch. **89**, 1—16 (1968).

— Neurohumors and neurohormones: Definitions and terminology. J. neuro-visc. rel., Suppl. **9**, 1—20 (1969).

— Kater, S. B.: Neurosecretion. XV. An electron microscopic study of the corpora cardiaca of *Periplaneta americana* after experimentally induced hormone release. Z. Zellforsch. **95**, 177—186 (1969).

Scharrer, E., Scharrer, B.: Neuroendocrinology. 289 pp. New York and London: Columbia Univ. Press 1963.

Scheffel, H.: Der Einfluß von Dekapitation und Schnürung auf die Häutung und die Anamorphose der Larven von *Lithobius forficatus* L. (Chilopoda) Zool. Jb., Abt. Physiol. **71**, 359—370 (1965a).

— Über die Wirkung implantierter Cerebraldrüsen auf die Larvenhäutungen von *Lithobius forficatus* L. (Chilopoda). Zool. Anz. **174**, 173—178 (1965b).

Schmekel, L., Wechsler, W.: Elektronenmikroskopische Untersuchungen an Cerebro-Pleural-Ganglien von Nudibranchiern. I. Die Nervenzellen. Z. Zellforsch. **89**, 112—132 (1968).

Schreiner, B.: Histochemistry of the A cell neurosecretory material in the milkweed bug, *Oncopeltus fasciatus* Dallas (Heteroptera: Lygaeidae), with a discussion of the neurosecretory material/carrier substance problem. Gen. comp. Endocr. **6**, 388—400 (1966).

Schuetz, A. W.: Chemical properties and physiological actions of a starfish radial nerve factor and ovarian factor. Gen. comp. Endocr. **12**, 209—221 (1969).

Seligman, M., Friedman, S., Fraenkel, G.: Bursicon mediation of tyrosine hydroxylation during tanning of the adult cuticle of the fly, *Sarcophaga bullata*. J. Insect Physiol. **15**, 553—562 (1969).

Simpson, L., Bern, H. A., Nishioka, R. S.: Examination of the evidence for neurosecretion in the nervous system of *Helisoma tenue* (Gastropoda Pulmonata). Gen. comp. Endocr. **7**, 525—548 (1966).

Smalley, K., Brown, C.: The effects of biogenic amines on water balance in the cockroach. Amer. Zool. **8**, 755 (1968).

Smith, N. A., Ralph, C. L.: Comparison of heart-accelerators from neuro-endocrine tissues of the american cockroach. Gen. comp. Endocr. (in press) (1970).

Smith, U., Smith, D. S.: Observations on the secretory processes in the corpus cardiacum of the stick insect, *Carausius morosus*. J. Cell Sci. **1**, 59—66 (1966).

Srivastava, K. P., Singh, H. H.: On the innervation of the prothoracic glands in *Papilio demoleus* L. (Lepidoptera). Experientia (Basel) **24**, 838—839 (1968).

Strumwasser, F.: Membrane and intracellular mechanism governing endogenous activity in neurons. In: Physiological and biochemical aspects of nervous integration, ed.: F. D. Carlson, p. 329—341. Englewood Cliffs, New Jersey: Prentice-Hall, Inc. 1968.

— Jacklet, J. W., Alvarez, R. B.: A seasonal rhythm in the neural extract induction of behavioral egg-laying in *Aplysia*. Comp. Biochem. Physiol. **29**, 197—206 (1969).

SZUDARSKI, M.: Neurosecretion of the central nervous system of the crab, *Rhithropanopeus harrisi* (Gould) subspecies *tridentata* (Maitl.). Acta Biol. Med. Soc. Sci. Gedan **7**, 1—32 (1963).

TEWARI, H. B., AWASTHI, V. B.: The identical topography of the distribution of alkaline phosphatase and neurosecretory material in the neuroendocrine organs of *Gryllodes sigillatus* (Walk). (Orthoptera, Gryllidae). Gen. comp. Endocr. **10**, 330—338 (1968).

THOMAS, A.: Recherches sur le contrôle neuro-endocrine de l'oviposition chez *Carausius morosus* Br. (Phasmides-Cheleutoptères). C. R. Acad. Sci. (Paris) **267**, Sér. D, 518—521 (1968).

THOMSEN, E.: Esterase in the cells of the hind-midgut of the *Calliphora* female, and its possible dependence on the medial neurosecretory cells of the brain. Z. Zellforsch. **75**, 281—300 (1966).

— LEA, A. O.: Control of the medial neurosecretory cells by the corpus allatum in *Calliphora erythrocephala*. Gen. comp. Endocr. **12**, 51—57 (1969).

THOMSEN, M.: The neurosecretory system of the adult *Calliphora erythrocephala*. IV. A histological study of the corpus cardiacum and its connections with the nervous system. Z. Zellforsch. **94**, 205—219 (1969).

TOEVS, L. A., BRACKENBURY, R. W.: Bag cell-specific proteins and the humoral control of egg laying in *Aplysia californica*. Comp. Biochem. Physiol. **29**, 207—216 (1969).

UDE, J., GERSCH, M.: Eine besondere Konfiguration membrangebundener Polysomen in neurosekretorischen Zellen des Zentralnervensystems eines Anneliden (*Enchytraeus albidus*). Gen. comp. Endocr. **10**, 429—433 (1968).

UNGER, H.: Der Einfluß der Neurohormone C und D auf die Farbstoffabsorptionsfähigkeit der Malpighischen Gefäße (und des Darmes) der Stabheuschrecke *Carausius morosus* (Br.) in vitro. Zool. Jb., Abt. Physiol. **71**, 710—717 (1965a).

— Der Einfluß körpereigener Wirkstoffe auf die Nerventätigkeit von *Periplaneta americana* L. Zool. Jb., Abt. Physiol. **71**, 727—740 (1965b).

VIGH-TEICHMANN, I., GOSLAR, H. G.: Enzymhistochemische Studien am Nervensystem. III. Das Verhalten einiger Hydrolasen im Nervensystem des Regenwurmes (*Eisenia foetida*). Histochemie **14**, 352—365 (1968).

VITZ, H.: Untersuchungen über die Steuerung des endokrinen Systems bei der Mehlmotte *Ephestia (Anagasta) kühniella* während des letzten Larvenstadiums. Wilhelm Roux' Arch. Entwickl.-Mech. Org. **159**, 1—30 (1967).

WAUTIER, J., PAVANS DE CECCATTY, M., RICHARDOT, M., BUISSON, B., HERNANDEZ, M. L.: Note sur les complexes neuro-endocriniens de *Gundlachia* sp. (Mollusque Ancylidae). Bull. Soc. Linnéenne Lyon **30**, 79—87 (1961).

WEITZMAN, M.: Ultrastructural study on the release of neurosecretory material from the sinus gland of the land carb, *Gecarcinus lateralis*. Z. Zellforsch. **94**, 147—154 (1969).

WILKENS, J. L.: The endocrine control of protein metabolism as related to reproduction in the fleshfly *Sarcophaga bullata*. J. Insect Physiol. **15**, 1015—1024 (1969).

WILLIAMS, C. M.: The present status of the brain hormone. In: Insects and physiology. Ed.: J. W. L. BEAMENT and J. E. TREHERNE, p. 133—139. Edinburgh and London: Oliver & Boyd 1967.

WYSS-HUBER, M., LÜSCHER, M.: Über die hormonale Beeinflußbarkeit der Proteinsynthese in vitro im Fettkörper von *Leucophaea maderae* (Insecta). Rev. suisse Zool. **73**, 517—521 (1966).

ZIMMERMANN, P.: Der „b-Zellen"-Komplex im Zentralnervensystem von *Lumbricus terrestris* L. Z. Zellforsch. **91**, 283—299 (1968).

# Neue Möglichkeiten zur fluorescenzmikroskopischen Darstellung neurosekretorischer Zellen*

Peter Zimmermann

Anatomisches Institut der Universität Gießen, Lehrstuhl I (West-Germany)
(Direktor: Prof. Dr. A. Oksche)

**Key words:** Neurosecretion — Invertebrate — Fluorescence microscopy.

Die Untersuchung der Absorptions- und Luminescenzeigenschaften von histologischen Schnittpräparaten hat als Methode der Struktur- und Bausteinanalyse den Vorteil, daß sie eine exakte Lokalisation der untersuchten Substrate erlaubt. Jede Substanz läßt sich durch ihre Lichtabsorption und -emission charakterisieren; dies beruht auf der Anwesenheit von chromophoren Gruppen, d.h. von Atomverbänden, die Lichtquanten im Ultraviolettbereich des Spektrums absorbieren. Die Chromophore der Proteinmakromoleküle lassen sich in monomere und polymere Formen unterteilen. Die erste Klasse wird von den 20 Aminosäuren eingenommen, die sowohl im freien Zustand als auch gebunden im Proteinpolymer durch Licht anregbar sind. Der Hauptanteil der Quantenabsorption im Bereich von 250–300 nm entfällt auf die aromatischen Aminosäuren Tyrosin und Tryptophan (s. Cowgill, 1963). Die Primärfluorescenz der Proteine stammt nur von diesen beiden Aminosäuren (Tyrosinfluorescenz: 304 nm; Tryptophanfluorescenz: 328—342 nm). Die polymeren Chromophore sind Atomgruppierungen, die nur bei der Verknüpfung von freien Aminosäuren zu Molekülverbänden entstehen, hierzu gehören Peptid- und Thioesterbindungen. Sie verschwinden, wenn das Makromolekül in seine Monomere aufgespalten wird. Die primäre Proteinfluorescenz ist relativ schwach. Sie läßt sich aber durch spezifische Kopplung der entsprechenden Aminosäurereste mit geeigneten Fluorochromen beträchtlich steigern. Neben der Bausteinanalyse (z.B. SH-Gruppen-Nachweis) kann man mit dieser Sekundär-Fluorescenzmethode auch Informationen über Sekundär- und Tertiärstrukturen von Proteinen sammeln, wie es die Arbeiten von Scheibe (1939) und Hoppe (1944) über Pseudoisocyanin beweisen. Die im folgenden Beitrag vorgelegten Befunde sollen als *Modell* einer mikrospektrographischen Analyse von spezifisch fluorochromierten neurosekretorisch aktiven Ganglienzellen im Nervensystem von *Lumbricus terrestris* L. verstanden werden.

Die Untersuchungen wurden mit 10 im Juli gefangenen Regenwürmern (*Lumbricus terrestris* L.) durchgeführt. Die formoldampffixierten 7 μm dicken Gefrierschnitte wurden 1. nativ und 2. nach Fluorochromierung mit einer $10^{-3}$ m Lösung von RF 500 bei pH 7 mit dem Mikrospektrographen der Firma Leitz, Wetzlar[1] analysiert. Filterkombination: BG 12, BG 38 und K 530.

* Mit Unterstützung durch die Deutsche Forschungsgemeinschaft.

1 Die mikrospektrographischen Messungen wurden mit dankenswerter Unterstützung durch die Firma Leitz, Wetzlar (Dr. Wasmund) durchgeführt.

Das Oberschlundganglion des Regenwurms eignet sich als Modellbeispiel besonders gut, da hier neben einfachen Ganglienzellen verschiedene Typen sekretorisch aktiver Neurone zwischen gut entwickelter faserhaltiger Glia vorkommen.

## 1. Native Gefrierschnitte

Die qualitativen und quantitativen Eigenschaften des untersuchten Cytoplasmas der verschiedenen Neurone bestimmen die Form der Absorptionskurven. Die Parameter sind Steilheit, Lage der Maxima und der Flächeninhalt der Kurven.

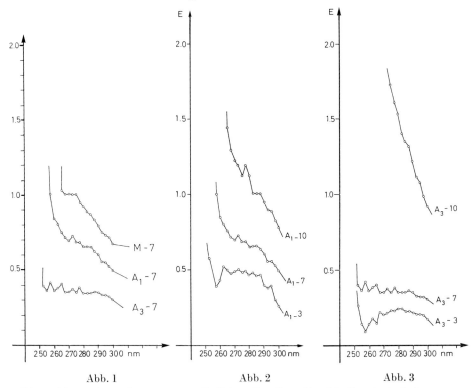

Abb. 1                    Abb. 2                    Abb. 3

Abb. 1. Absorptionsspektren von gewöhnlichen Ganglienzellen $(A_3\text{-}7)$, sekretorischen $A_1$-Neuronen $(A_1\text{-}7)$ und Zellen des sog. „b-Komplexes" $(M\text{-}7)$

Abb. 2. Absorptionskurven der neurosekretorischen Ganglienzellen bei verschiedenen pH-Werten. $A_1\text{-}3$ 2. Absorptionsmaximum von Tyrosin bei 295 nm kommt stärker bei pH 3 hervor. $A_1\text{-}10$ Bei pH 10 ist das 1. Maximum von Tyrosin (273 nm) besonders deutlich

Abb. 3. Absorptionsspektren von gewöhnlichen Ganglienzellen. Es fällt die starke Differenz zwischen den Kurven von pH 7 $(A_3\text{-}7)$ und pH 10 $(A_3\text{-}10)$ auf

Abb. 1 zeigt, daß die gewöhnlichen Ganglienzellen bei pH 7 am stärksten in dem Wellenlängenbereich von 250—300 nm absorbieren. Die Zellen des sog. „b-Komplexes", die zu den Mastzellen gerechnet werden müssen[2], nehmen die wenigsten Lichtquanten auf, und der Beginn der Absorptionskurve ist am weitesten in den langwelligen Bereich verschoben. Die Absorptionsmaxima der aro-

---

[2] Vgl. ZIMMERMANN (1968).

matischen Aminosäuren (Tyrosin 273 nm, Tryptophan 280 nm) treten nur in den Ganglienzellen auf, sie fehlen in den ,,b-Komplexen". Eine weitere Differenzierung gelingt durch Messung bei unterschiedlichen pH-Werten. In Abb. 2 erkennt man, daß eine Alkalisierung des Milieus eine Absorptionsabnahme zur Folge hat. Außerdem werden die Kurven der neurosekretorisch aktiven Ganglienzellen stärker

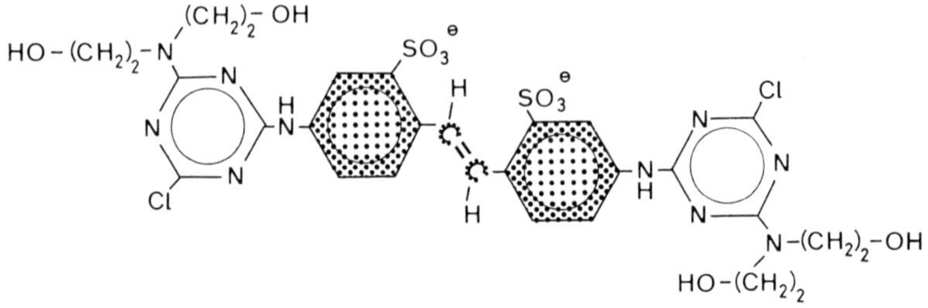

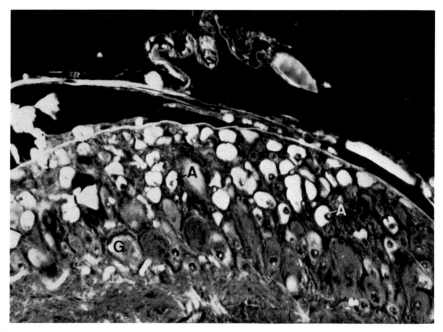

Abb. 4. RF 500 — 4,4′-Bis-(2-Chlor-4-diäthanolamino-1,3,5-triazinyl-(6)-amino)-stilben-2,2″-disulfonsaures Natrium

Abb. 5. Ausschnitt aus dem Oberschlundganglion von *Lumbricus terrestris*. Fluorochromierung mit RF 500. $A$-$A_1$ Neurone, $G$ einfache Ganglienzellen. Vergr. 550fach

gegliedert. Das 1. Maximum der Tyrosinabsorption wird verstärkt, während sich die relative Extinktion von Tryptophan — bezogen auf die Einzelkurve — nicht verändert. Bei pH 3 tritt das 2. Absorptionsmaximum von Tyrosin gut hervor. Ganz anders verhalten sich die einfachen Ganglienzellen (s. Abb. 3). Die Dissoziation der Absorptionskurven zwischen pH 7 und 10 ist viel ausgeprägter. Das 2. Maximum von Tyrosin kommt nicht zur Darstellung; auch der Tryptophan-

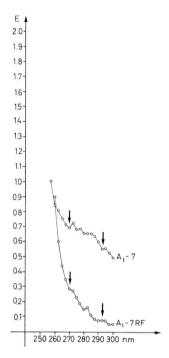

Abb. 6. Absorptionskurven von sekretorischen $A_1$-Neuronen vor ($A_1$-7) und nach ($A_1$-7 RF) Fluorochromierung mit RF 500. ↓ Maxima der Tyrosinabsorption. Sie verschwinden nach der Fluorochromierung

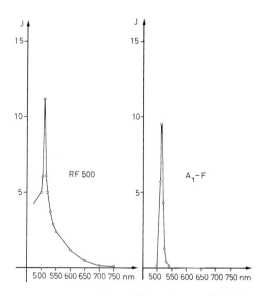

Abb. 7. Fluorescenzspektren des kristallinen Fluorochroms (RF 500) und der fluorochromierten $A_1$-Ganglienzelle ($A_1$-F). In beiden Kurven liegt das Maximum bei 510 nm

anteil des Absorptionsspektrums ist nur schwach ausgebildet. Diese wenigen Bei-
spiele demonstrieren, daß sich die Absorptionsmessungen für die Charakterisierung
bestimmter Zelltypen, besonders im Verlauf von Sekretionscyclen, gut eignen.
Man stellt sich mit dem Monochromator einen Wellenlängenabschnitt ein, in dem
der gesuchte Zelltyp am intensivsten absorbiert und kann so das ganze Schnitt-
präparat durchmustern, um die Verteilung dieser Zellform zu studieren.

## 2. Fluorochromierte Gefrierschnitte

RF 500, das mir freundlicherweise von Dr. H. HARMS, Leverkusen, zur Ver-
fügung gestellt wurde, gehört zu den Reaktivfluorochromen (Abb. 4). Das zentrale
Stilbenmolekül liegt in der allein fluorescenzfähigen planaren trans-Isomerform
vor. Die beiden Triazinringe sind als Träger der Kopplungsgruppen (Cl-) anzusehen. Die spektralphotometrischen Daten, breite Absorptions- und Fluorescenzspektren sowie hohe Intensitäten, zeichnen dieses Fluorochrom aus. RF 500
fluorochromiert sowohl Faserglia als auch neurosekretorisch aktive Ganglienzellen ohne vorherige Oxydation. Hierfür eignen sich besonders gut die $A_1$-Neurone
von *Lumbricus terrestris* (Abb. 5). Dies hängt mit dem Gehalt an freien SH-
Gruppen zusammen, die in den $A_1$-Zellen in hoher Konzentration vorliegen, wie
es TEICHMANN, AROS und VIGH (1966) mit der DDD-Methode zeigen konnten.
Außer den Sulfhydrylgruppen sind die OH-Reste von Tyrosin an der Kopplungs-
reaktion beteiligt. Nach einer Blockierung der SH-Gruppen mit 0,1 m Monojod-
acetat ist noch ein Randsaum des $A_1$-Cytoplasmas fluorochromierbar. Einige der
$A_1$-Neurone nehmen RF 500 auch trotz Blockierung elektiv auf. Außerdem rea-
gieren sie positiv mit der Millonschen Reaktion zum Tyrosinnachweis. Eleganter
gelingt dies mit der mikrospektrographischen Analyse (Abb. 6). Neben der ver-
stärkten Absorption der $A_1$-Zellen nach Fluorochromierung mit RF 500 beobachtet man eine selektive Abnahme der Tyrosin-Absorptionsmaxima. Da RF 500
erst bei 400 nm zu absorbieren beginnt, kann von einer unspezifischen Absorptions-
zunahme der $A_1$-Proteine nicht gesprochen werden, zumal das Maximum der
Tryptophan-Absorption nicht beeinflußt wird. Durch die Kopplung des Fluorochroms müssen Energie-Austauschvorgänge zwischen RF 500 und den kovalent
gebundenen Tyrosinresten infolge der UV-Anregung stattfinden. Die Analyse des
Fluorescenzspektrums der $A_1$-Neurone nach Fluorochromierung mit RF 500 ergab
einen weiteren interessanten Befund: Das Fluorescenzmaximum liegt bei 510 nm
und entspricht dem des kristallinen Fluorochroms (Abb. 7). Ob RF 500 mit den
Cytoplasmaproteinen ebenfalls kristallartige Verbindungen eingeht, läßt sich nicht
mit Sicherheit sagen, da die Empfindlichkeit der Methodik noch nicht ausreicht.

Die vorgelegten Befunde beweisen, daß die $A_1$-Neurone des Oberschlund-
ganglions von *Lumbricus terrestris* L. sowohl Tyrosin als auch Cystein in hoher
Konzentration enthalten. Der prozentuale Anteil der beiden Aminosäuren variiert
je nach Funktionszustand; dies läßt sich durch Fluorochromierung mit RF 500
nach Blockierung der SH-Gruppen nachweisen. Der Einsatz eines Mikrospektrographen zur Struktur- und Bausteinanalyse von Cytoplasmabestandteilen erübrigt
komplizierte histochemische Nachweisverfahren und schont das zu untersuchende
Präparat. Eine exakte biochemisch-physikalische Charakterisierung verschiedener
Zelltypen und ihrer Funktionen ist möglich.

## Literatur

Cowgill, R. W.: Fluorescence and the structure of proteins. I. Effects of substituents on the fluorescence of indole and phenole compounds. Arch. Biochem. **100**, 36—44 (1963).

Hoppe, W.: Beziehungen zwischen Struktur und Lichtabsorption der reversiblen Polymerisate der Pseudoisocyaninreihe. Kolloid.-Z. **109**, 21—27 (1944).

Scheibe, G.: Die Stereoisomere organischer Farbstoffe und ihr Zusammenhang mit der Konstitution und Eigenschaften reversibler polymerer Farbstoffe. Angew. Chem. **52**, 631—642 (1939).

Teichmann, I., Aros, B., Vigh, B.: Histochemical studies on Gomori-positive substances. III. Examination of the earthworms neurosecretory system (*Lumbricus herculeus, Eisenia foetida*). Acta biol. Acad. Sci. hung. **17**, 329–357 (1966).

Zimmermann, P.: Der „b-Zellen"-Komplex im Zentralnervensystem von *Lumbricus terrestris* L. Z. Zellforsch. **91**, 283—299 (1968).

# The Mechanism of Hormone Release from Neurosecretory Axon Endings in the Insect *Calliphora erythrocephala*

Tom Christian Normann

Institute of General Zoology, University of Copenhagen (Denmark)

**Key words:** Neurosecretion — Neurohormone release — *Calliphora erythrocephala*.

The corpus cardiacum of the blowfly *Calliphora erythrocephala* contains neurosecretory cells (the c.n.c.) axons of which together with some extrinsic n.s. axons occupy a medullary portion, the c. card. neuropile. Here n.s. substances are stored and—upon appropriate stimulation—released into the haemolymph (Normann, 1965, 1969; Normann and Duve, 1969).

This neurohaemal organ offers two main advantages for the study of structural features of neurohormone release: 1) The phase of extrusion of material contained in n.s. granules, though short lived, is of sufficient duration for allowing the "omega-appearance" characteristic of exocytosis to be "frozen" by fixation. 2) The location and size of the c. card. permits viewing as well as rapid fixation at any chosen moment during stimulation (cf. Normann and Duve, 1969).

Exocytosis seems to be a rather fundamental mechanism since it occurs in many, perhaps all, the merocrine gland cells, in which the secretory product is delivered as membrane-surrounded packages from the Golgi apparatus, and for which plain evidence as to the mode of secretion has been obtained. Moreover, n.s. neurons probably conduct nervous impulses and so offer particular possibilities for the investigation of the induction of exocytosis, the "stimulus-secretion coupling". It thus appeared desirable to take advantage of the above-mentioned special properties of the blowfly c. card in order to obtain a more detailed analysis of the cellular events from the onset of exocytosis to the later phases of the secretory process. Besides, such an analysis might help to clarify the essential dissimilarities—if any—existing between the phenomena apparently connected with exocytosis in some n.s. cells, and those structural indications of release-processes observed in n.s. cells where exocytosis is held not to occur.

## Materials and Methods

Four day old female *Calliphora* kept at 25°C and fed sugar and water ad libitum were used for all experiments.

A standard procedure for electron microscopy has been described elsewhere (Normann, 1969) together with a method of quantitative evaluation by counting the cases of exocytosis ("E") and vesicle clusters ("VC") as well as all n.s. axon profiles in sections of the c. card. neuropile. The frequency of exocytosis and vesicle clusters was calculated as counts per 100 axon profiles: E/100 a and VC/100 a.

*Electrical Stimulation*

The stimulating electrodes—electrolytically pointed steel semi-microelectrodes, lacquer-insulated to the tip and mounted in a micromanipulator, were placed in front of and behind the c. card. The front electrode was inserted between oesophagus and aorta and touched the "cardiac-recurrent nerve", which innervates the gland. A stimulus current of 5–15 μA was delivered as 0.5 msec, 5 V rectangular pulses, 3/sec for 30–45 sec. After that period fixative was applied, the stimulator, however, not being switched off until the movements of visceral muscles below the c. card. had ceased. This lasted a few seconds during which period fixative must have penetrated the c. card.

*Depolarization Experiments*

Acetylcholine-chloride ($10^{-4}$ M) together with eserine ($10^{-5}$ M) were dissolved in Ringer (composition see NORMANN and DUVE, 1969). After exposure of the c. card. by removal of the neck membrane and some small muscles and tracheae, the ACh-solution was applied. This resulted in vigorous movements of visceral muscles (aorta and oesophagus). After 30–60 sec this liquid was replaced by fixative. Five such specimens were inspected with the electron microscope.

Earlier unpublished observations on corpora cardiaca, which had been immersed in the same Ringer for up to 5 min had indicated that no essential structural alterations were brought about by the use of this liquid. Therefore no controls were used in these preliminary experiments.

Loading with potassium consisted in the application of a Ringer with $K^+$ contents raised to 100 mM and $Ca^{++}$ to 5 mM. After exactly two minutes this fluid was replaced by fixative. Only two specimens were examined.

*Stress-Experiments*

Flies were subjected to "stress" by shaking them in a flask for a few minutes, whereupon they were etherized, dissected and the c. card. fixed for electron microscopy. Since fixation obviously could not take place until about one minute after "stimulation", and since it is practically impossible to quantify this treatment only two specimens were investigated.

# Results

## I. Membrane Phenomena

In a preliminary report on experimentally induced exocytosis of n.s. granules (NORMANN, 1969), it was suggested that granule liberation might consist of a sequence of cellular events starting with the formation of a contact between granule membrane and axolemma. Hence exocytosis, in the sense of a complex dynamic phenomenon, will appear differently on electron micrographs depending on the actual phase preserved by fixation. The successive stages, including that of extrusion of granule contents, and also the vesicle clusters probably representing fragmentation products of granule membranes following exocytosis, are here illustrated by the electron micrographs of Fig. 1a–f, the legend of which summarizes the hypothesis.

### A. Electrical Stimulation

To obtain more precise information especially on the relation between exocytosis and the vesicle clusters than the above mentioned study could provide, more well-defined stimulation conditions appeared desirable. Certain factors of relevance for the selection of stimulus parameters will later be discussed in relation to the functioning of the n.s. system. At this point, however, some observations made during the work of selecting the experimental conditions used for the present study should be mentioned. Incidentally, such pilot work together with a large

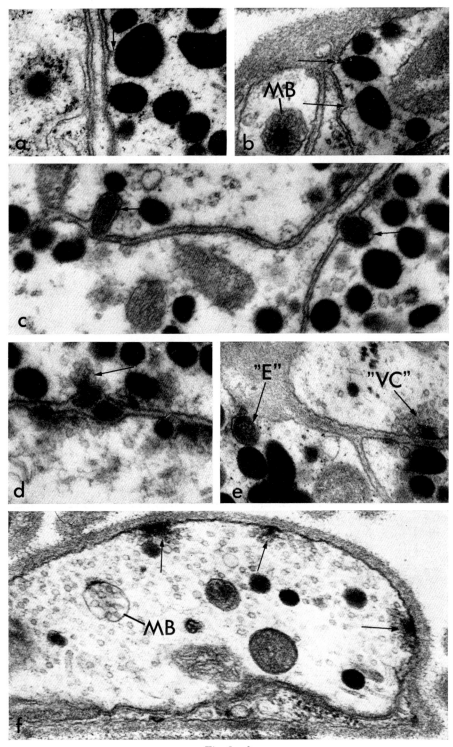

Fig. 1 a–f

material from earlier studies provided a basis for detecting for example electro-lytical artifacts and to obtain a morphologically satisfactory experimental material.

Firstly, direct stimulation of the c. card. brings about a release of hyper-glycemic neurohormone comparable to that caused by indirect stimulation via the brain, as described by NORMANN and DUVE (1969). A sensitive spectrophoto-metrical method for quantitative determination of hemolymph trehalose sup-ported the results obtained by thin layer chromatography (DUVE, unpublished).

Secondly, stimulation for longer periods ($>$ 1 minute) brought about a more or less complete disappearance from the c. card. neuropile of the bluish-white tint, so characteristic of n.s. granules in living cells and axons. The c.n.c. peri-karya, however, were not readily depleted. Such corpora cardiaca upon fixation and embedding for electron microscopy appeared less dark than usual owing to the disappearance of osmiophilic material, and in the E.M. many n.s. axons appeared depleted of granules. On the other hand they usually contained abundant small vesicles (300–500 Å) and also several multilamellate bodies (cf. NORMANN, 1969).

Ten specimens, which had been stimulated for 30–45 sec and in good state of preservation, were carefully inspected, and they supported the interpretation of structural indications of secretion previously given. The main purpose was to investigate the possible covariance of "exocytosis" and vesicle clusters. Here the term exocytosis is used in the more restricted sense of the phase appearing as an "omega-figure" (Fig. 1 c, e). The result of the quantitative analysis is given in Fig. 2, where the solid circles relate the frequency of exocytosis and of vesicle clusters for these specimens. The open circles represent the controls from the previous study (NORMANN, 1969). As is readily seen, there exists a high positive linear correlation, and statistical analysis shows a correlation coefficient of 0.946 in this material, which may be regarded as normally functioning cells. Of greater interest is the regression equation which is given in the legend of Fig. 2 and indicated in the plot as the solid line.

The most obvious interpretation of these data seems to be that the vesicle clusters persist more than twice as long as the omega-figures of exocytosis and therefore are found in greater numbers. From the equation can also be seen that —statistically—there is a good probability of finding vesicle clusters in n.s. axons not engaged in exocytosis at the very moment of fixation.

Fig. 1 a–f. *Consecutive stages of exocytosis in electrically stimulated c. card.* All magnifications ×50,000. a The newly established connection between granule membrane and axolemma appears as a very delicate membrane. b At membrane fusion the axolemma is drawn inward (arrows). *MB* multivesicular body. c Omega-figures typical of exocytosis (arrows). The con-tents of the extruded granules show substructure before dissolution. d The empty granule membrane collapses and ruptures, the remnants rounding up to form tiny vesicles (arrow). e Typical omega figure ("*E*") and vesicle cluster ("*VC*"). Only structures which without doubt could be identified as either "E" or "VC" were counted and calculated (cf. Fig. 2). f Nearly depleted axon ending. Most n.s. granules have been replaced by small vesicles. Three vesicle clusters at release sites are still present (arrows). Gradually, however, the vesicles disperse in the axoplasm. Some may be enclosed in multivesicular bodies (*MB*). Occasionally multilamellate bodies are formed (not shown)

*Synapses and "Synaptoid Structures"*

Since some uncertainty exists with regard to the existence of synapses in the c. card. and the terms "synaptic" and "synaptoid" junctions have now and then been used to indicate structures related to release phenomena rather than to impulse transmission (see Discussion), the author wishes to emphasize the following observations:

The small vesicles occurring at release sites mostly have the same size range as synaptic vesicles. However, whereas vesicle clusters may be found wherever

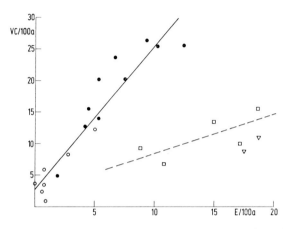

Fig. 2. *Frequency of omega-figures (E/100 a) and vesicle clusters (VC/100 a)* in corpora cardiaca electrically stimulated for 30–45 sec were plotted as solid circles; controls (see text) open circles; specimens depolarized with acetylcholine, squares; and potassium-loaded c. card., triangles. The controls and the electrically stimulated c. card. (thought to be normally functioning) were statistically treated as one group ($n = 17$). High positive linear correlation is present ($r = 0.946$) and the regression equation (solid line): $\bar{Y}_c = 2.68 + 2.31\,E$ indicates that the vesicle clusters though transient persist much longer than the "E", and the Y intercept (2.68) shows that there is—statistically—good probability of finding vesicle clusters in non-stimulated material. The broken line represents the regression equation for the ACh-specimens. The high frequency of omega-figures and the different slope of the line are discussed in the text

release of a granule has been taking place (e.g. opposite glial or stromal envelopes or opposite other axons) and only occasionally give rise to structural modifications at the outer side of the axolemma in the form of dense n.s. substance not dissolved at the moment of fixation, the synapses have additional structural features, notably a more regular thickening of pre- and postsynaptic membranes and the presence of a typical subsynaptic web (cf. NORMANN, 1965). In addition, in the *Calliphora* c. card. the synapses always consist of a presynaptic axon containing smaller (800–1,400 Å) and more round granules, whereas the postsynaptic axon always belongs to an intrinsic n.s. cell (c.n.c.) and contains larger (up to 3,000 Å) and often more elongate granules. Occasionally it may be difficult to decide whether a small aggregation of vesicles represents a release site or part of a synapse, more peripherally sectioned. Such cases were not included in the counts of vesicle clusters.

## B. The Effect of Depolarizing Agents

Since n.s. cells probably have electrophysiological properties such as resting and action potentials in common with other neurons, and since secretion from their axon endings may be closely linked with their impulse-activity, it appeared of interest to examine ultrastructurally the secretory phenomena under conditions of membrane-depolarization. Relatively high concentrations of both acetylcholine and potassium were used, because little information exists on the normal ionic milieu of these cells, and because the purpose was to obtain a massive effect within a short period. This could in fact be recorded before visible osmotic damage began to occur. In view of the findings of Beaulaton (1967) with regard to the cholin-esterase-content of the *Rhodnius* c. card., eserine was added to the Ringer containing acetylcholine.

Under the influence of ACh the n.s. axons show an exocytosis activity far exceeding any, which has yet been recorded in electrically stimulated corpora cardiaca. Fig. 2 contains five plots of specimens exposed to ACh for 30–60 sec (open squares). The regression equation shown as a broken line results from the analysis of that material. The two potassium-loaded specimens, which seem to react very similarly (triangles) were not included in the analysis, since after all exocytosis in these might have been provoked by a more or less different mecha-nism. The correlation coefficient with regard to exocytosis and vesicle clusters for the five ACh-preparations is 0.73.

The axons of the corpora cardiaca thought to be depolarized by the two above-mentioned methods share some special structural features. Firstly, in non-stimulated or "normal" electrically stimulated c. card., fusion of membranes from two or more n.s. granules practically never occurs (neither does fusion of granule membrane with axolemma apparently take place, unless some stimulating impulse has reached the axon ending). In this material, however, the following phenomenon might be observed: One n.s. granule had started an exocytosis, its membrane being continuous with the axolemma as usual. On another part of the granule membrane a second granule had made a similar fusion to start exocytosis so to say into the first one (see Fig. 3). In a few cases several granules were thus in mutual connection with the cell membrane. This may well be meaningful in terms of a possible relation between membrane polarity and membrane inter-actions and will be dealt with in the Discussion.

A second difference between this material and "normally" secreting axon endings is evident from Fig. 2. The relation between occurrence of exocytosis and vesicle clusters is significantly different, exocytosis being found in a greater number of cases in c. card. subjected to $K^+$ or ACh-treatment. It is the author's impression that this is due both to a more effective induction of exocytosis and to a longer persistence of the "omega-structure" relative to the duration of the "vesicle cluster"-phase.

## C. "Stressed" Flies

Under certain conditions which perhaps may be regarded as discomfort and which cause a sudden rise in expenditure of energy for movement, termed "stress", the insect c. card. apparently releases substances such as hyperglycemic and heart-accelerating substances (see e.g. HODGSON and GELDIAY, 1959). Stressing of blowflies was attempted by shaking them in a flask for several minutes. Afterwards they were etherized and processed as usual for electron microscopy. For the reasons already mentioned only two specimens were examined, and quantitative analysis was not undertaken at that time. Exocytosis was not observed, whereas vesicle clusters were abundant, and many axons contained high numbers of small vesicles (300–600 Å) and could be more or less depleted of n.s. granules. It may perhaps be concluded, that since stimulation had ceased when fixation could take place, only the later stages of the secretory process could be observed.

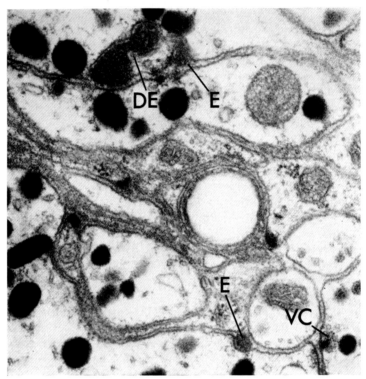

Fig. 3. *N.s. axons in ACh-depolarized c. card.* One vesicle cluster and some extruded granules E and DE) are present. A n.s. granule membrane has fused with one, already engaged in exocytosis (DE). The substructure is becoming visible in the exteriorized contents. ×80,000

## II. The Contents of the N.S. Granules

In well-preserved material the granule membrane which, incidentally, has typical unit membrane structure [termed a "double-membrane" by BARGMANN and v. GAUDECKER (1969)], and which is originally a Golgi-membrane, encloses a seemingly homogeneous, electron opaque substance.

At high magnification a certain granularity may be seen, but normally actual geometrical order is not visible. However, under special circumstances it may be revealed that the n.s. material present in the c. card. has a regular substructure, consisting of filaments with a less electron dense core, which makes them resemble tubules.

The length of these filaments often corresponds to the long axis of the granules, but sometimes they appear more or less bent or even folded and then may have a greater length. Their outer diameter (as measured on sectioned material) is

120–140 Å. In cross-sections they appear as circles (Fig. 4), but no reason seems to exist for identifying or even comparing them with cytoplasmatic microtubules. Neither do they have anything in common with membranous' vesicles. Groups of small vesicles enclosed within a larger vesicle, the so-called "multivesicular bodies" present in several cell types including n.s. cells, are thus different pheno-

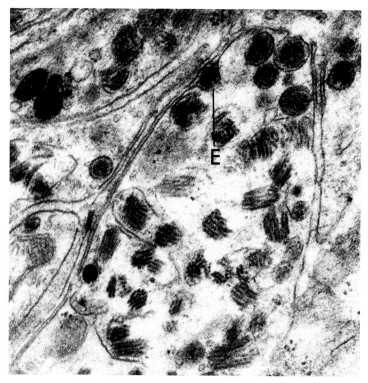

Fig. 4. *The internal structure of n. s. granules* —not normally visible (cf. text) —revealed because of electrolytical artifacts in the form of osmotic swelling. The subunits consist of long thin filaments with a less electron dense core. They run parallel in bundles. ×80,000

mena. In Fig. 1 c and e, may be seen the subunits of n.s. granules, here engaged in exocytosis, whereas multivesicular bodies are present in Fig. 1 b and f.

The filamentous subunits in n.s. granules may be arranged in one or a few bundles, each consisting of a number of parallel filaments; they are often oriented in different directions (Fig. 4).

This substructure is hardly visible in intact, intraaxonal granules. During exocytosis after opening of the granule membrane it may show up, apparently before actual dissolution has started. This is the case both when exocytosis has been induced by electrical stimulation and by depolarization (Fig. 3).

In granules still inside axons the substructure only becomes conspicuous under conditions which to all appearance are somewhat abnormal, and which in drastic cases appears to involve osmotic swelling and even disrupture of granule membranes. It has, however, also been observed in some axon endings in a c. card.

which has been indirectly stimulated (via the brain). This particular specimen was included in the material previously described (NORMANN, 1969) and had the code letter "J". The relation between E/100 a and VC/100 a differed considerably from the rest, and if plotted in Fig. 2 would rather be found among the depolarization experiments. Upon reexamination including the quantitative analysis of many additional sections the data formerly obtained were found to be valid; nevertheless, the impression was that some axons, perhaps because of fatigue, had not been able to maintain normal ionic balance. The structural alterations, however, were not nearly as conspicuous as those seen in Fig. 4. The latter specimen, on the other hand, still seems to have been able to function since exocytosis is occurring. It may be concluded that the granule membrane has the ability to keep the contents tightly packed. When its function as a barrier between neurohormone and surrounding milieu is over at exocytosis, or when abnormal conditions interfere with this property, the subunits temporarily spread and stand out before actual dissolution commences.

## Discussion

The results of this study support the hypothesis of a functional relationship between different structural features, each of which in its own way have been related to release processes.

Ultrastructural studies of insect n.s. systems have led to two different interpretations of the mode of release, either that exocytosis was the responsible mechanism (NORMANN, 1965; SMITH and SMITH, 1966; MADDRELL, 1966; BRADY and MADDRELL, 1967; FINLAYSON and OSBORNE, 1968), or that "intracellular fragmentation" of granules resulted in the formation of vesicle clusters or "synaptoids" (JOHNSON, 1966; B. SCHARRER, 1968; B. SCHARRER and KATER, 1969).

At this point it may be mentioned that vesicle clusters were occasionally observed in the material described earlier (NORMANN, 1965); no role could, however, be ascribed to them at that time.

The concept of exocytosis as a dynamic sequence of cellular events (NORMANN, 1969) accounts for the fate of the granule membrane after extrusion of its contents, and brings the above-mentioned observations into agreement.

It must be realized that since exocytosis involves transient phases, the chance of observing one or the other of these depends on time in more than one way. Firstly, preservation of "omega-figures" requires their presence at the very moment of fixation. Therefore B. SCHARRER and KATER (1969), who disregard the possibility of exocytosis, may not have observed it because their material was fixed at least several seconds after delivering the last pulse of stimulation. Incidentally, the period of stimulation found to be necessary for obtaining a physiologically measurable output of hormone (for example 15 min) may be out of proportion to the duration of the underlying cellular events, and probably the omega-phase lasts only a small fraction of a second. The exact duration of this particular phase cannot be determined by the present material; it is, however, sufficiently long in relation to the time required in *Calliphora* by the penetrating fixative to preserve this structural configuration.

This then is the second time-dependent factor. The time required for the action of fixative is not infinitesimal. Therefore in some n.s. systems an omega-phase may be too short-lived to be preserved by the fixation methods now available. Besides, the granule membrane at this stage appears especially unstable, and arriving fixative might precipitate fragmentation and vesiculation.

Anyway, it is interesting that in so many n.s. axons, where evidence for exocytosis is lacking, including much vertebrate material "configurations analogous to sites of hormone release in neurosecretory neurons of insects" occur and similarly "show clusters of small vesicles and deposits of electron dense material close to the axolemma in certain focal areas of neurohemal organs" (B. SCHARRER, 1968). The term "synaptoid", sometimes used to denote such configurations, seems less appropriate, since it may suggest a more direct relation to impulse transmission (cf. p. 34).

The author wishes to point out once again that no particular locations of the membrane of n.s. axon endings in *Calliphora* appear to be specialized release sites (cf. p. 34 and NORMANN, 1965). The occasional occurrence of a n.s. granule released into a synaptic cleft (from the postsynaptic cell), mentioned by B. SCHARRER (1968) when arguing against views put forward in the above-mentioned study, and which later work has corroborated, may well be a rare phenomenon, but certainly not inconsistent with any of my interpretations.

On the other hand, it seems worthwhile to note that "synaptic" or "synaptoid" contacts described in the vertebrate hypophysis [for example by KNOWLES and VOLLRATH (1966), see also survey by KNOWLES (1967)] are not only found opposite other axons or endocrine cells but also at pituicytes or basement membranes of perivascular spaces. If such structures, or at least some of them, represent release sites the similarity to the conditions in insects is striking. In view of the findings of PALAY (1957) and later by several others that "synaptic" vesicles might arise by fragmentation of n.s. granules, it may be suggested that the possible differences between arthropods and vertebrates as to the mode of secretion may be of minor importance and largely consist in differences as to the exact manner of fragmentation. An important similarity, however, would be that the process occurs at the —probably impulse-conducting—axolemma.

Configurations like that shown in Fig. 1 d are most readily interpreted as intermediate stages between "omega-structures" and the vesicle clusters; this and the statistical correlation between the occurrence of these phenomena evidently indicate a functional connection. An alternative view, that two (or more) different mechanisms are operating in the same cells, would demand explanation of the fact that they so often occur at the same release sites. Besides, it is difficult to conceive of any advantage for such cells of using and having to control different mechanisms responsible for the same effect.

The greater number of vesicle clusters than of omega-figures normally found in fixed material, indicates longer persistence of the former. Further, as Fig. 2 shows there is a certain probability of observing vesicle clusters in corpora cardiaca fixed during low secretory activity, e.g. in non-stimulated specimens. Whether this reflects some basal rate of secretion, or is due to stimulation in the form of mild stress caused by handling the flies before fixation (cf. NORMANN and DUVE, 1969), cannot be determined.

It may be mentioned that although the excess of vesicle clusters could be explained otherwise, e.g. by a formation of several crowds of vesicles from each granule membrane, this is not in keeping with the actual observations and would, besides, involve an unexpected and probably expensive membrane synthesis in connection with exocytosis. Some geometrical considerations may be relevant to that point. If exocytosis proceeds without appreciable alterations of the total membrane area, the membrane of a spherical n.s. granule with a diameter of 2,000 Å may be transformed into 25 vesicles of 400 Å. Depending on the size of the n.s. granule and of the resulting small vesicles, clusters of up to 40 (but often of less than 20) may occur, these estimated figures being consistent with the actual observations on single vesicle clusters. Consider, similarly the hypothetical case of a spherical axon ending with a diameter of 1 μ and containing 500 n.s. granules, all measuring 1,800 Å. If, by exocytosis of all these, the membrane remnants were not pinched off again, the axolemma would have to incorporate in it an amount of membrane material corresponding to about 16 times its own area. The abundance of small vesicles actually found in depleted axon endings, however, accounts for this material (Fig. 1f).

In certain axons exocytosis of n.s. granules does not involve the formation of small vesicles. In such cases (exceptional in *Calliphora*, but perhaps common in other n.s. systems) granule membranes are pinched off without fragmentation to form larger, more or less greyish empty vesicles. This is not inconsistent with the hypothesis (NORMANN, 1969) since the prevailing physico-chemical conditions in particular axons may influence the structural results of membrane coalescence.

With the above considerations in mind it is tempting to suggest that exocytosis may also occur in n.s. systems, where direct evidence is lacking. The physiological results obtained by DOUGLAS (1967) on mammalian neurohypophysis seem particularly pertinent to that idea. In arthropods it not only occurs in insects, but has been beautifully demonstrated in crustacean material (BUNT and ASHBY, 1967, 1968; WEITZMAN, 1969). WEITZMAN in fact arrived at the same conclusion with regard to the formation of synaptic-type vesicles from rearrangement of membranes temporarily fused at the release site.

As earlier mentioned, the selection of stimulus conditions may be problematic since those suitable for provoking a physiologically detectable hormone output may not be ideal for studying the morphology of cellular mechanisms. This to some degree applies to the material previously published (NORMANN, 1969), but apparently has been overcome by the present work. It has further become evident that the pulse repetition rate formerly used (10/sec) may have been somewhat too high, and that 3/sec is more appropriate. Perhaps we are dealing with impulses having particularly long refractory periods.

Anyway, even though less ideal stimulus parameters were used when stimulating via the brain, n.s. granules were released from the intrinsic n.s. cells of the c. card., this liberation being dependent on an intact nervous connection from brain to c. card. (NORMANN and DUVE, 1969). This indication of impulse transmission in the n.s. system is consistent with the finding that the c.n.c. are postsynaptic cells, whereas the postsynaptic axons to all appearance belong to a group of brain n.s. cells (of B fibre-type).

The finding of a substructure in the granules of the c.n.c. (apparently also in some granules of extrinsic origin) is difficult to interpret at present. It appears different both to that already described by KNOWLES (1960) and to the subunits described by BARGMANN and v. GAUDECKER (1969). There exists some evidence that the hormone(s) of the intrinsic n.s. cells is a peptide of small molecular size (see for example BROWN, 1965; MORDUE and GOLDSWORTHY, 1969). However, until more is known about the biochemistry of this hormone—not to mention the question of "carrier proteins"—it remains impossible to interpret these "hollow" filaments in molecular terms. It should be mentioned that similar structural details are found in newly formed granules in the Golgi region and in n.s. granules that have reached the axon endings.

In a hypothesis on the coupling between stimulus and secretion (NORMANN, 1965) it was mentioned that the n.s. granules by their apparently random movements often touch the axolemma without being engaged in exocytosis. It was suggested that only as long as the axolemma temporarily had changed properties, viz. during the passage of an action potential, could an actual contact be established between granule membrane and axolemma. This hypothesis gains support by the results of stimulation, and also becomes attractive in view of the effect of depolarizing agents. Firstly, this more permanent effect could explain the greater occurrence of exocytosis in such material. Cases like that shown in Fig. 3, where the granule membrane continuous with the axolemma fuses with a new granule membrane likewise point to a relation between membrane polarity and membrane interactions. The disturbed relationship between the omega-figures and the vesicle clusters seen in Fig. 2, points to a longer duration of the omega-phase. It is tempting to suggest, that even as membrane depolarization appears necessary for induction of exocytosis, the coalescence and rearrangement of membrane remnants may depend to some degree on the restitution of normal membrane polarity in these axons.

## Summary

Secretion of neurohormones from corpora cardiaca of *Calliphora* was induced by 1) electrical stimulation in vivo, 2) depolarization with acetylcholine + eserine or with potassium, and 3) by "stress". Electron microscopy of secreting n.s. axon endings provided evidence supporting the view that some seemingly different structural expressions of secretory activity are functionally connected.

Thus in *Calliphora* swarms of small vesicles at the axolemma, resembling the so-called "synaptoid contacts", but different from the synapses, represent fragmentation products of granule membranes during exocytosis.

Numerical analysis of occurrence of "exocytosis" and "vesicle clusters" indicates that in normally functioning secretory neurons the latter persist longer than the "omega-figures" and may—in terms of statistical probability—be observed in cases of low secretory rate or when stimulation has ceased before fixation.

Significant deviations from normal duration of the particular phases of the liberation process occur upon permanent depolarization and are discussed in terms of membrane-interaction.

The material contained in the granules has a tubular substructure not normally conspicuous. It occasionally becomes visible at exocytosis, when dissolution begins, but may also be observed in neurons the inside ionic milieu of which may have become abnormally altered.

# References

BARGMANN, W., GAUDECKER, BR. V.: Über die Ultrastruktur neurosekretorischer Elementargranula. Z. Zellforsch. **96**, 495–504 (1969).

BEAULATON, J.: Sur la localisation ultrastructurale d'une activité cholinestérasique dans le corps cardiaque de *Rhodnius prolixus* Stal. (Hétéroptère, *Reduvidae*) aux quatrième et cinquième stades larvaires. J. Microscopie **6**, 65–80 (1967).

BRADY, J., MADDRELL, S. H. P.: Neurohaemal organs in the medial nervous system of insects. Z. Zellforsch. **76**, 389–404 (1967).

BROWN, B. E.: Pharmacologically active constituents of the cockroach corpus cardiacum. Resolution and some characteristics. Gen. comp. Endocr. **5**, 387–401 (1965).

BUNT, A. H., ASHBY, E. A.: Ultrastructure of the sinus gland of the crayfish, *Procambarus clarkii*. Gen. comp. Endocr. **9**, 334–342 (1967).

— — Ultrastructural changes in the crayfish sinus gland following electrical stimulation. Gen. comp. Endocr. **10**, 376–382 (1968).

DOUGLAS, W. W.: Stimulus-secretion coupling in the adrenal medulla and the neurohypophysis: Cellular mechanisms of release of catecholamines and posterior pituitary hormones. In: Neurosecretion. IV. Internat. Symposium on Neurosecretion (ed. F. STUTINSKY), p. 178–190. Berlin-Heidelberg-New York: Springer 1967.

FINLAYSON, L. H., OSBORNE, M. P.: Peripheral neurosecretory cells in the stick insect (*Carausius morosus*) and the blowfly larva (*Phormia terrae-novae*). J. Ins. Physiol. **14**, 1793–1801 (1968).

HODGSON, E. S., GELDIAY, S.: Experimentally induced release of neurosecretory materials from roach corpora cardiaca. Biol. Bull. **117**, 275–283 (1959).

JOHNSON, B.: Ultrastructure of probable sites of release of neurosecretory materials in an insect, *Calliphora stygia* Fabr. (Diptera). Gen. comp. Endocr. **6**, 99–108 (1966).

KNOWLES, F. G. W.: A highly organized structure within a neurosecretory vesicle. Nature (Lond.) **185**, 710–711 (1960).

— Neuronal properties of neurosecretory cells. In: Neurosecretion. IV. Internat. Symposium on Neurosecretion (ed. F. STUTINSKY), p. 8–19. Berlin-Heidelberg-New York: Springer 1967.

— VOLLRATH, L.: Neurosecretory innervation of the pituitary of the eels *Anguilla* and *Conger*. Phil. Trans. B **250**, 311–342 (1966).

MADDRELL, S. H. P.: The site of release of the diuretic hormone in *Rhodnius*—A new neurohaemal system in insects. J. exp. Biol. **45**, 499–508 (1966).

MORDUE, W., GOLDSWORTHY, G. J.: The physiological effects of corpus cardiacum extracts in locusts. Gen. comp. Endocr. **12**, 360–369 (1969).

NORMANN, T. C.: The neurosecretory system of the adult *Calliphora erythrocephala*. I. The fine structure of the corpus cardiacum with some observations on adjacent organs. Z. Zellforsch. **67**, 461–501 (1965).

— Experimentally induced exocytosis of neurosecretory granules. Exp. Cell Res. **55**, 285–287 (1969).

— DUVE, H.: Experimentally induced release of a neurohormone influencing hemolymph trehalose level in *Calliphora erythrocephala* (Diptera). Gen. comp. Endocr. **12**, 449–459 (1969).

PALAY, S. L.: The fine structure of the neurohypophysis. In: Ultrastructure and cellular chemistry of neural tissue (H. WAELSCH, ed.), p. 31–49. New York: Hoeber-Harper 1957.

SCHARRER, B.: Neurosecretion. XIV. Ultrastructural study of sites of release of neurosecretory material in blattarian insects. Z. Zellforsch. **89**, 1–16 (1968).

— KATER, S. B.: Neurosecretion. XV. An electron microscopic study of the corpora cardiaca of *Periplaneta americana* after experimentally induced hormone release. Z. Zellforsch. **95**, 177–186 (1969).

SMITH, U., SMITH, D. S.: Observations on the secretory processes in the corpus cardiacum of the stick insect, *Carausius morosus*. J. Cell Sci. **1**, 59–66 (1966).

WEITZMAN, M.: Ultrastructural study on the release of neurosecretory material from the sinus gland of the land crab *Gecarcinus lateralis*. Z. Zellforsch. **94**, 147–154 (1969).

# Investigations on Neurosecretion in the Central and Peripheral Nervous System of the Pulmonate Snail *Lymnaea stagnalis* (L.)

Some Preliminary Results*

S. E. WENDELAAR BONGA

Department of Zoology, Free University, Amsterdam (The Netherlands)

**Key words:** Neurosecretion — Invertebrate — Central nervous system — Peripheral nervous system — Pulmonates.

In all central ganglia, except for the buccal and pedal, of the pond snail *Lymnaea stagnalis* neurosecretory cell groups have been described using the classic neurosecretory stains paraldehyde fuchsin and chrome haematoxylin (LEVER et al., 1961). In each of the cerebral ganglia a group of phloxinophilic cells in addition to two groups of Gomori-positive cells has been studied in some detail by light microscopy (JOOSSE, 1964; BOER, 1965) as well as by electron microscopy (BOER et al., 1967).

However, the selectivity of the Gomori methods has limitations for studying neurosecretory materials, because other substances like glycogen, lysosomes and connective tissue elements also take up the stains (SIMPSON et al., 1966). Therefore the Alcian blue/Alcian yellow technique, which has been introduced for the identification of neurosecretion—in the preoptic-neurohypophyseal tract in *Rana temporaria*—by PEUTE and VAN DE KAMER (1967), was applied with slight modifications. After oxydation with potassium permanganate the Alcian blue solution was used at pH 0.5 for staining strong acid groups and the Alcian yellow solution at pH 2.5 for identifying weak acid groups. It appeared that in this way the neurosecretory materials in this snail could be easily distinguished from other Gomori-positive tissue elements. Furthermore it was demonstrated that there exist at least three different types of Gomori-positive cells staining light-green, yellow-green and dark-green, respectively. The colours indicate that the ratio of strong acid groups to weak acid groups is different in the neurosecretory substances concerned. In addition to these cells, two Gomori-negative cell types which were not regarded as neurosecretory before, were found. The one stained strongly with Alcian yellow and the lipid stain Sudan black B, while the other could be identified by an affinity for phloxin and a moderate reaction with Sudan black B.

With the electron microscope it was established that each of the types of histochemically different neurosecretory materials consisted of elementary granules of characteristic size and appearance.

---

* This study is supported by a grant of the Netherlands Organization for the Advancement of Pure Research.

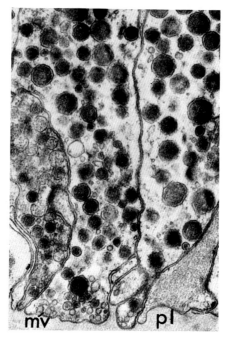

Fig. 1. Axon endings in the periphery of a visceral nerve containing elementary granules of the phloxinophilic type of neurosecretion. The occurrence of transparent granules (axon at the left) and microvesicles (*mv*) indicates release; *pl* perineurial layer. ×20,500

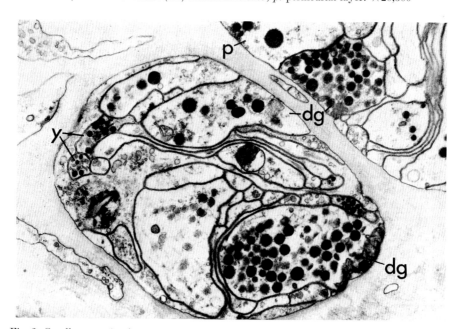

Fig. 2. Small nerves in the connective tissue capsule near the parietal ganglion. The axons contain elementary granules of the "dark-green" (*dg*), "yellow" (*y*), and phloxinophilic (*p*) type of neurosecretion. ×14,000

Apparently the periphery of the lip nerves and the intercerebral commissure serve as neurohaemal areas for the neurosecretory cell groups in the cerebral commissure (JOOSSE, 1964; BOER *et al.*, 1967). Storage of neurosecretory material at the periphery of connectives and nerves appears to be a general phenomenon at least in this snail. Axon endings of the neurosecretory cell groups in the pleural, parietal and visceral ganglia were observed in the peripheral regions of the connectives between these ganglia and especially of the parietal and visceral nerves. Indications of release of neurosecretory material were frequently found (Fig. 1).

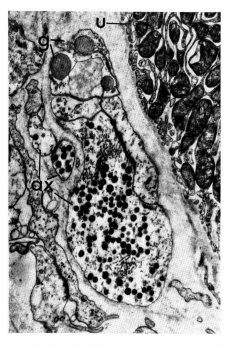

Fig. 3. Axons (*ax*) containing the "yellow" type of neurosecretory elementary granules in the connective tissue near the ureter epithelium; *g* glial cell; *u* basal infoldings of ureter cells.
×17,200

Neurohaemal zones in *Lymnaea stagnalis* seem to be even more extensive since it was further observed that tiny nerves containing several types of stainable materials penetrate the perineurial layer around the ganglia and nerves, forming a network near blood vessels, blood spaces and capillaries in the connective tissue capsule surrounding the central nervous system and the proximal parts of the nerves (Fig. 2). In this capsule also release generally occurs.

Moreover accumulations of neurosecretory material were observed in peripheral parts of the nervous system as far as the nerve endings in some effector organs. Axons containing the "yellow" type of neurosecretion were observed in the visceral nerve and in the branches of this nerve which innervate the kidney. These axons are ending non-synaptically in the connective tissue between the folds of the ureter epithelium (Fig. 3). This part of the kidney is assumed to be involved in transport of salts and water (WENDELAAR BONGA and BOER, 1969). Release of the contents of the elementary granules in this area appeared to take place in a neurosecretory way.

In order to investigate whether this material might have a direct hormonal effect upon the ureter, groups of three animals were exposed to solutions of different osmolarity (de-mineralized water, a 0.56% NaCl sol., and tap water) and studied at the electron microscope level. After two hours the percentage of axon profiles showing release phenomena in the group exposed to de-mineralized water when compared to animals in tap water increased from about 20% to approximately 70%. In snails placed in the saline solution there was a slight decrease. Per snail 450 axons were examined. This result suggests that this type of peripherally released neurosecretion exerts an influence on the water balance in this species.

## References

Boer, H. H.: A cytological and cytochemical study of neurosecretory cells in Basommatophora, with particular reference to *Lymnaea stagnalis* L. Arch. néerl. Zool. **16**, 313–386 (1965).
— Douma, E., Koksma, J. M. A.: Electron microscope study of neurosecretory cells and neurohaemal organs in the pond snail *Lymnaea stagnalis*. Symp. zool. Soc. Lond. **22**, 237–256 (1967).
Joosse, J.: Dorsal bodies and dorsal neurosecretory cells of the cerebral ganglia of *Lymnaea stagnalis* L. Arch. néerl. Zool. **16**, 1–103 (1964).
Lever, J., Kok, M., Meuleman, E. A., Joosse, J.: On the location of Gomori-positive neurosecretory cells in the central ganglia of *Lymnaea stagnalis*. Proc. kon. ned. Akad. Wet., Ser. C **64**, 640–647 (1961).
Peute, J., van de Kamer, J. C.: On the histochemical differences of Aldehyd-fuchsin positive material in the fibres of the hypothalamo-hypophyseal tract of *Rana temporaria*. Z. Zellforsch. **83**, 441–448 (1967).
Simpson, L., Bern, H. A., Nishioka, R. S.: Survey of evidence for neurosecretion in Gastropod molluscs. Amer. Zool. **6**, 123–138 (1966).
Wendelaar Bonga, S. E., Boer, H. H.: Ultrastructure of the reno-pericardial system in the pond snail *Lymnaea stagnalis* (L.). Z. Zellforsch. **94**. 513–529 (1969).

# Innervation of the Cephalopod Optic Gland

RICHARD S. NISHIOKA, HOWARD A. BERN and DAVID W. GOLDING*

Department of Zoology and its Cancer Research Genetics Laboratory,
University of California, Berkeley (U.S.A.)

**Key words:** Neurosecretion — Cephalopod optic gland — Innervation.

The optic glands of cephalopods are endocrine organs secreting a gonadotropic hormone under the control of the brain (WELLS, 1964; DURCHON and RICHARD, 1967). Light is inhibitory to optic gland function in octopods, and this inhibition

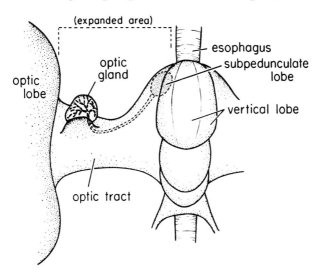

Fig. 1. Diagram to show approximate relations of optic gland and its nerve supply to the brain in *Octopus*

is mediated by a complex neural pathway from the retina to the subpedunculate lobe of the brain and thence to the optic gland itself. A prominent nerve can be seen entering the gland (BOYCOTT and YOUNG, 1956; MESSENGER, 1966, personal communication; BONICHON, 1967) (Fig. 1).

Although the optic gland has been examined ultrastructurally (BJÖRKMAN, 1963; DEFRETIN and RICHARD, 1967) and is reported to resemble typical glandular tissue, no data on the nature of the nerve supply have been presented. In view of the increasing interest in the innervation of endocrine tissues, and in the problem of "neurosecretory innervation" generally (cf. KNOWLES and BERN, 1966), a com-

* Present address: Dove Marine Laboratory, Cullercoats, North Shields (Northumberland), United Kingdom.

bination of light, fluorescence and electron microscope observations has been used
to elucidate the nature of the nerve to the optic gland.

## Materials and Methods

*Octopus bimaculatus* from the Los Angeles area, *O. apollyon* from Bodega Bay, and the
squid *Loligo opalescens* from Monterey Bay, all in California, were used in this study. The

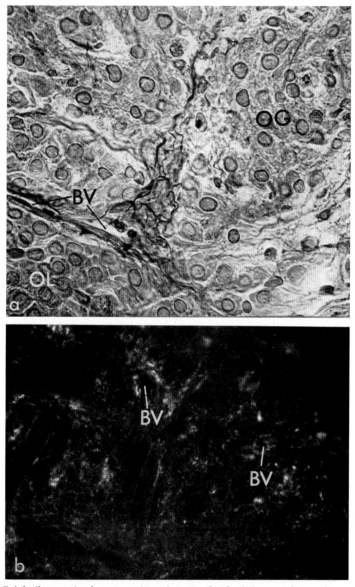

Fig. 2. a Cajal silver-stained preparation of optic gland of *Octopus bimaculatus*. Branch of
nerve enters optic gland (*OG*) from region of a large blood vessel (*BV*) situated between optic
gland and olfactory lobe (*OL*). ×480. b Fluorescence microscopy of optic gland. Larger
fluorescent loci are adjacent to dark areas representing blood vessels (*BV*). ×340

octopi weighed between $1/_4$ and 1 pound and were in various states of reproductive activity. The squids were part of the seasonal breeding migration into Monterey Bay. At least 8 specimens of each species were fixed for histologic examination. A modified Cajal silver technique (SERENI and YOUNG, 1932) was used on material from four *O. bimaculatus* and three *L. opalescens*.

The basic fluorescence technique of FALCK and OWMAN (1965) was employed on tissues from the two *Octopus* species. After freezing, the tissues were transferred to a prechilled small desiccator containing phosphorus pentoxide, which was attached to a lyophilizer with a dry ice/isopropyl alcohol cold finger, and allowed to dry for 5 days. The tissues were then treated for 3 hours with formaldehyde at 60° C. After vacuum embedding in paraffin, the tissues were cut at 10 microns and mounted on slides with n-butyl alcohol with or without subsequent warming. Sections were examined with a Reichert fluorescence microscope, equipped with a cardioid condenser.

Most of the electron-microscope data were obtained on *O. bimaculatus*. Tissues were fixed in veronal-acetate buffer (pH 7.7) and osmium tetroxide. Between 300 and 325 mg/ml of sucrose were added to raise the osmolarity of the fixative. Other fixatives and lower concentrations of sucrose did not yield adequate ultrastructural preservation. The seemingly impervious and tough capsule made immersion fixation difficult; dissection into smaller pieces was precluded owing to the tendency of the tissue to evert; and perfusion was only partially successful owing to the viscosity of the fixative. Ten *O. bimaculatus* and four *L. opalescens* provided tissues for electron microscopy.

## Results

The predominant cell type (stellate or chief cells) of the optic gland of *Octopus* and *Loligo* possesses a large nucleus containing a prominent nucleolus. These cells are characterized by having many small mitochondria and one or more cell processes (Fig. 3). Although the processes have not been fully traced, they appear to become closely apposed to processes or somata of other stellate cells, or to axonal processes (Fig. 4a and c). In some cells there are many Golgi centers; their cisternae often appear to contain dense material. Adjacent to the Golgi area, many vesicles are frequently present in addition to some small granules. The endoplasmic reticulum is irregularly organized. Larger inclusions of several types are present: homogeneous bodies often with a pale center; bodies containing dense material and stacks of membranes or filaments; membranous systems organized into stacks and whorls (Fig. 3).

The second cell type is presumably glial. These cells and their processes are characterized by pale, "empty"-appearing cytoplasm and are found between the stellate cells and their processes (Figs. 3 and 4).

The majority of fiber profiles encountered in optic gland sections are undoubtedly processes from stellate cells. They contain organelles and inclusions identical with those found in the stellate cell-body, although Golgi centers are absent. Occasionally some of these processes contain a few dense granules and vesicles. It is difficult to distinguish cross-sections of small stellate cell processes from small neuronal processes (Fig. 4a and c). Some stellate cell processes penetrate the cytoplasm of the cell-body of other stellate cells (Fig. 4c).

In silver-stained preparations, a major bundle of nerve fibers enters the optic gland through the olfactory lobe below the optic gland. This nerve tract is usually adjacent to a major blood vessel supplying the gland and ramifies in parallel with the extensive capillary bed (Fig. 2a).

Green-yellow fluorescence is demonstrable along the nerve tracts in *Octopus*, both leading to and inside the optic gland. One tract is usually discrete and

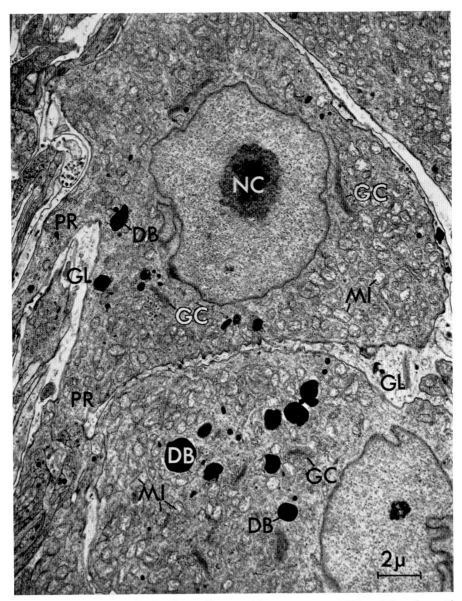

Fig. 3. Electron micrograph of stellate cells, one with two processes (*PR*) and the other with several large dense bodies (*DB*). Cytoplasm contains many mitochondria and several Golgi systems with vesicles and small granules. Glial processes (*GL*) with clear cytoplasm are between stellate cells. Note prominent nucleolus (*NC*), numerous Golgi centers (*GC*) and mitochondria (*MI*)

strongly fluorescent, whereas the others are more diffuse. Within the optic gland, fluorescent loci are most numerous around blood vessels (Fig. 2b).

Neuronal processes are relatively few in number and are generally associated with the numerous blood vessels in the optic gland in both *O. bimaculatus* and

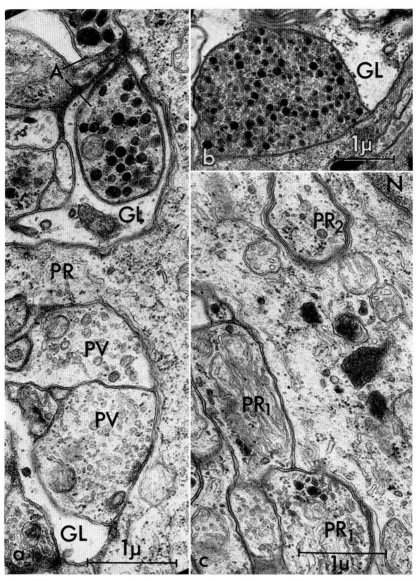

Fig. 4a–c. Electron micrographs of processes of several types. a Two axons (A) contain large granules. Two processes containing vesicles (PV) adjacent to stellate cell and process (PR) may themselves represent processes of stellate cells. GL glial process. b Axon with many granules (aminergic?) with loose limiting membrane. Processes with this type of granule are most numerous within optic gland. GL glial process. c Two stellate-cell processes (PR₁) are adjacent to stellate cell-body; another process (PR₂) is surrounded by stellate cell cytoplasm. N nucleus

*L. opalescens.* The more common type of axonal process contains granules measuring 800–1,600 Å in diameter, which have a loosely applied, often crenated limiting membrane (Fig. 4 b). Some of these processes are seen in close proximity to stellate cell-bodies but generally they are found among stellate cell-processes. A few axon-

4*

like processes containing larger dense granules, 1,000–3,000 Å or more in diameter, are also evident. Here, the granule-limiting membranes are smooth and filled with dense material (Fig. 4a). Both types of axonal processes also contain vesicles in some sections.

True synapses are not encountered in the optic gland. An occasional contact of a process with another process or cell soma exhibits slightly darker membranes at the point of apposition (Fig. 4a), but neither dense material attached to the membrane nor associated vesicles are generally observed. Synapses typical of octopus (Gray, 1964, 1969) occur in other parts of the nervous system of *O. bimaculatus*.

The neurons of the olfactory lobe directly adjacent to the optic gland are more uniform than the stellate cells of the optic gland. They contain extensive stacks of endoplasmic reticulum and well-developed Golgi systems. Many small vesicles and granules occur near the Golgi region.

## Discussion

The physiology of the optic gland suggests an analogy with the pituitary gland (Wells and Wells, 1969). There are further bases for a more specific analogy of the optic gland with the rostral pars distalis of the teleost pituitary in that both are under inhibitory control and in that the relation of nerve fibers to glandular elements in both appears to be non-synaptic. Control is presumably accomplished by diffusion of a substance from axon endings to nearby cells (Zambrano et al., 1970).

The electron-microscope data showing neuronal processes containing dense-cored granules closely parallel the fluorescence localization. Granules of this type have been described as being adrenergic, and endings containing them have been shown to become fluorescent after formaldehyde treatment.

The cells of origin of the optic gland fibers (aminergic ?) are presumably located in the subpenduculate lobe (Wells, 1960). Recent examination reveals some green-yellow fluorescent neurons at the periphery of this lobe (Nishioka, unpublished). Olfactory lobe neurons, located immediately subjacent to the optic gland in *Octopus*, are highly secretory in appearance, and could be confused with optic gland secretory cells. However, this lobe enjoys no evident functional relation with the optic gland.

All of the optic glands examined include at least some stellate cells with large dark inclusion bodies. Although we did not attempt to induce experimentally enlargement of the optic glands, animals which had partially enlarged optic glands had stellate cells that contained many dense bodies with stacks of membranes or filaments. These dense bodies may correspond to "the droplets of yellow secretion" described by Wells (1960) in enlarged optic glands of octopus.

The ease of confusion of processes of the stellate cells (which are themselves of neural origin—Boycott and Young, 1956; Björkman, 1963) with nerve fibers is reminiscent of the mediodorsal body problem in gastropod molluscs. In several pulmonates, a mass of granule-containing, axon-like fibers was initially interpreted as a neurosecretory neuropil (Simpson, Bern and Nishioka, 1966) originating from the brain. It has since been established that these fibers are in fact processes of the mediodorsal body cells, projecting toward the cerebral ganglia (BOER *et al.*, 1968; SIMPSON, 1969). This experience has dictated caution in estimating the extent of nerve fiber ramification throughout the optic glands.

# Summary

The cephalopod optic gland and the nerve supplying it were selected for study by light, fluorescence, and electron microscopy, as an example of an innervated endocrine organ. The optic gland of *Octopus* and *Loligo* is composed largely of stellate cells with axon-like processes. Glial elements and numerous blood vessels are also present. A nerve from the brain showing considerable fluorescence (aminergic?) ramifies among the stellate cells in close association with capillaries. Most nerve fiber profiles contain small, adrenergic-type, dense-cored granules. Other nerve fibers contain larger electron-dense granules. Although nerve fibers abut against stellate cells, no synaptoid structures were evident. The control exerted by the nerve supply over the optic gland would seem to be by diffusion of the inhibitory material from nerve fibers lying among the secretory stellate cells.

*Acknowledgements.* We express our thanks to our colleagues at the Bodega Marine Laboratory of the University of California for collection of *Octopus apollyon*. We are grateful to Dr. DAVID ZAMBRANO and Mrs. MARILYN MIYAMOTO for advice on fluorescence microscopy, to Mrs. ANNE MOS for microtechnical assistance, to Mr. JOHN UNDERHILL for photographic help, and to Mrs. EMILY REID for the diagram. The research was supported by NSF Grant GB 6424.

## References

BJÖRKMAN, N.: On the ultrastructure of the optic gland in octopus. J. Ultrastruct. Res. **8**, 195 (1963).

BOER, H. H., SLOT, J. W., ANDEL, J. VAN: Electron microscopical and histochemical observations on the relation between medio-dorsal bodies and neurosecretory cells in the basommatophoran snails *Lymnaea stagnalis*, *Ancylus fluviatilis*, *Australorbis glabratus* and *Planorbarius corneus*. Z. Zellforsch. **87**, 435–450 (1968).

BONICHON, A.: Contribution à l'étude de la neurosécrétion et de l'endocrinologie chez les Céphalopodes. I. *Octopus vulgaris*. Vie et Milieu, Sér. A **18**, 227–263 (1967).

BOYCOTT, B. B., YOUNG, J. Z.: The subpedunculate body and nerve and other organs associated with the optic tract of cephalopods. Bertil Hanström: Zool. Papers in Honour of His 65th Birthday. Zool. Inst., Lund, Sweden. K. G. WINGSTRAND (ed.), p. 76–105 (1956).

DEFRETIN, R., RICHARD, A.: Ultrastructure de la glande optique de *Sepia officinalis* L. (Mollusque Céphalopode). Mise en évidence de la sécrétion et de son contrôle photopériodique. C. R. Acad. Sci. (Paris) **265**, 1415–1418 (1967).

DURCHON, M., RICHARD, A.: Étude, en culture organotypique, du rôle endocrine de la glande optique dans la maturation ovarienne chez *Sepia officinalis* L. (Mollusque Céphalopode). C. R. Acad. Sci. (Paris) **264**, 1497–1500 (1967).

FALCK, B., OWMAN, C.: A detailed methodological description of the fluorescence method for the cellular demonstration of biogenic monoamines. Acta Univ. Lund., Sect. II **7**, 1–23 (1965).

GRAY, E. G.: The fine structure of normal and degenerating synapses of the central nervous system. Arch. biol. **75**, 285–299 (1964).

— Electron microscopy of the glio-vascular organization of the brain of *Octopus*. Phil. Trans. B **255**, 13–32 (1969).

KNOWLES, F., BERN, H. A.: The function of neurosecretion in neuroendocrine regulation. Nature (Lond.) **210**, 271–272 (1966).

SERENI, E., YOUNG, J. Z.: Nervous degeneration and regeneration in cephalopods. Publ. Staz. zool. Napoli **12**, 173–208 (1932).

SIMPSON, L.: Morphological studies of possible neuroendocrine structures in *Helisoma tenue* (Gastropoda: Pulmonata). Z. Zellforsch. **102**, 570–593 (1969).
— BERN, H. A., NISHIOKA, R. S.: Examination of the evidence for neurosecretion in the nervous system of *Helisoma tenue* (Gastropoda Pulmonata). Gen. comp. Endocr. **7**, 525–548 (1966).
WELLS, M. J.: Optic glands and the ovary of *Octopus*. Symp. Zool. Soc. Lond. **2**, 87–107 (1960).
— WELLS, J.: Pituitary analogue in the octopus. Nature (Lond.) **222**, 293–294 (1969).
ZAMBRANO, D., NISHIOKA, R. S., BERN, H. A.: Comparison of the innervation of the pituitary of two euryhaline teleost fishes, *Gillichthys mirabilis* and *Tilapia mossambica*, with special reference to the origin and nature of type "B" fibres. Mem. Soc. Endocrin. U.K. Vol. *19* (1970) (in press).

# Adrenergic Neurons

## Adrenergic Neurons in Mammals with Special Reference to Fluorescence Microscopical Studies

Annica Dahlström*

Department of Histology, Institute of Neurobiology, University of Göteborg,
Göteborg (Sweden)

**Key words:** Adrenergic neurons — Mammals — Fluorescence microscopy

Before the end of the 19th century it was proposed that two antagonistic systems, the sympathetic and the parasympathetic, were involved in mammalian autonomic nervous control (Gaskell, 1886). In the year of 1900 Langley (1900) was able to show that the autonomic nervous system was built up of 2 sets of neurons, one preganglionic and one postganglionic.

The possible function of adrenaline (A) as a transmitter substance in sympathetic nerves was proposed as early as 1905 by Elliot (1905), and 1909 by Dixon and Hamill (1909). Experimental evidence for this view was given by Loewi (1921) and by Cannon and Uridil (1921). At that time only A was discussed as the possible transmitter, and during the following decade many investigators helped to establish the false identity of A as the sympathetic transmitter in mammals.

In 1933 Cannon and Rosenblueth (1933) noted clear differences in action between A and the substance liberated at sympathetic nerve stimulation. They proposed therefore the presence of two so-called "sympathins", one of which Bacq in the following year (1934) proposed to be equivalent to noradrenaline (NA).

The necessity of a new classification of the two antagonistic autonomic systems became evident in 1934, when Dale and Feldberg (1934) discovered that some *sympathetic* postganglionic systems, in addition to the parasympathetic ones, used acetylcholine (ACh) as transmitter instead of "sympathin". The new terms "cholinergic" and "adrenergic" were introduced for nerves which liberated ACh and A-like substances, respectively.

The enzyme 3,4-dihydroxyphenylalanine (DOPA)-decarboxylase was discovered in mammalian tissue by Holtz, Heise and Ludtke (1938). This enzyme was found to convert DOPA to dopamine (DA), and in the following year Blascko (1939) postulated the synthesis chain: tyrosine—DOPA—DA—NA—A, to occur in mammalian tissues.

During the next decade von Euler (1946), Holtz, Credner and Kroneberg (1947), and Schmiterlöw (1948) identified the main catecholamine (CA) present

* Some of the work described in this paper was supported by grants from the Swedish Medical Research Council (No: B69-14X-2207–03, B70-14X-2207–04), from Magnus Bergwall's Foundation, from Gustav and Majen Lindgren's Foundation, and from Wilhelm and Martina Lundgren's Foundation.

in mammalian tissues and urine as NA. In 1948 von Euler (1948) showed that this naturally occurring NA was the l-isomer. In the same decade it was demonstrated that NA was released from splenic nerves and sympathetically innervated organs after postganglionic nerve stimulation (e.g. Peart, 1949; West, 1950; Mann and West, 1950, 1951; Outschoorn, 1952; Outschoorn and Vogt, 1952).

Nowadays NA is generally accepted as the sympathetic adrenergic transmitter in mammalian peripheral tissues. In the experiments of Loewi (1921), the results of which caused A to be considered as the sympathetic transmitter in mammals, frog hearts were used. As shown by Falck, Häggendal and Owman (1963) (see also Angelakos, Glassman, Millard and King, 1965; McLean, Bell and Burnstock, 1967) frogs in contrast to mammals, use A instead of NA as sympathetic transmitter. Thus, Loewi was in fact right that in his preparation A was the transmitter.

The NA content found in the brain and spinal cord was long thought to be localized in nerve endings of the blood vessels of the brain. In 1954 Vogt (1954) demonstrated that the distribution of NA was quite unequal in different regions of the brain, which should not be the case if NA was bound to the blood vessels. She proposed that NA could play some role in neurotransmission in the brain, a role that most investigators now agree on. Also DA, earlier regarded only as a precursor of NA, was found to be unequally distributed in the brain (see Carlsson, Lindqvist, Magnusson and Waldeck, 1958). In some regions, e.g. the caudate nucleus, the concentration of this amine even exceeded that of NA, indicating a particular action of this amine.

Apart from NA and DA, also serotonin (5-HT) was for many years known to occur in significant amounts in the central nervous system (CNS) (Twarog and Page, 1953; Amin, Crawford and Gaddum, 1954), but up to 1962 very little was known about the localization of these three amines. Thus, it was not generally accepted that these three amines in the CNS were localized within nerve cells.

With the introduction of the histochemical fluorescence method of Hillarp, Falck and coworkers in 1962 (for references and detailed description of the method see Dahlström and Fuxe, 1964a; Norberg and Hamberger, 1964; Falck and Owman, 1965; Corrodi and Jonsson, 1967; Eränkö, 1967) new possibilities of studying the localization, distribution and morphology of amine containing neurons opened up. During the treatment of the tissues according to the method strongly fluorescent products are formed from the amines and formaldehyde. The products of CA appear green to yellowgreen in the microscopic reaction used, while the reaction product of 5-HT is yellow. It is thus possible to differentiate between CA and 5-HT in the microscope. The method is not quantitative, but within the lower ranges of amine concentration the fluorescence intensity is correlated to the concentration of the amine in the structures studied. The histochemical method may, therefore, be used also in certain pharmacological and physiological studies when evaluating relative changes of transmitter content or distribution in adrenergic neurons (cf. Malmfors, 1965). However, it is sometimes preferable to combine the histochemical method with a quantitative method for assay of NA. Many of the results described in the present review were obtained with a combination of the histochemical fluorescence method, and the modified trihydroxyindole (THI) method (Häggendal, 1963).

## Morphology of Adrenergic Neurons

The *sympathetic adrenergic neuron* consists of a cell body (perikaryon), a nerve fibre (axon) and a nerve terminal network (Fig. 1). The cell body is usually located in an autonomic ganglion (Fig. 2), but may also be found intramurally, e.g. in the bladder wall (NORBERG and HAMBERGER, 1964). From the ganglion un-myelinated axons of about 0.2–1 µ in diameter pass, often in bundles within the

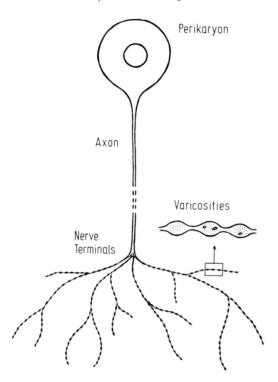

Fig. 1. Schematic drawing of an adrenergic neuron. Noradrenaline (NA) distribution in rat and cat adrenergic neurons: *Cell body*: NA concentration about 10–100 µg/g w.w. (NORBERG and HAMBERGER, 1964; DAHLSTRÖM and HÄGGENDAL, 1966a). NA content on the average about 0.4 pg/cell body (DAHLSTRÖM and HÄGGENDAL, 1966a). *Nerve terminals:* Total content of NA per neuron about 300 times that of the cell bodies, i.e. 0.12 ng (DAHLSTRÖM and HÄG-GENDAL, 1966a). NA concentration in varicosities about 3,000 µg/g w.w. NA content per average varicosity about 0.005 pg (DAHLSTRÖM, HÄGGENDAL and HÖKFELT, 1966). The added lengths of the nerve terminals belonging to the average neuron in the order of 10–30 cm (*cf.* DAHLSTRÖM, 1966)

same Schwann cell, to the area to be innervated. When approaching this area the usually rather smooth axons become slightly varicose, and in the innervated tissue the axons, now clearly varicose, branch to form an extensive nerve terminal net-work (Fig. 3a, b) the added lengths of which may be of the order of 10–34 cm/neu-ron (DAHLSTRÖM, 1966). These nerve terminals have a characteristic appearance with small so-called varicosities (diameter about 1–2 µ), separated by much thin-ner interparts. The nerve terminal fibres of one neuron usually run in bundles

together with fibres of other neurons, to form the "ground plexus" described by
HILLARP (1946, 1959).

Adrenergic nerve terminals have been discovered in most peripheral tissues
containing smooth muscles or glandular components. In the iris a dense net of
varicose terminals innervates the blood vessels and the smooth muscles of the
dilator and constrictor muscle (Fig. 3a) (EHINGER, 1964; MALMFORS, 1965; LATIES
and JACOBOWITZ, 1966). The salivary glands, particularly the submandibular
gland, contain in addition to a vessel innervation also thin varicose nerve terminals
arranged in basket-like formations around the acini (NORBERG and HAMBERGER,

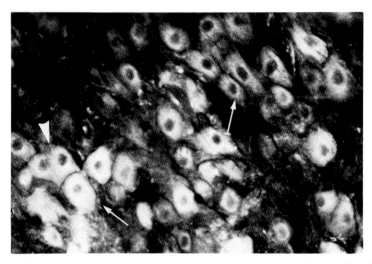

Fig. 2. Ganglion from the lumbar sympathetic chain in normal rat. Nerve cell bodies with
fluorescent cytoplasm are seen. Some cells have a strong fluorescence intensity ($\rightarrow$) while
others have a lower fluorescence intensity ($\mapsto$), indicating variations in NA content in the
different cell bodies. One binuclear ganglion cell is seen ($\triangleright$). Fluorescence microphotograph,
$\times 290$

1964). Cardiac muscle contains small varicose fibres running along the muscle
cells, and especially in the atria the innervation is dense (ANGELAKOS, FUXE and
TORCHIANA, 1963; DAHLSTRÖM, FUXE, MYA-TU and ZETTERSTRÖM, 1965). Also
adipose tissue appears to receive adrenergic innervation (e.g. WIRSÉN, 1965). The
NA found in skeletal muscle (0.1 µg/g, SEDVALL, 1964) is probably localized in the
adrenergic nerve terminals of the blood vessels. No sign of a direct adrenergic
innervation to the skeletal muscle cells or muscle spindles has so far been observed
(FUXE and SEDVALL, 1965). For detailed description and references of adrenergic
innervation, see review by NORBERG (1967).

The adrenergic nerve terminals of sympathetic adrenergic neurons are mostly
situated close to the smooth muscles, cardiac muscles or glands, often forming
basket-like arrangements around the innervated structures. There appears to be
little doubt that the nerve terminal varicosities are the presynaptic structures
from which the NA is released at nerve activity (cf. IVERSEN, 1967; ANDÉN,
CARLSSON and HÄGGENDAL, 1969).

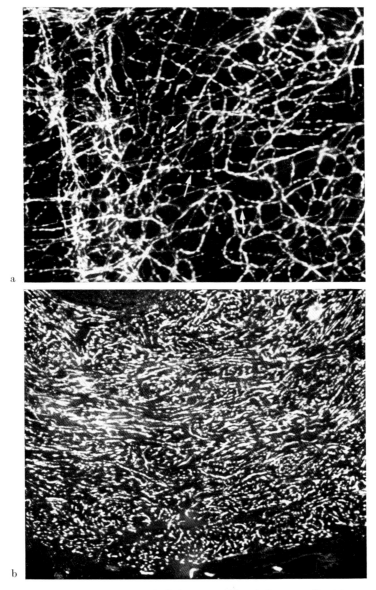

Fig. 3a and b. Adrenergic nerve terminals in rat peripheral tissues. a Stretch preparation of iris. A dense plexus of adrenergic nerve terminals with strongly fluorescent varicosities (→) is seen in the dilator muscle. To the left is a small artery with adrenergic nerve terminals in the wall. Fluorescence microphotograph, ×280. b Adrenergic nerve terminals in the muscle layers of vas deferens. Cross section. The lumen is at the top of the figure. Fluorescence microphotograph, ×130

In the *CNS* the monoamine (MA) neurons have a morphology which is similar to that of the peripheral NA neurons. The cell bodies have been found in the brain stem, while the nerve terminals are spread throughout the whole brain with few exceptions (e.g. DAHLSTRÖM and FUXE, 1964a; FUXE, 1965). The 5-HT cell bodies seem to occupy mainly mid-line positions in different raphe nuclei, while the CA cell bodies have mainly lateral positions (DAHLSTRÖM and FUXE, 1964a, 1965; ANDÉN, DAHLSTRÖM, FUXE, LARSSON, OLSON and UNGERSTEDT, 1966). As in the sympathetic adrenergic neuron (see below) the fluorescence intensity of the cell bodies in the CNS is low to medium, while the varicosities of the nerve terminals show strong fluorescence intensities, indicating a higher amine concentration.

The nerve terminals of the MA neurons are often seen surrounding, and very close to, non-fluorescent cell bodies. The fluorescent microscopical localization of the terminals is thus highly suggestive of synaptic contact between the two structures. Whether the contact may be of a direct or indirect type cannot be judged in the fluorescence microscope. However, electronmicroscopic studies from brain areas, rich in CA nerve terminals, have failed to reveal the presence of the indirect type of contact (axo-axonic); only the direct type (axo-somatic or axo-dendritic) has been found (e.g. FUXE, HÖKFELT and NILSSON, 1965; HÖKFELT, 1968). Electrical stimulation of CNS regions, containing MA nerve cell bodies or axons, causes a release of MA from the nerve terminals of the stimulated neurons (e.g. ANDÉN, CARLSSON, HILLARP and MAGNUSSON, 1964, 1965; FUXE and GUNNE, 1964; DAHLSTRÖM, FUXE, KERNELL and SEDVALL, 1965). It is thus probable that also in the CNS the MA varicosities are the presynaptic structures, releasing MA on nerve activity (cf. ANDÉN, CARLSSON and HÄGGENDAL, 1969) and that the action of these terminals is exerted directly on other nerve cells.

## Mapping out of Peripheral Adrenergic Neurons

Experimental methods, like denervation and/or axotomy, together with fluorescence histochemical studies have been used in the mapping out of peripheral adrenergic neurons. Removal of the cell bodies of an adrenergic neuron system (e.g. removal of a ganglion) or axotomy cause a degeneration and disappearance of the adrenergic terminals within 1–2 days (e.g. MALMFORS and SACHS, 1965). The cutting or ligation of a peripheral nerve also indicates the direction of the adrenergic nerve fibres, which has been of great value in studying the connections between the sympathetic ganglia in the peripheral nervous system (PNS). After a cut or ligation large amounts of NA, easily detectable in the fluorescence microscope, rapidly accumulate on the proximal side of the nerve (Fig. 4) (DAHLSTRÖM and FUXE, 1964b; DAHLSTRÖM, 1965; KAPELLER and MAYOR, 1965), while only minute amounts of, or no, NA accumulate on the distal side (DAHLSTRÖM, 1965).

This combination of experimental techniques has been used by e.g. HAMBERGER and NORBERG (1965) in their study on the connections of the abdominal ganglia in the cat. Their results indicate that adrenergic nerve terminals in the *small intestine* are mainly derived from cell bodies in the coeliac ganglion, while the adrenergic supply to the colon has its origin mainly in the inferior mesenteric ganglion. The adrenergic nerve terminals in the colon were observed lying mainly around non-fluorescent (probably cholinergic) intramural ganglion cells, while only very few fibres ended on the smooth muscles. An important part of the sympathetic inner-

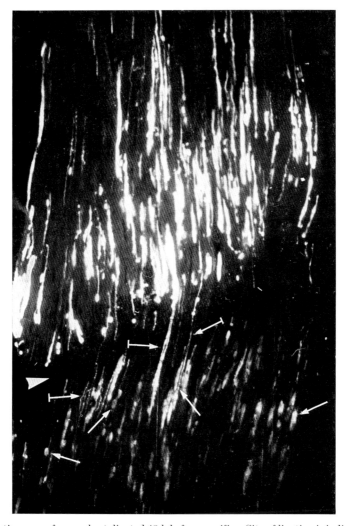

Fig. 4. Sciatic nerve of normal rat, ligated 48 h before sacrifice. Site of ligation is indicated (▷). Proximal to the ligation (upper part of the figure) is seen a large number of adrenergic axons with large amounts of accumulated fluorescent material (NA). The axons are enlarged and bulging. Note the differences in amount of accumulated NA in the different axons. Below the ligation signs of the small retrograde NA accumulations are seen, often as spheroids (→). Outgrowing sprouts, containing fluorescent material and slightly varicose, can be seen penetrating the zone of ligation, growing down into the distal part (↦). Fluorescence microphotograph, ×180

vation to this organ seems to involve *three neurons* in a chain: One preganglionic cholinergic (from the spinal cord) to the inferior mesenteric ganglion, one postganglionic adrenergic neuron from this ganglion to the intestine, and finally one cholinergic intramural neuron in the wall of the colon. This intimate connection between adrenergic and cholinergic autonomic neurons was previously unknown.

# Mapping out of Central Monoamine Neuron Systems

The MA containing nerve cell bodies in the CNS are situated mainly in the lower brain stem (see above). These cells give rise to the NA, DA and 5-HT terminals in the whole brain and spinal cord. The mapping out of these neuron systems has been done by combining the technique of brain lesions with fluorescence histochemistry and chemical assay. Three types of approaches have been

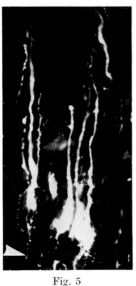

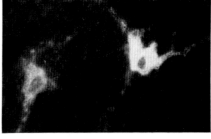

Fig. 5                                          Fig. 6

Fig. 5. From the spinal cord of a normal rat, transsected 24 h before sacrifice. Longitudinal section. Accumulations of strongly fluorescent material (NA) can be seen accumulated in distended axons in the white matter above the lesion (▷). Fluorescence microphotograph, ×460

Fig. 6. From the medulla oblongata of a rat, the spinal cord of which was sectioned 24 h before sacrifice. Two NA containing nerve cell bodies are seen. The one to the left has a normal appearance with a medium fluorescence intensity in the cytoplasm. The right one shows retrograde cell body changes, like an increased fluorescence intensity in the cytoplasm and a displaced nucleus. The appearance is slightly swollen. Fluorescence microphotograph, ×310

used: 1) Destruction of the cell bodies, which results in a complete degeneration and disappearance of the nerve terminals belonging to the group of cell bodies destroyed. 2) Cutting or coagulation of axon-containing areas. In the CNS three phenomena are usually observed after axotomy in MA containing neurons, namely a) accumulations of the transmitter substance in enlarged axons proximal to the lesions (Fig. 5) (Dahlström and Fuxe, 1964c), b) disappearance of the fluorescent nerve terminals distal to the lesion within some days, c) retrograde cell body changes occurring after 20–24 h, observed as increased fluorescence intensity, a swollen appearance, and often a displaced nucleus (Fig. 6) (e.g. Dahlström and Fuxe, 1965). 3) Removal of terminal areas by suction or lesion techniques. This results in a) accumulations of the transmitter substance in the afferent axons and b) retrograde cell body changes. By making series of lesions and observing the mentioned phenomena a gross outline of the MA neuron systems in the CNS has been obtained. Thus, it was found that most NA and 5-HT cell bodies in the medulla oblongata send axons down to the spinal cord. Most of the NA and 5-HT cell bodies in the pons and a few in the medulla oblongata send ascending axons, which pass in and close to the median forebrain bundle (MFB) to innervate the hypothalamus, thalamus, limbic forebrain and neocortex (see *e.g.* ANDÉN, DAHLSTRÖM, FUXE, LARSSON, OLSSON and UNGERSTEDT, 1966). The 5-HT neurons from these areas also seem to innervate the neo- and palaeostriatum. The DA cell bodies in the mesencephalon send a few fibres down to the pons and the medulla oblongata, but the majority of fibres ascend just lateral to the MFB to innervate the limbic forebrain and the neostriatum. The nerve cell bodies of the terminals inner-vating the neostriatum are found in the substantia nigra in the lateral mesence-phalon (*e.g.* ANDÉN, DAHLSTRÖM, FUXE and LARSSON, 1965). This last mentioned pathway has also been verified with silver-stain techniques (FINK and HEIMER, 1967).

# Effect of Nerve Growth Factor and Immunosympathectomy on Adrenergic Neurons

The specific nerve growth factor (NGF) purified by LEVI-MONTALCINI (1964) has been found to stimulate growth of sympathetic and sensory neurons (LEVI-MONTALCINI, 1964; EDWARDS, FENTON, KAKARI, LARGE, PAPADAKI and ZAIMIS, 1966). The *antiserum of the NGF* on the other hand caused marked decrease and destruction of sympathetic ganglia (ZAIMIS, BERK and CALLINGHAM, 1965). Fluorescence histochemical studies by OLSON (1967) of peripheral tissues in NGF treated mice have shown a marked increase of size and fluorescence intensity of sympathetic ganglion cells. The usually comparatively small number of varicose nerve terminals in ganglia were increased in NGF treated mice and seen around every nerve cell in basket-like arrangements. The nerve terminals in *e.g.* iris and submandibular gland had increased markedly in number of fibres running together. Also areas normally devoid of terminals showed adrenergic innervation in these animals (OLSON, 1967).

After immunosympathectomy a pronounced decrease in the number of fluores-cent adrenergic nerve terminals was observed. Also, most of the sympathetic ganglia showed signs of atrophy and contained mainly small, very weakly fluorescent nerve cell bodies (HAMBERGER, LEVI-MONTALCHINI, NORBERG and SJÖQVIST, 1965; OLSON, 1968).

## Intraneuronal Distribution of NA

When studied in the fluorescence microscope the different parts of the neuron show different fluorescence intensities (see Fig. 2), indicating varying concentra-tions of the amine. The cytoplasm of the cell bodies (the nucleus is dark) has in normal mammals a low to medium fluorescence intensity indicating a fairly low NA concentration (*e.g.* NORBERG and HAMBERGER, 1964). Most nerve cells in sym-pathetic ganglia have been shown to contain NA induced fluorescence and the few nerve cells without this fluorescence have instead a high acetylcholinesterase (AChE) activity, probably being cholinergic (*cf.* HAMBERGER, NORBERG and SJÖQvist, 1965). The non-terminal axons have low NA concentrations, as indicated by the very low to low intensity of fluorescence (e.g. Dahlström and Fuxe, 1964 b). The varicosities of the nerve terminals show a very strong fluorescence intensity, while the thinner interparts have low fluorescence intensities. Thus, the varicosities appear to be the parts of the neuron which contain the highest concentration of the transmitter (e.g. Norberg and Hamberger, 1964; Malmfors, 1965). Also in central MA neurons similar concentration differences appear to exist as judged from studies in the fluorescence microscope (e.g. Dahlström and Fuxe, 1964 a, 1965; Fuxe, 1965; Hillarp, Fuxe and Dahlström, 1966).

By combining the histochemical fluorescence technique with a quantitative method for chemical assay of NA (the THI method as modified by Häggendal, 1963) more accurate data on the intraneuronal distribution of NA in the sympathetic adrenergic neuron were obtained. The studies were performed in rat and cat. The cytoplasm of the adrenergic nerve cell bodies was found to hold a NA concentration of 10–100 µg/g w.w. (Dahlström and Häggendal, 1966a), a figure earlier proposed on the basis of the fluorescence intensity found in the cell bodies (Norberg and Hamberger, 1964). The concentration in the non-terminal axons is probably of the same magnitude as in the cell bodies, as may be judged from the fluorescence intensities (e.g.Norberg and Hamberger, 1964; Dahlström, 1966). The average NA content per nerve cell body was calculated to be about 0.4 pg (Dahlström and Häggendal, 1966a), which is in good agreement with the earlier proposed figure of 0.7pg (Norberg and Hamberger, 1964). Since the different perikarya within a ganglion show very different flourescence intensities (probably due to variations in the degree of activity), it must be remembered that the figures for both NA concentration and NA contents given above, are average figures and that the content of NA in the cell bodies varies in different neurons.

In the varicosities of the nerve terminals the NA content was found to be about 0.005 pg of NA per average varicosity in the rat iris. The NA concentration in these structures was calculated to be about 1,000–3,000 µg/g w.w. (Dahlström, Häggendal and Hökfelt, 1966).

The NA distribution within the adrenergic neuron probably also indicates the relative distribution of amine storage granules. von Euler and Hillarp (1956) found that NA in peripheral tissues was localized in small subcellular particles, the so-called amine storage granules. Pharmacological evidence indicates that NA in the normal animal is, at least to the major part, bound within these granules (e.g. Carlsson, 1965; Malmfors, 1965; Iversen, 1967; Andén, Carlsson and Häggendal, 1969). If the amine is not stored in the granules it appears to be readily deaminated by monoamine oxidase (MAO), presumably located in the mitochondria (cf. Axelrod, 1963). For further information and references on the pharmacology of adrenergic neurons, see e.g. Iversen (1967), Andén, Carlsson and Häggendal (1969).

Recent electronmicroscopical studies on adrenergic neurons (Hökfelt, 1969), using the potassium permanganate fixation technique (Richardsson, 1966), have demonstrated that the cell bodies contain a medium density of granulated vesicles (probably corresponding to the amine storage granules; for references and discussion see Hökfelt, 1968). The pre-terminal axons were shown to contain few, scattered, granulated vesicles, while the axon enlargements (probably corresponding to the varicosities) contained very high numbers of this structure. Thus, the electronmicroscopical distribution of dense-cored vesicles showed a good correlation with the intraneuronal distribution of NA (HÖKFELT, 1969).

Attempts to calculate the number of amine storage granules within one varicosity were made earlier (DAHLSTRÖM, HÄGGENDAL and HÖKFELT, 1966), based on a) the NA concentration figures in the varicosities, b) the presumption that at least the major part of NA in the varicosities is stored within the storage granules, c) on the assumption that the amine storage granules may hold the same concentration of NA as the suprarenal medullary granules, i.e. 43,000 µg/g w.w. (HILLARP and NILSSON, 1965), and d) on the assumption that the amine storage granules correspond to the small dense-cored vesicles with a diameter of 500 Å. The average number of granules in the varicosities was calculated to be about 1,000. Electronmicroscopical studies on the rat iris have revealed that the average number of dense-cored vesicles within the varicosities was about 320, varying between 45 and 850 (HÖKFELT, 1969). About 2 per cent of the dense cored vesicles in the nerve terminal varicosities of the rat iris were found to be of the large type (diameter more than 750 Å), which may also be connected to amine storage (cf. HÖKFELT, 1968).

## Axonal Transport of Amine Storage Granules in Adrenergic Neurons

The concept of axoplasmic flow was introduced in 1948 by WEISS and HISCOE (1948). According to WEISS (1961) the neuron is perpetually growing, in that proteins, continously formed in the cell body, are transported proximo-distally to supply the axon and the nerve endings with material, needed for maintenance and growth. Since that time numerous investigations have reported phenomena in constricted or cut nerve fibres that give strong support to this theory. Also in uninterrupted nerves evidence for proximo-distal flow was obtained by the use of labelled amino acids (for ref. see e.g. LUBIŃSKA, 1964; DAHLSTRÖM and HÄGGEN-DAL, 1970).

The above mentioned studies were performed mostly on myelinated nerve fibres. During the last years evidence for axonal transport in sympathetic adrenergic neurons has also been obtained. When a peripheral nerve containing sympathetic adrenergic nerve fibres is ligated or compressed, NA accumulates rapidly above the lesion, in the nerve part connected to the perikarya (Fig. 4) (e.g. DAHLSTRÖM and FUXE, 1964b; DAHLSTRÖM, 1965; DAHLSTRÖM and HÄGGENDAL, 1966b, 1967; KAPELLER and MAYOR, 1965, 1967). In the fluorescence microscope the onset of accumulation of NA induced fluorescence in enlarged adrenergic axons may be seen as early as 5–10 min after ligation (DAHLSTRÖM, 1965). The amount of specific NA fluorescence rapidly increases with time, the axons just above the ligations becoming more and more enlarged, bulging and distorted (Fig. 4). The height of the accumulations increases gradually, rarely, however, reaching a level above 1 cm proximal to the ligation. Quantitative assays have shown that the amount of NA accumulated follows approximately a straight line with the time after ligation up to at least 24 h (DAHLSTRÖM and HÄGGENDAL, 1966a, 1967; BOYLE and GILLES-PIE, 1968; GEFFEN and RUSH, 1968; LADURON and BELPAIRE, 1968a).

Results obtained after drug treatments have provided evidence that the accumulating NA is, at least to the greater part, probably stored within amine storage granules (*e.g.* Dahlström, 1965, 1967a). Also, electronmicroscopic studies have revealed that above the ligation a considerable increase in the number of dense-cored vesicles occurs (Kapeller and Mayor, 1966; Dahlström and Hök-felt, unpublished data). The observation that the accumulating NA is probably stored in amine storage granules, together with the rapid onset of accumulation, and the approximately linear time curve for NA accumulation, supported the idea that the ligation had arrested a continous down-transport in the axons of amine storage granules, probably formed in the perikarya (*e.g.* Dahlström, 1965, 1966; Dahlström and Häggendal, 1966b).

By quantitative assays of the accumulated amount of NA, compared to the NA amount found in unligated nerve, the rate of transport of the amine storage granules was calculated. In the adrenergic axons of the sciatic nerve the figure obtained was about 5 mm/h in rat, about 10 mm/h in cat, and about 3 mm/h in rabbit (Dahlström and Häggendal, 1966b, 1967). Studies in the cat splenic nerve have given a figure of about 3 mm/h (Boyle and Gillespie, 1968; Geffen and Rush, 1968). These figures probably represent the average rate of transport in the adrenergic axons of the nerve studied. The different axons in ligated nerves show clear variations in the amount of NA accumulated (Fig. 4), indicating different degrees of activity in the different neurons.

Other techniques to study transport of NA containing granules have been used. Thus, Laduron and Belpaire (1968a) studied the accumulation of DA-$\beta$-hydroxylase, probably localized within the amine storage granules (*e.g.* Kaufmann and Friedmann, 1965). DA-$\beta$-hydroxylase was found to accumulate approximately in parallel to NA in dog splenic nerve. Calculations on the rate of transport of DA-$\beta$-hydroxylase (probably amine storage granules) in this neuron system gave a figure of about 5 mm/h (Laduron and Belpaire, 1968a). By following the transport in the axons of [14]C-NA and [14]C-leucine labelled protein, Livett, Geffen and Austin (1968) obtained a figure of 5 mm/h for the rate of transport of amine storage granules in cat splenic nerve.

It may be that the average rate of transport of granules may vary in different neuron systems, also within the same animal. The size of the nerve terminal network, and the length of the preterminal axons may be of importance in this connection. In the spinal cord of rat, for instance, the rate of transport of NA containing granules in the bulbo-spinal NA neuron system appeared to be much lower (less than 1 mm/h, Häggendal and Dahlström, 1969) than in the sciatic nerve of the same species (5 mm/h, Dahlström and Häggendal, 1966b).

Some observations indicate that the amount of granules transported down the axons to the nerve terminals—and perhaps also the rate of transport—can increase under certain conditions. For instance, during the third to sixth day after the administration of one large dose of reserpine (10 mg/kg i.p.) to rats, the amounts of NA accumulated above a ligation of the sciatic nerve was significantly increased above normal (Dahlström and Häggendal, 1969). This indicates that during this time interval after reserpine the amount of granules produced in the perikarya (see below) and transported down the axons, is increased above normal. The basis for such an increase in production of the protein containing granules may be an increased nerve activity, which, according to e.g. HYDÉN (1960), induces an increased protein synthesis in neurons. Such an increased nerve activity in the sympathetic autonomic nervous system after reserpine has been observed earlier in cats (IGGO and VOGT, 1960).

## Site of Synthesis of Amine Storage Granules

Since the amine storage granules appear to be complex structures, containing a specific storage protein [probably the same as that in the suprarenal medullary granules, chromogranin A (BANKS, HELLE and MAYOR, 1969)], the enzyme DA-$\beta$-hydroxylase, and ATP (e.g. KAUFMANN and FRIEDMAN, 1966) and having a well developed membrane (e.g. HÖKFELT, 1968), it appears reasonable to believe that they are synthetized in the perikaryon, where high concentrations of RNA are found (e.g. HYDÉN, 1960).

Several observations support this view.

1. Nerve ligation causes an accumulation of presumably amine storage granules on the proximal side of the lesion (see above). The same accumulation of granules appears to develop regardless of the level of the ligation. When the ligation is placed just below a ganglion, the accumulation of NA, presumably bound to storage granules, can be seen to develop at about the same rate as when the ligation is performed at a lower level. The accumulations of NA induced fluorescence have been seen to reach the perikarya and cause an increased fluorescence in the cytoplasm (DAHLSTRÖM, unpublished observations). This may indicate that the NA storage granules are formed in the cell bodies.

2. In double ligated nerves, i.e. two ligations performed on the same nerve simultaneously with a certain distance between the ligations, the NA in the separated nerve part is shifted towards the distal ligature, but no clear change in the net amount of NA has so far been observed in nerves treated this way (DAHLSTRÖM, 1967b; DAHLSTRÖM and HÄGGENDAL, 1966b; BANKS, MAGNALL and MAYOR, 1969). This may probably be explained in the following way: no granules can pass through the high ligature to the separated nerve part, and no local synthesis of amine storage granules has taken place. In the nerve part connected to the cell bodies, however, a steady increase in NA containing granules takes place due to axonal transport (DAHLSTRÖM, 1967b; BANKS, MAGNALL and MAYOR, 1969).

3. After a large dose of reserpine, which blocks the storage mechanism of the granules for a long time (e.g. CARLSSON, HILLARP and WALDECK, 1963; CARLSSON, 1965), the monoamine stores in the CNS and PNS are depleted. The first signs of recovery of NA, both in the CNS and in the PNS, can be seen in a small ring just around the nucleus in the cell bodies of the MA containing neurons (DAHLSTRÖM, FUXE and HILLARP, 1965; DAHLSTRÖM and FUXE, 1965b; NORBERG and HAMBERGER, 1964; DAHLSTRÖM, 1967a). The reason for this may be that new granules, not affected by reserpine, are formed in this perinuclear area, where also the Golgi-complex is situated.

4. Electronmicroscopic studies have revealed the presence in the cell body cytoplasm of a comparatively high number of granulated vesicles, both small and large (HÖKFELT, 1969). The granulated vesicles were often found near components

5*

of the Golgi-complex. Since dense-cored vesicles, which probably correspond to amine storage granules, have been demonstrated also in the perikarya of adrenergic neurons, it seems reasonable to believe that at least the dense-cored vesicles observed in the perikaryon had been manufactured there and not in any other part of the neuron. No direct evidence for a centripetally directed flow of amine storage granules exists so far (e.g. Banks, Magnall and Mayor, 1969).

Even if it may appear clear that the amine storage granules (mature or immature) are synthesized, at least to the major part, in the perikarya, the electron-microscopical appearance of the granules need not necessarily be the same just after the formation as it is in the nerve terminals. In the varicosities a certain proportion (a few per cent) of the dense-cored vesicles appear to be of the large type, while in the axons and in the perikarya the relative number of large dense cored vesicles appears to be higher (cf. Hökfelt, 1969). It is not yet clearly demonstrated that also the large type vesicle is involved in amine storage, but if this is the case, it would not appear unreasonable that the large type vesicle may correpond to the young storage granule. In view of recent preliminary observations, indicating that old and new granules may have different properties, especially regarding the capacity to take up exogenous NA, it seems reasonable that morphological differences may exist (cf. Häggendal and Dahlström, 1970).

## Mechanisms of Transport

In the adrenergic neuron, the amine storage granules appear to be transported proximo-distally at a high rate (see above). Other intra-axonal particles, e.g. the mitochondria, appear to be transported much slower, as judged from electron-microscopical studies (Banks, Magnall and Mayor, 1969) and studies on the behavior after ligation of different enzymes presumably localized within the mito-chondria, e.g. MAO (Dahlström, Jonason and Norberg, 1970) and cytochrome oxidase (Banks, Magnall and Mayor, 1969). DOPA-decarboxylase, believed to be localized extragranularly (possibly in the endoplasmic reticulum), accumulates slower than storage granules, but faster than the mitochondria (Dahlström and Jonason, 1969). Thus, different constituents of the neuron appear to be transported down the axon at entirely different rates. Obviously, the transport mechanisms for the different constituents may be different.

The appearance of the axons just above a constriction, with beaded parts, separated by "bottlenecks", gave the impression that some peristaltic mechanism was involved in the transport (e.g. Weiss, 1961). This idea was supported by the observation, that Schwann cells in tissue culture showed pulsative activities (Ernyei and Young, 1966). However, the possible participation of Schwann cells in transport mechanisms, would not explain the transport of material in CNS neurons (cp. Figs. 4 and 5), since Schwann cells are not found in the CNS, and the glia are arranged in a different way.

The mechanism for transport of amine storage granules in the axons is quite independent of both cell body and nerve terminals, as demonstrated in the double ligation experiments (see above, Dahlström, 1967b; Banks, Magnall and Mayor, 1969), where a proximo-distal transport of about the same rate was found in the separated nerve as in the nerve part connected to the cell body. The mechanism for this transport thus appears to be connected to some structure in the axon itself.

Recently, the neurotubules were suggested to be the subcellular structures connected to fast transport. In most cells where fast transport occurs microtubules are found in high numbers (for ref. see SCHMITT, 1968). The substance colchicine, used as mitotic inhibitor, due to its depolymerizing effect on the tubules of the mitotic spindle, has been found to destroy also the microtubules in the same

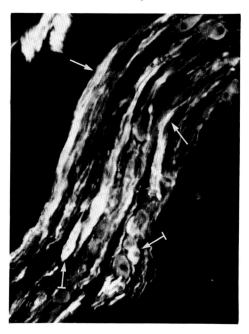

Fig. 7. From the lumbar sympathetic chain of a rat. Colchicine (2 per cent) was applied locally 24 h before death on the lower part of the chain in the figure. Accumulations of strongly fluorescent material (NA) can be observed within many enlarged adrenergic axons (→). Some nerve cell bodies with increased fluorescence intensities can also be observed (↦). Fluorescence microphotograph, ×310

manner. Colchicine applied locally to the sympathetic chain ganglia or injected locally into the sciatic nerve, appears to inhibit the fast transport of amine granules from the cell body, down the axons (Fig. 7) (DAHLSTRÖM, 1968). Similar results have been obtained with vinblastine, another mitotic inhibitor (DAHL-STRÖM, 1970). Injected into the sciatic nerve colchicine also inhibits the fast transport of AChE in myelinated axons (KREUTZBERG, 1969). In the optic nerve inhibition of transport of the fast moving protein components is caused by colchicine injection into the eye (KARLSSON and SJÖSTRAND, 1969). Since colchicine destroys the neurotubules, it is thought that these observations indicate that neurotubules participate in the mechanism of fast transport (see SCHMITT, 1968).

It may appear evident that the slowly moving components are flowing down in the stream of perpetuously out-growing axoplasmic bulk, and that certain structures, e.g. the amine storage granules, are transported by a mechanism connected to the neurotubules. However, it has recently been reported that higher doses of colchicine interrupt also the slow transport (e.g. Davison, 1970).

## Life-Span of Amine Storage Granules

A steady down-transport of amine storage granules to the nerve terminals appears to take place, as mentioned above. A corresponding number of granules must consequently be destroyed and disappear from the nerve terminals, if an over-loading of the system is to be prevented. It appears, thus, that the amine storage granules may have a limited life-span in the nerve terminals. This life-span was calculated to about 5 weeks in the rat, and about twice that time in the cat (Dahl-ström and Häggendal, 1966b). The figure was based on the assumption that the granules in all parts of the adrenergic neuron contain similar amounts of NA.

However, in a recent study (Dahlström and Häggendal, 1970) factors of importance for life-span calculations, e.g. the degree of NA loading of the granu-les in the different parts of the neuron, have been considered in more detail. The granules in the nerve terminals appear not to be fully loaded in the normal ani-mal, since preganglionic denervation causes an increase in the nerve terminal NA content of about 25 per cent (Sedvall, 1964; Almgren, 1969). Also, it ap-pears that the amine granules in the axon can increase their NA content to about 160 per cent of what they contain when transported down the axon. Incor-porating these factors in the calculations of life-span of amine storage granules in the rat sympathetic nervous system, will give a figure of about 3 weeks (Dahlström and Häggendal, 1970).

It is to be noticed that the calculations on the rate of transport and life-span of granules in the adrenergic system refer not to the NA itself, but to the *factories* for NA synthesis. It has been demonstrated that the NA synthesis can take place in all parts of the neuron, which appears reasonable, since the storage granules, containing the enzyme for the last step in the NA synthesis, DA-$\beta$-hydroxylase, are present in the whole neuron (cf. Iversen, 1967). Therefore, the down-trans-port of NA in the granules does probably not play any important role for the economy of the NA stores in the nerve terminals. It has been demonstrated that the NA turnover in the nerve terminals is fast, of the order of hours or days (e.g. Björling and Waldeck, 1965; Iversen, 1967), and it may therefore be concluded that the local synthesis and reuptake of NA in the nerve terminals is of major importance for the maintenance of the NA stores in the nerve terminals.

## Noradrenaline Release from Nerve Terminals

The site of function of the amine storage granules is, presumably, the nerve terminal varicosities, where they synthesize, store and take up NA. They also appear to be essential for the release of the transmitter at nerve activity, since extragranular NA appeared not to be released by nerve stimulation, in experi-ments by Häggendal and Malmfors (1968).

Very little is so far known about the mechanism by which the transmitter is released at nerve activity. It has been speculated that also in the adrenergic system, as has been proposed for the cholinergic one (e.g. Katz, 1962), the transmitter release would take place in the form of "quanta", i.e. the NA content in one granulum would be released to produce one miniature end plate potential, and that several such quanta (i.e. several granules) would have to be released to induce an action potential (e.g. BURNSTOCK and HOLMAN, 1962). This release of a NA quantum packet would also imply the release of the protein content in the granules, by so called exocytosis.

However, it may appear unlikely that the release of NA at adrenergic nerve terminals would take place by exocytosis. Primarily, the life-span of the granules in the nerve terminals appears to be of the order of several weeks (see above), while the turn-over of NA in the nerve terminals is at most 1–2 days (BJÖRLING and WALDECK, 1965; cf. IVERSEN, 1967). Secondly, why should the granules have such a special and efficient machinery for synthesis of NA if they were only used once? Thirdly, the release of the whole content of proteins, formed in the perikarya and transported down by a probably complicated transport mechanism, may appear to be an unnecessarily wasteful procedure.

Some attempts to study the amounts of NA released per nerve impulse per nerve terminal varicosity have been made. FOLKOW and HÄGGENDAL (1967), and FOLKOW, HÄGGENDAL and LISANDER (1967) studied the NA released from vaso-constrictor nerves in the hindlimb of cat after stimulation of the sympathetic chain. They used whole blood from the cat to perfuse their system, and prevented vasoconstriction by simultaneous stimulation of the motor nerves to the area. Recapture of the released NA back into the nerve terminals was prevented by membrane pump blockers (desmethylimipramine or Lu-030–10). The authors cal-culated from their results, that, assuming that all varicosities were reached by the nerve impulses, and that each varicosity contained about 1,000 storage gra-nules, the equivalent of a *few per cent of the NA content of one granulum*, was released per varicosity per nerve impulse. These results appear to contradict the view on exocytosis as the mechanism of release. For discussion of the assumptions made, see FOLKOW, HÄGGENDAL and LISANDER (1967).

Another attempt to study the NA release from cats' hind limb was performed by STJÄRNE, HEDQVIST and BYGDEMAN (1969). They used an artificial perfusion fluid instead of whole blood, and phenoxybenzamine as inhibitor of recapture and of vasoconstriction. The figure obtained by these authors cannot directly be compared to the figure of FOLKOW, HÄGGENDAL and LISANDER (1967) because of the differences in experimental conditions. For instance, phenoxybenzamine, probably not a satisfactory inhibitor of the membrane pump (e.g. MALMFORS, 1965) but possibly interfering with the NA overflow by other mechanisms (see below), was used by STJÄRNE, HEDQVIST and BYGDEMAN (1969). However, these authors arrived at a figure only 3–4 times higher than that of FOLKOW, HÄGGEN-DAL and LISANDER (1967). Thus, also the results of STJÄRNE, HEDQVIST and BYG-DEMAN (1959) support the view that true exocytosis of granules is not likely to occur at nerve activity.

It has been demonstrated recently that chromogranin A is released together with CA from the suprarenal medulla after nerve stimulation, indicating that exocytosis takes place in this organ (BANKS and HELLE, 1965; KIRSHNER, SAGE, SMITH and KIRSHNER, 1966; BLASCHO, COMLINE, SCHNEIDER, SILVER and SMITH, 1967). Also, it has been shown that chromogranin A is one of the main protein constituents of the amine storage granules in the adrenergic nerves (BANKS, HELLE and Mayor, 1969). By analogy, it would appear reasonable to assume that the same release of chromogranin A takes place in the adrenergic nerve terminals. However, differences exist between the two cells, the suprarenal medullary cell and the sympathetic adrenergic neuron, that may induce doubts about the validity of such an assumption by analogy. For instance, the suprarenal medullary cells may be compared only to the perikarya of the adrenergic neurons. The blood vessels may correspond to the adrenergic nerve terminals, since the released CA reaches the effector cells via the circulatory system in the case of the adrenal medullary cells, and via the nerve terminals in the case of the adrenergic neurons.

Recent experiments on the NA release process in sheep spleen after stimulation of the splenic nerve, appear to indicate that small amounts of chromogranin A may be released together with NA at nerve stimulation (Livett, personal communication). The ratio between chromogranin-A and NA estimated in the effluent was much less than the ratio obtained in the adrenal gland studies. Experiments on calf spleen indicate that both chromogranin A and DA-$\beta$-hydoxylase are released together with NA, the ratio of proteins to NA being much less in the effluent than in the NA storage vesicles (de Potter, Shaepdryver, Moerman and Smith, 1969). This indicates that exocytosis of whole granules probably does not exist in adrenergic nerves. Possibly the adrenergic nerves may use a release procedure which permits a small percentage of the granular protein content to be released at nerve activity. If this is the case, small repeated losses of protein may be responsible for the aging of the granules, and may explain why new granules appear to have e.g. a higher ability to take up exogenous NA than have the old ones (cf. Häggendal and Dahlström, 1970).

An interesting hypothesis on the NA release mechanism in monoaminergic nerves has recently been discussed (Häggendal, 1969, and personal communication). The hypothesis mainly concerns the mechanism which regulates the amounts of transmitter liberated per nerve impulse. It was suggested that a local feed-back mechanism connected to the effector cell response and acting via the synaptic gap, may regulate the amount of transmitter released per nerve impulse. The transmitter release would thus continue until effector cell response is brought about. A shift of electrolytes—or some hypothetical substance—in the synaptic gap occurring at the response of the effector cell (e.g. contraction of the smooth muscle cells) would then switch off the release. Thereafter the reverse mechanism—reuptake by the "membrane pump"—takes over to eliminate the transmitter in the synaptic gap. This hypothesis has so far no direct experimental evidence, but may feasibly explain certain peculiar results obtained with the use of drugs which affect the effector cells, e.g. α-receptor blocking drugs like phenoxybenzamine. The remarkably increased overflow of NA obtained in organs pretreated with these α-receptor blockers would, according to this theory, be due to the decreased excitability of the effector cells, which would imply that the offswitch of transmitter release, depending upon the response of the effector cell, is considerably delayed. Such a hypothetical mechanism may seem adequate for the adrenergic neurons, with their very widespread terminal networks, since a local impairment of the effector cell-response would not have to cause a compensatory increased impulse activity in the whole neuron but only a local adjustment of the amounts of transmitter released per nerve impulse (Häggendal, 1970).

Recently it has been shown that stimulation of the splenic nerves causes a release of prostaglandin from the spleen in cat and dog (DAVIES, HORTON and WITHINGTON, 1967; GILMORE, VANE and WYLLIE, 1968). It has also been demonstrated that prostaglandin $E_2$ may reduce the NA overflow from stimulated spleen (HEDQVIST, 1969a), and that prostaglandin $E_2$, when administered together with phenoxybenzamine could inhibit the effect of phenoxybenzamine on the NA overflow (HEDQVIST, 1969b). It is thus possible that prostaglandin $E_2$ liberated from the tissue at nerve activity may—at least in the spleen—act as a brake on the NA release from the nerve terminals by a negative feed-back mechanism (HEDQVIST, 1969a). It remains to be demonstrated e.g. that the liberation of prostaglandin $E_2$ occurs *from the effector cells* and only *at onset of or during their response* (e.g. contraction) at nerve activity, to make prostaglandin $E_2$ identical to the hypothetical key-substance proposed by HÄGGENDAL (1969, 1970).

## Summary

The paper deals with studies mainly on the sympathetic adrenergic neuron, with special reference to work done with the use of the histochemical fluorescence method for cellular localization of catecholamines and serotonin. The distribution, synthesis, transport and life-span of amine storage granules is discussed as well as some aspects of the mechanisms of axonal transport and transmitter release.

## References

ALMGREN, O.: Personal communication (1969).

AMIN, A. H., CRAWFORD, T. B. B., GADDUM, J. H.: Distribution of substance P and 5-hydroxytryptamine in the central nervous system of dog. J. Physiol. (Lond.) **126**, 596–618 (1954).

ANDÉN, N.-E., CARLSSON, A., HÄGGENDAL, J.: Adrenergic mechanisms. Ann. Rev. Pharmacol. **9**, 119–134 (1969).

— — HILLARP, N.-Å., MAGNUSSON, T.: 5-Hydroxytryptamine release by nerve stimulation of the spinal cord. Life Sci. **3**, 473–478 (1964).

— — — — Noradrenaline release by nerve stimulation of the spinal cord. Life Sci. **4**, 129–132 (1965).

— DAHLSTRÖM, A., FUXE, K., LARSSON, K.: Further evidence for the presence of nigronoestriatal dopamine neurons in the rat. Amer. J. Anat. **116**, 329–333 (1965).

— — — — OLSON, L., UNGERSTEDT, U.: Ascending monoamine neurons to the telencephalon and diencephalon. Acta physiol. scand. **67**, 313–326 (1966).

ANGELAKOS, E., FUXE, K., TORCHIANA, M.: Chemical and histochemical evaluation of the distribution of catecholamines in the rabbit and guinea pig hearts. Acta physiol. scand. **59**, 184–192 (1963).

— GLASSMAN, T., MILLARD, P. M., KING, M.: Regional distribution and subcellular localization of catecholamines in the frog heart. Comp. Biochem. Physiol. **15**, 313–324 (1965).

AXELROD, J.: The formation, metabolism, uptake and release of noradrenaline and adrenaline. In: The clinical chemistry of monoamines (VARLEY-GOWENLOCK, ed.), p. 5–18. Amsterdam: Elsevier Publ. Co. 1963.

BACQ, Z. M.: La pharmacologie du système nerveux autonome, et particulièrement du sympathique, d'après la théorie neurohumorale. Ann. Physiol. **10**, 467–528 (1934).

BANKS, P., HELLE, K.: The release of protein from the stimulated adrenal medulla. Biochem. J. **97**, 40C (1965).

— HELLE, K. B., MAYOR, D.: Evidence for the presence of a chromogranin-like protein in bovine splenic nerve granules. Molec. Pharmacol. **5**, 210–212 (1969).

— MANGNALL, D., MAYOR, D.: The re-distribution of cytochrome oxidase, noradrenaline and adenosine triphosphate in adrenergic nerves constricted at two points. J. Physiol. (Lond.) **200**, 745–762 (1969).

BJÖRLING, M., WALDECK, B.: The disappearance of 1-$^{14}$C-nor-adrenaline formed from $^{14}$C-dopamine *in vivo*. Life Sci. **4**, 2239–2242 (1965).

BLASCHKO, H.: The specific action of L-dopa decarboxylase. J. Physiol. (Lond.) **96**, 50–51 P (1939).

— COMLINE, R. S., SCHNEIDER, F. H., SILVER, M., SMITH, A. D.: Secretion of a chromaffine granule protein, chromogranin, from adrenal gland after splanchnic stimulation. Nature (Lond.) **215**, 58–59 (1967).

BOYLE, F. C., GILLESPIE, J. S.: Relationship between the accumulation of noradrenaline and the development of fluorescence above a constriction in cat splenic nerves. J. Physiol. (Lond.) **195**, 27–28 P (1968).

BURNSTOCK, G., HOLMAN, M. E.: Spontaneous potentials at sympathetic nerve endings in smooth muscle. J. Physiol. (Lond.) **160**, 446–480 (1962).

CANNON, W. B., ROSENBLUETH, A.: Sympathin-E and sympathin-I. Amer. J. Physiol. **104**, 557–574 (1933).

— URIDIL, J. E.: Studies on the conditions of activity in endocrine glands. VIII. Some effects on the denervated heart of stimulating the nerves of the liver. Amer. J. Physiol. **58**, 353–354 (1921).

CARLSSON, A.: Drugs which block the storage of 5-hydroxytryptamine and related amines. In: Handbuch der experimentellen Pharmakologie (V. ERSPARMER, ed.), p. 529–592. Berlin-Heidelberg-New York: Springer 1965.

— HILLARP, N.-Å., WALDECK, B.: Analysis of the Mg$^{++}$-ATP dependent storage mechanism in the amine granules of the adrenal medulla. Acta physiol. scand. **59**, Suppl. 215, 1–38 (1963).

— LINDQVIST, M., MAGNUSSON, T., WALDECK, B.: On the presence of 3-hydroxytryptamine in brain. Science **127**, 471 (1958).

CORRODI, H., JONSSON, G.: The formaldehyde fluorescence method for the histochemical demonstration of biogenic amines. A review on the methodology. J. Histochem. Cytochem. **15**, 65–78 (1967).

DAHLSTRÖM, A.: Observations on the accumulation of noradrenaline in the proximal and distal parts of peripheral adrenergic nerves after compression. J. Anat. (Lond.) **99**, 677–689 (1965).

— The intraneuronal distribution of noradrenaline and the transport and life-span of amine storage granules in the sympathetic adrenergic neuron. M. D. Thesis, Stockholm (1966).

— The effect of reserpine and tetrabenazine on the accumulation of noradrenaline in the rat sciatic nerve after ligation. Acta physiol. scand. **69**, 167–179 (1967a).

— The transport of noradrenaline between two simultaneously performed ligations of the sciatic nerves of rat and cat. Acta physiol. scand. **69**, 158–166 (1967b).

— Effect of colchicine on transport of amine storage granules in sympathetic nerves of rat. Europ. J. Pharmacol. **5**, 111–113 (1968).

— The effects of drugs on axonal transport of amine storage granules. In: New Aspects of Storage and Release Mechanisms of Catecholamines. Bayer Symposium II. Berlin-Heidelberg-New York: Springer 1970 (in press).

— FUXE, K.: Evidence for the existence of monoamine containing neurons in the central nervous system. I. Demonstration of monoamines in the cell bodies of brain stem neurons. Acta physiol. scand. **62**, Suppl. 232, 1–55 (1964a).

— — A method for the demonstration of adrenergic nerve fibres in peripheral nerves. Z. Zellforsch. **62**, 602–607 (1964b).

— — A method for the demonstration of monoamine containing nerve fibres in the central nervous system. Acta physiol. scand. **60**, 293–294 (1964c).

— — Evidence for the existence of monoamine containing neurons in the central nervous system. II. Experimentally induced changes in the intraneuronal amine levels of bulbospinal neuron systems. Acta physiol. scand. **64**, Suppl. 247, 1–36 (1965).

— — HILLARP, N.-Å.: Site of action of reserpine. Acta pharmacol. (Kbh.) **22**, 277–292 (1965).

— — KERNELL, D., SEDVALL, G.: Reductions of the monoamine stores in the terminals of bulbospinal neurons following stimulation in the medulla oblongata. Life Sci. **4**, 1207–1212 (1965).

DAHLSTRÖM, A., FUXE, K., MYA-TU, M., ZETTERSTRÖM, B. E. M.: Some observations on the adrenergic innervation of the dog's heart. Amer. J. Physiol. **209**, 689–692 (1965).
— HÄGGENDAL, J.: Some quantitative studies on the noradrenaline content in the cell bodies and terminals of a sympathetic adrenergic neuron system. Acta physiol. scand. **67**, 271–277 (1966a).
— — Studies on the transport and life-span of amine storage granules in a peripheral adrenergic neuron system. Acta physiol. scand. **67**, 278–288 (1966b).
— — Studies on the transport and life-span of amine storage granules in the adrenergic neuron system of the rabbit sciatic nerve. Acta physiol. scand. **69**, 153–157 (1967).
— — Recovery of noradrenaline in adrenergic axons of rat sciatic nerves after reserpine treatment. J. pharm. pharmacol. **21**, 633–638 (1969).
— — Axonal transport of amine storage granules in sympathetic adrenergic neurons. In: Biochemistry of Simple Neuronal Models (E. COSTA and E. GIACOBINI, eds.). New York: Raven Press 1970a (in press).
— — A reevaluation of the life-span of amine storage granules with regard to their capacity to store endogenous noradrenaline in adrenergic nerve terminals of the rat. (In preparation) (1970).
— — HÖKFELT, T.: The noradrenaline content of the varicosities of sympathetic adrenergic nerve terminals in the rat. Acta physiol. scand. **67**, 287–294 (1966).
— HÖKFELT, T.: Unpublished observations.
— JONASON, J.: DOPA-decarboxylase activity in sciatic nerves of the rat after constriction. Europ. J. Pharmacol. **4**, 377–383 (1968).
— — NORBERG, K.-A.: Monoamine oxidase activity in rat sciatic nerves after constriction. Europ. J. Pharmacol. **6**, 248–254 (1969).
DALE, H. H., FELDBERG, W.: The chemical transmission of secretory impulses to the sweat glands of the cat. J. Physiol. (Lond.) **82**, 121–128 (1934).
DAVIES, B. N., HORTON, E. W., WITHRINGTON, P. G.: The occurrence of prostaglandin $E_2$ in splenic venous blood of the dog following splenic nerve stimulation. J. Physiol. (Lond.) **188**, 38P–39P (1967).
DAVISON, P.: Neurotubules and neurofilaments: possible implications in axoplasmic flow. In: Biochemistry of Simple Neuronal Models (E. COSTA and E. GIOCOBINI, eds.). New York: Raven Press 1970 (in press).
DIXON, W. E., HAMILL, P.: The mode of action of specific substances with special reference to secretin. J. Physiol. (Lond.) **38**, 314–336 (1909).
EDWARDS, D. C., FENTON, E. L., KAKARI, S., LARGE, B. J., PAPADAKI, L., ZAIMIS, E.: Effects of nerve growth factor in new-born mice, rats and kittens. J. Physiol. (Lond.) **186**, 10P–12P (1966).
EHINGER, B.: Distribution of adrenergic nerves to orbital structures. Acta physiol. scand. **62**, 291–292 (1964).
ELLIOT, T. R.: The action of adrenaline. J. Physiol. (Lond.) **32**, 401–467 (1905).
ERNYEI, A., YOUNG, M. R.: Pulsatile and myelinforming activities of Schwann cells *in vitro.* J. Physiol. (Lond.) **183**, 469–480 (1966).
ERÄNKÖ, O.: The practical histochemical demonstration of catecholamines by formaldehyde—induced fluorence. J. roy. micr. Soc. **87**, 259–276 (1967).
EULER, U. S. VON: A specific sympathomimetic ergone in adrenergic nerve fibres (sympathin) and its relations to adrenaline and noradrenaline. Acta physiol. scand. **12**, 73–97 (1946).
— Identification of the sympathomimetic ergone in adrenergic nerves of cattle (sympathin N) with laevonoradrenaline. Acta physiol. scand. **16**, 63–74 (1948).
— HILLARP, N.-Å.: Evidence for the presence of noradrenaline in submicroscopic structures of adrenergic axons. Nature (Lond.) **177**, 44–45 (1956).
FALCK, B., HÄGGENDAL, J., OWMAN, C.: The localization of adrenaline in adrenergic nerves in the frog. Quart. J. exp. Physiol. **48**, 253–257 (1963).
— OWMAN, C.: A detailed methodological description of the fluorescence method for the cellular demonstration of biogenic monoamines. Acta Univ. Lund., sect. II, **7**, 1–23 (1965).
FINK, R. P., HEIMER, L.: Two methods for selective silver impregnation of degenerating axons and their synaptic endings in the central nervous system. Brain Res. **4**, 369–374 (1967).

Folkow, B., Häggendal, J.: Quantitative studies on the transmitter release at adrenergic nerve endings. Acta physiol. scand. **70**, 453–454 (1967).
— — Lisander, B.: Extent of release and elimination of noradrenaline at peripheral adrenergic nerve terminals. Acta physiol. scand., Suppl. 307, 1–38 (1967).
Fuxe, K.: Evidence for the existence of monoamine containing neurons in the central nervous system. IV. The distribution of monoamine nerve terminals in the central nervous system. Acta physiol. scand. **64**, Suppl. 247, 38–85 (1965).
— Gunne, L.-M.: Depletion of the amine stores in brain catecholamine terminals on amygdaloid stimulation. Acta physiol. scand. **62**, 493–494 (1964).
— Hökfelt, T., Nilsson, O.: A fluorescence and electronmicroscopic study on certain brain regions rich in monoamine terminals. Amer. J. Anat. **117**, 33–46 (1965).
— Sedvall, G.: The distribution of adrenergic nerve fibres to the blood vessels of skeletal muscle. Acta physiol. scand. **64**, 75–86 (1965).
Gaskell, W. H.: On the structure, distribution and function of the nerves which innervate the visceral and vascular systems. J. Physiol. (Lond.) **7**, 1–80 (1886).
Geffen, L. B., Rush, R. A.: Transport of noradrenaline in sympathetic nerves and the effect of nerve impulses on its contribution to transmitter stores. J. Neurochem. **15**, 925–930 (1968).
Gilmore, N., Vane, J. R., Wyllie, J. H.: Prostaglandins released by the spleen. Nature (Lond.) **218**, 1135–1140 (1968).
Häggendal, J.: An improved method for the fluorimetric determination of small amounts of adrenaline and noraderenaline in plasma and tissue. Acta physiol. scand. **59**, 242–254 (1963).
— On release of transmitter from adrenergic nerve terminals at nerve activity. Acta physiol. scand., Suppl. 330, 29 (1969).
— A hypothetical feed-back mechanism regulating the noradrenaline release from adrenergic nerves at nerve activity. In: New Aspects of Storage and Release Mechanisms of Catecholamines. Bayer Symposium. II Berlin-Heidelberg-New York: Springer 1970 (in press).
— Dahlström, A.: The transport and life-span of amine storage granules in bulbospinal noradrenaline neurons of the rat. J. Pharm. Pharmacol. **21**, 55–57 (1969).
— — The recovery of noradrenaline in adrenergic nerve terminals of the rat after reserpine treatment. J. pharm. pharmacol. (in press) (1970a).
— — Uptake and retention of ³H-noradrenaline in adrenergic nerve terminals after reserpine and axotomy. Europ. J. Pharmacol. (in press) (1970b).
— Malmfors, T.: The effect of nerve stimulation on actecholeamines taken up in adrenergic nerves after reserpine pretreatment. Acta physiol. scand. **75**, 33–38 (1969).
Hamberger, B., Levi-Montalcini, R., Norberg, K.-A., Sjöqvist, F.: Monoamines in immunosympathectomized rats. Int. J. Neuropharmacol. **4**, 91–95 (1965).
— Norberg, K.-A.: Studies on some systems of adrenergic synaptic terminals in the abdominal ganglia of the cat. Acta physiol. scand. **65**, 235–242 (1965).
— — Sjöqvist, F.: Correlated studies of monoamines and acetylcholinesterase in sympathetic ganglia, illustrating the distribution of adrenergic and cholinergic neurons. In: Pharmacology of Cholinergic and Adrenergic Transmission (G. B. Koelle, W. W. Douglas and A. Carlsson), vol. 3, p. 41–54. Oxford: Pergamon Press 1965.
Hedqvist, P.: Modulating effect of prostaglandin $E_2$ on noradrenaline release from isolated cat spleen. Acta physiol. scand. **75**, 511–512 (1969a).
— Antagonism between prostaglandin $E_2$ and phenoxybenzamine on noradrenaline release from the cat spleen. Acta physiol. scand. **76**, 383–384 (1969b).
Hillarp, N.-Å.: Structure of the synapse and the peripheral innervation apparatus of the autonomic nervous system. M. D. Thesis, Acta anat. (Basel) **2**, Suppl. 4, 1–153 (1946).
— The construction and functional organization of the autonomic innervation apparatus. Acta physiol. scand. **46**, Suppl. 157, 1–38 (1959).
— Fuxe, K., Dahlström, A.: Central monoamine neurons. In: Mechanisms on release of biogenic amines (U.S. v. Euler, S. Rosell and B. Uvnäs, eds.), p. 31–37. Pergamon Press 1966.
— Nilson, B.: The structure of the adrenaline and noradrenaline containing granules in the adrenal medullary cells with reference to the storage and release of the sympathomimetic amines. Acta physiol. scand. **31**, Suppl. 113, 79–107 (1954).

HOLTZ, P., CREDNER, K., KRONEBERG, G.: Über das sympathicomimetische pressorische Prinzip des Harns (Urosympathin). Naunyn-Schmiedebergs Arch. exp. Path. Pharmak. **204**, 228–243 (1947).
— HEISE, R., LUDTKE, K.: Fermentativer Abbau von 1-dioxyphenylalanin (DOPA) durch die Niere. Naunyn-Schmiedebergs Arch. exp. Path. Pharmak. **191**, 87–118 (1938).
HYDÉN, H.: The neuron. In: The Cell (J. BRACHET and A. MIRSKY, eds.), vol. IV, p. 215–323. New York-London: Academic Press 1960.
HÖKFELT, T.: In vitro studies on central and peripheral monoamine neurons at the ultra-structural level. Z. Zellforsch. **91**, 1–74 (1968).
— Distribution of noradrenaline storage particles in peripheral adrenergic neurons as revealed by electron microscopy. Acta physiol. scand. **76**, 427–440 (1969).
IGGO, A., VOGT, M.: Preganglionic sympathetic activity in normal and in reserpine-treated cats. J. Physiol. (Lond.) **150**, 114–133 (1960).
IVERSEN, L. L.: The uptake and storage of noradrenaline in sympathetic adrenergic nerves. London: Cambridge University Press 1967.
KAPELLER, K., MAYOR, D.: Accumulation of noradrenaline proximal to the site of constriction of sympathetic nerves. J. Physiol. (Lond.) **182**, 44–45 P (1965).
— — Ultrastructural changes proximal to a constriction in sympathetic axons during first 24 hours after operation. J. Anat. (Lond.) **100**, 439–441 (1966).
— — The accumulation of noradrenaline in constricted sympathetic nerves as studied by fluorescence and electron microscopy. Proc. roy. Soc. B **167**, 282–292 (1967).
KARLSSON, J.-O., SJÖSTRAND, J.: The effect of colchicine on the axonal transport of protein in the optic nerve and tract of the rabbit. Brain Res. **13**, 617–619 (1969).
KATZ, B.: The transmission of impulses from nerve to muscle, and the subcellular unit of synaptic action. Proc. roy. Soc. B **155**, 455–479 (1962).
KAUFMANN, S., FRIEDMAN, S.: Dopamine-$\beta$-hydroxylase. Pharmacol. Rev. **17**, 71–100 (1965).
KIRSHNER, N., SAGE, H. J., SMITH, W. J., KIRSHNER, A. G.: Release of catecholamines and specific protein from adrenal glands. Science **154**, 529–531 (1966).
KREUTZBERG, G.: Neuronal dynamics and axonal flow. IV. Blockage of intra-axonal enzyme transport by colchicine. Proc. nat. Acad. Sci. (Wash.) **62**, 722–728 (1969).
LADURON, P., BELPAIRE, F.: Transport of noradrenaline and dopamine-$\beta$-hydroxylase in sympathetic nerves. Life. Sci. **7**, 1–7 (1968a).
— — Evidence for an extragranular localization of tyrosine hydroxylase. Nature (Lond.) **217**, 1155–1156 (1968b).
LANGLEY, J. N.: The sympathetic and other related systems of nerves. Textbook of physiology (E. A. SCHÄFER, ed.), vol. 2, p. 616–696, 1900.
LATIES, A., JACOBOWITZ, A.: A comparative study of the autonomic innervation of the eye in monkey, cat and rabbit. Anat. Rec. **156**, 383–396 (1966).
LEVI-MONTALCINI, R.: The nerve growth factor. Ann. N.Y. Acad. Sci. **118**, 149–170 (1964).
LIVETT, B. G., GEFFEN, L. B., AUSTIN, L.: Proximo-distal transport of $^{14}$C-noradrenaline and protein in sympathetic nerves. J. Neurochem. **15**, 931–939 (1968).
LOEWI, O.: Über humorale Übertragbarkeit der Herznervenwirkung. Pflügers Arch. ges. Physiol. **189**, 239–242 (1921).
LUBIŃSKA, L.: Axoplasmic streaming in regenerating and in normal nerve fibres. In: Mechanisms of Neuronal Regeneration. Progr. brain res. (M. SINGER and J. P. SCHADÉ, eds.), vol. 13, p. 1–71. Amsterdam: Elsevier Publishing Co. 1964.
MALMFORS, T.: Studies on adrenergic nerves. The use of rat and mouse iris for direct observations on their physiology and pharmacology at cellular and subcellular levels. Acta physiol. scand. **64**, Suppl. 248, 1–93 (1965).
— SACHS, C.: Direct studies on the disappearance of the transmitter and the changes in the uptake-storage mechanisms of degenerating adrenergic nerves. Acta physiol. scand. **64**, 211–223 (1965).
MANN, M., WEST, G. B.: The nature of hepatic and splenic sympathin. Brit. J. Pharmacol. **5**, 173–177 (1950).
— — The nature of uterine and intestinal sympathin. Brit. J. Pharmacol. **5**, 173–177 (1951).

McLean, J. R., Bell, C., Burnstock, G.: Histochemical and pharmacological studies of the innervation of the urinary bladder of the frog. *(Rana temporaria).* Comp. Biochem. Physiol. **21**, 383–392 (1967).

Norberg, K.-A.: Transmitter histochemistry of the sympathetic adrenergic nervous system. Brain Res. **5**, 125–170 (1967).

— Hamberger, B.: The sympathetic adrenergic neuron. Some characteristics revealed by histochemical studies on the intraneuronal distribution of the transmitter. Acta physiol. scand. **63**, Suppl. 238, 1–42 (1964).

Olson, L.: Outgrowth of sympathetic adrenergic neurons in mice treated with a nerve-growth factor (NGF). Z. Zellforsch. **81**, 155–173 (1967).

— Unpublished observations (1968).

Outschoorn, A. S.: The hormones of the adrenal medulla and their release. Brit. J. Pharmacol. **7**, 605–615 (1952).

— Vogt, M.: The nature of cardiac sympathin in the dog. Brit. J. Pharmacol. **7**, 319–324 (1952).

Peart, W. S.: The nature of splenic sympathin. J. Physiol. (Lond.) **108**, 491–501 (1949).

Richardson, K. C.: Electron microscopic identification of autonomic nerve endings. Nature (Lond.) **210**, 756 (1966).

Schmiterlöv, C. G.: The nature and occurrence of pressor and depressor substances in extracts from blood vessels. Acta physiol. scand. **16**, Suppl. 56 (1948).

Schmitt, F. O.: The molecular biology of neural fibrous proteins. Neurosci. Res. Progr. Bull. **6**, 119–144 (1968).

Sedvall, G.: Noradrenaline storage in skeletal muscle. Acta physiol. scand. **60**, 39–50 (1964).

Stjärne, L., Hedqvist, P., Bygdeman, S.: Neurotransmitter quantum released from sympathetic nerves in cat's skeletal muscle. Life Sci. **8**, 189–196 (1969).

Twarog, B. M., Page, I. H.: Serotonin content of some mammalian tissues and urine and methods for its determination. Amer. J. Physiol. **175**, 157–161 (1953).

Weiss, P.: The concept of perpetual neuronal growth and proximo-distal substance convection. In: Regional Neurochemistry (S. S. Kety and J. Elkes, eds.), p. 220. New York: Pergamon Press 1961.

— Hiscoe, H.: Experimentals on the mechanism of nerve growth. J. exp. Zool. **107**, 315–396 (1948).

West, G. B.: Further studies on sympathin. Brit. J. Pharmacol. **5**, 165–172 (1950).

Wirsén, C.: Distribution of adrenergic nerve fibres in brown and white adipose tissue. In: Handbook of physiology (A. E. Renold and C. F. Cahill, eds.), sect. 5, Adipose Tissue. Baltimore 1965.

Vogt, M.: The concentration of sympathin in different parts of the central nervous system under normal conditions and after the administration of drugs. J. Physiol. (Lond.) **123**, 451–481 (1954).

Zaimis, E., Berk, L., Callingham, B.: Morphological, biochemical and functional changes in the sympathetic nervous system of rats treated with NGF-antiserum. Nature (Lond.) **206**, 1221–1222 (1965).

# Electron Microscopic Studies on Peripheral and Central Monoamine Neurons*

Tomas Hökfelt

Department of Histology, Karolinska Institutet, Stockholm (Sweden)

Key words: Monoamine neurons — Peripheral — Central — Ultrastructure.

Monoamines are considered as putative transmitter substances both in the peripheral and central nervous system. This view is supported by a huge number of studies using different types of techniques (for references see monograph by Iversen, 1967). However, electron microscopic studies on this topic have until recently been hampered by difficulties in visualizing monoamines and monoamine storage sites at the ultrastructural level (see e.g. Fuxe et al., 1965).

In the present paper results will be summarized on studies using potassium permanganate (KMnO₄) as a fixative (Richardson, 1966) concerning the ultrastructural localization of monoamines and certain properties of peripheral and central monoamine neurons (see also Hökfelt, 1967 a, b, c, 1968 a, b, 1969; Hökfelt and Jonsson, 1968; Hökfelt and Ungerstedt, 1969).

## A. Identification of Monoamine Neurons at the Ultrastructural Level

After *KMnO₄ fixation* a special type of neurons can be identified both in the peripheral and central nervous system. These neurons are characterized by so called granular or dense core vesicles, *i.e.* vesicles containing an electron dense core (Figs. 1–4). Two types of granular vesicles can be distinguished (*cf.* Grillo and Palay, 1962): The *small granular vesicles* with a diameter of about 500 Å and the *large granular vesicles* with a diameter of about 1,000 Å (see section "D"). It has, however, to be pointed out that neurons containing these two types of vesicles after KMnO₄ fixation usually constitute only a small percentage of all neurons, especially in the central nervous system (see section "D"). Thus, also after KMnO₄ fixation the majority of nerve endings[1] and boutons contains only agranular or empty vesicles (so called synaptic vesicles) of various sizes.

* The investigation has been supported by grants from Karolinska Institutet (Reservationsanslaget), by research grants from the Swedish Medical Research Council (12 X-715–01, 12 X-715–02, 12 X-715–03, 12 X-715–04 A, B 70–14 X-2887–01) and by grants from "Stiftelsen G. och T. Svenssons Minne", "Stiftelsen Therese och Johan Anderssons Minne", "Magnus Bergwalls Stiftelse", "C.-H. Nathorsts Stiftelse", "Svenska Livförsäkringsbolags nämnd för medicinsk forskning" and "Ollie och Elof Ericssons Stiftelse".

1 The term nerve ending will be used synonymously with the terms axonal enlargement (peripheral nervous system) and bouton (central nervous system) for axonal processes containing high numbers of vesicles.

There is now good evidence that the *small* granular vesicles are characteristic of monoamine neurons and that after $KMnO_4$ fixation their dense core represents a precipitate formed by a reaction between $KMnO_4$ and the amine. Thus, *the dense core probably reflects the presence of the amine at the moment of fixation.* The evidence for this view may be summarized as follows:

1. Monoamines react with $KMnO_4$ to form a precipitate in *test tube experiments*. Using labelled amines in these experiments up to 95% of the radioactivity is present in the precipitate provided that high $KMnO_4$ concentrations are used. However, calculations on the amount of radioactivity present *in tissues* (rat iris) after $KMnO_4$ fixation reveal that only about 50% is retained, indicating rather high losses during fixation-dehydration procedure.

2. The intensity of the reaction between amine and $KMnO_4$ in test tubes is dependent on the molecular structure of the amine. Thus, no precipitate could be observed after mixing monoamine analogues without hydroxyl groups (*e.g. β-phe-nylethylamine*) and $KMnO_4$.

3. Studies on the neuronal uptake of monoamines *in vivo* and *in vitro* in combination with pharmacological experiments using *e.g.* depleting agents, such as reserpine and metaraminol, or inhibitors of the nerve-membrane uptake, such as cocaine, all support the view that the dense core is correlated to the presence of the amine in the vesicle at the moment of fixation. As an example the following results may be mentioned. Reserpine in a high dose (10 mg/kg, i.p.) is known to cause an almost complete depletion of monoamine stores, probably depending on an impaired granular uptake-storage mechanism (see CARLSSON, 1966). In accordance with this all vesicles appear empty in the electron microscope. Administration of exogenous amines *in vivo* or *in vitro* in moderate doses does not cause the reappearance of a dense core in the vesicles although concomitant fluorescence microscopic studies reveal that high amounts of amines have been taken up in the nerves and are present intraneuronally. Since the *granular* ("vesicular") storage mechanism is impaired and prevents the *granular* ("vesicular") storage of amines, the amines in the nerves are at least mainly localized *extragranularly* ("extra-vesicularly"). However, if extremely high concentrations of amines are used [10 μg/ml of α-methyl-noradrenaline (α-methyl-NA) for dopamine (DA) boutons in the caudate nucleus, 100 μg/ml of α-methyl-NA for noradrenaline (NA) nerve endings in the iris dilator muscle] dense cores indeed reappear demonstrating a so called *reserpine-resistant granular uptake.* A similar uptake and storage has been described previously *e.g.* by LUNDBORG (1967) and is probably not using the ATP-Mg++ dependent uptake and storage mechanism of intact storage granules (see CARLSSON *et al.*, 1963; EULER and LISHAJKO, 1963a, b).

4. Studies on the regional distribution, frequency and size of monoamine nerve terminals and boutons in the peripheral nervous system and various brain regions reveal a good correlation between fluorescence histochemical results (method of FALCK and HILLARP) and electron microscopic results obtained in $KMnO_4$ fixed tissues.

Recent data indicate that not only the small granular vesicles but also the large granular vesicles *in monoaminergic neurons* may contain an amine—probably the same one as the small granular vesicles—and that the dense core also of the large vesicles as revealed *after KMnO₄ fixation* reflects the presence of the amine at the moment of fixation. This question will be discussed under section "D".

Although the evidence summarized above seems to offer a good basis for identification of monoamine neurons some recent investigations present *seemingly* conflicting results. Thus, autoradiographic studies on $KMnO_4$ fixed tissues have failed to demonstrate increased numbers of grains over nerve endings or boutons containing small granular vesicles (TAXI, 1968; DESCARRIES and BLOOM, personal communication). Similar studies on glutaraldehyde-OsO₄ fixed tissues, on the other hand, reveal high numbers of grains over certain boutons, in which the *small* vesicles only are of the *agranular* type (see *e.g.* AGHAJANIAN and BLOOM, 1966a; DESCARRIES and DROZ, 1968). Thus, there seems to be a lack of correlation between the presence of grains (radioactivity, NA levels) and small granular vesicles. Apart from a number of technical reasons, which could complicate autoradiographic studies on $KMnO_4$ fixed tissues, the following points should be considered:

1. The amount of radioactivity retained in tissues (*e.g.* rat iris) is considerably lower after $KMnO_4$ fixation (about 50%) than after glutaraldehyde fixation (about 70%) (HÖKFELT and JONSSON, 1968). Studies on vas deferens have revealed still larger differences (DEVINE and LAVERTY, 1968). Thus, glutaraldehyde-OsO₄ fixation should *a priori* be more favourable for autoradiography.

2. Only little is known about the reaction between $KMnO_4$ and amines and the resulting reaction product. It is reasonable to assume that the dense core as observed in the electron microscope represents a precipitate of mainly manganese dioxide caused by a reduction of $KMnO_4$ by the amine. The oxidized amine is probably not chemically bound to the precipitate on a molar basis, but rather retained to a certain extent within the precipitate. In addition the possibility may be considered that the dense precipitate surrounding the labelled, oxidized amine may in fact prevent the radiation to reach the emulsion. This would explain the comparatively high losses of amine during the fixation-embedding procedure and the difficulties to perform autoradiographic studies on $KMnO_4$ fixed tissues. It is therefore only possible to state—as done in this and previous papers—that the dense core reflects the presence of amines *at the moment of fixation*.

3. Using $KMnO_4$ fixation small dense core vesicles can be demonstrated in adrenergic nerves in iris of rats treated with a synthesis inhibitor to almost about the same extent as in normal rats (HÖKFELT, 1967a, 1968b). Since this treatment reduces the NA levels to approximately 15–20% of the normal values (JONSSON, 1969) comparatively small amounts of amines are required for the formation of dense cores in these neurons. This indicates that the dense core not necessarily means that high amounts of amines (labelled amines) are present in the vesicles. Furthermore, it may be concluded that quantitative studies based on the small dense core vesicles are possible only to a very limited extent and under special conditions.

4. The possibility has to be kept in mind that the vigorous reaction between $KMnO_4$ and the amine may indeed partly "destroy" the amine molecule. Thus, labelled groups may be split off and lost during the fixation and embedding procedures. Test tube experiments with ¹⁴C-NA, however, indicate losses of about the same magnitude also with this isotope (HÖKFELT and JONSSON, 1968).

The results summarized above have been obtained with KMnO$_4$ fixation. However, also a number of previous studies on peripheral adrenergic neurons using OsO$_4$ or combined glutaraldehyde-OsO$_4$ fixation have given evidence for the close correlation between small granular vesicles and noradrenaline (DE ROBERTIS and PELLEGRINO DE IRALDI, 1961a, b; TAXI, 1961a, b, 1965; WOLFE et al., 1962; RICHARDSON, 1962, 1964; BLOOM and BARRNETT, 1966; BONDAREFF, 1966; ORDEN et al., 1966, 1967; TRANZER and THOENEN, 1967a).

Finally, it should be pointed out that other methods are available for the identification of monoamine and monoamine storage sites, such as autoradiography (WOLFE et al., 1961; AGHAJANIAN and BLOOM, 1966a, b, 1967; TAXI and DROZ, 1966a, b; DEVINE, 1967; DESCARRIES and DROZ, 1968; BUDD and SALPETER, 1969). Furthermore, 5-hydroxy-dopamine (5-OH-DA), a DA analogue which is taken up specifically into both small and large vesicles of adrenergic neurons and "adds" electron opacity to them (TRANZER and THOENEN, 1967b) and also specific cytochemical methods for the demonstration of CA (COUPLAND et al., 1964; TRAMEZZANI et al., 1964; WOOD and BARRNETT, 1964; WOOD, 1966) and 5-hydroxytryptamine (5-HT) (JAIM-ETCHEVERRY and ZIEHER, 1968) have been very useful tools in ultrastructural studies on monoamine containing tissues.

## B. Peripheral Adrenergic Neurons

Both small and large granular vesicles can be found in all parts of peripheral adrenergic neurons as indicated in studies on cell bodies in the superior cervical ganglion (Fig. 1), on axons in the internal carotid trunk and on nerve endings in the dilator muscle of rat iris (Fig. 2). The highest amounts are found in the axonal enlargements of the *axon terminals*, where up to 800 vesicles per enlargement can be seen. As revealed in serial sectioning, however, such enlargements may vary considerably in size and may contain down to 50 vesicles. These findings indicate that the axonal enlargements or "varicosities" at least in rat dilator muscle, may not be considered as "standardized" units, and that the question even may be raised whether these enlargements should be considered as static structures or whether they represent a "snapshot" of a dynamic event. The *axons* contain only few granular vesicles whereas the *cell bodies* as judged from single ultrathin sections seem to contain varying amounts of granular vesicles, which are localized in the highest amounts in the peripheral parts of the cell body, often where the cell processes leave the cell body (Fig. 1). The granular vesicles can, however, also be found in the neighbourhood of the Golgi apparatus and even in probable dendrites, sometimes just below synapses between preganglionic cholinergic nerve endings and dendrites. This distribution parallels the distribution of NA as revealed in fluorescence microscopic studies (see e.g. NORBERG and HAMBERGER, 1964; DAHLSTRÖM, 1966).

The proportions of small and large granular vesicles in the various parts of neurons are only incompletely known. In the axonal enlargements of the rat dilator muscle only about 2% of the vesicles are of the large type, in rat vas deferens they constitute about 4% according to FARRELL (1968). As to the non-terminal parts of the axons studies on the proximal part of ligated axons of cats seem to indicate that mainly large granular vesicles are present in the axons (KAPELLER and

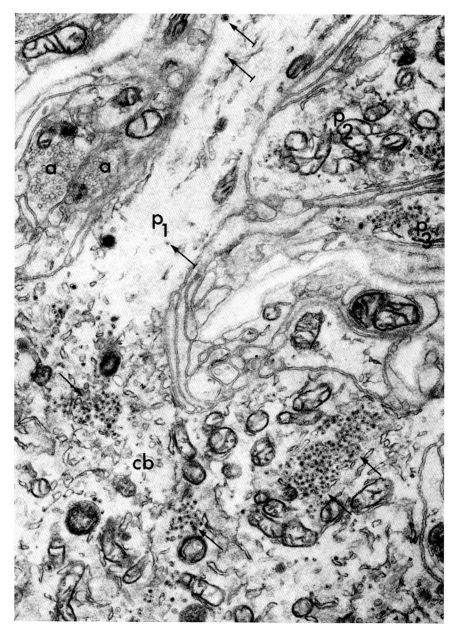

Fig. 1. Superior cervical ganglion, untreated rat. The peripheral part of a cell body (c b) is seen. Large numbers of mainly small granular vesicles can be seen in the cytoplasm ( ⤢ ) often aggregated in clusters. In a cell process ($p_1$) in continuity with the cell body a few granular vesicles can be seen ( ⤢ ). Note high numbers of granular vesicles in cell processes $p_2$ and $p_3$. Two preganglionic, cholinergic axonal enlargements are seen, characterized by agranular vesicles (a). ×32,000

MAYOR, 1967, 1969). Preliminary studies on the internal carotid trunk of rat indicate that single vesicles in the axons mainly are of the large type. However, clusters of small granular vesicles may be seen in single axons. In the cell body clusters of small granular vesicles are seen mainly in the peripheral part of the cell body, whereas in the neighbourhood of the Golgi apparatus comparatively few, probably mainly large granular vesicles are seen. The significance of these results will be discussed below (see section "D").

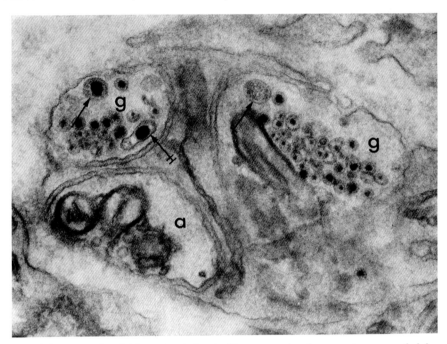

Fig. 2. Dilator muscle of iris, untreated rat. Three axonal enlargements surrounded by a Schwann cell are seen. Dense core vesicles are present in two of them (*g*). The majority of the vesicles are of the small type. Two large vesicles are seen, one of which ( ⌁ ) contains a dense core, while the other one ( ⌁ ) has an interior of a very low electron density. Note that a third large granular vesicles ( ⌁ ) is elongated, which could indicate a "dynamic" event. The third enlargement (*a*) contains a few agranular vesicles characteristic of cholinergic axons. ×58,000

# C. Central Monoaminergic Neurons

So far boutons containing small granular vesicles can be found consistently only in regions known to contain NA nerve terminals. However, if thin slices from brain regions containing DA or 5-HT are incubated in amine containing buffer solutions, thus increasing intraneuronal and intravesicular amine levels, small granular vesicles can be seen also in probable DA and 5-HT neurons. Together with the small granular vesicles also large granular vesicles are mostly seen in all three types of monoamine neurons. Thus, both small and large granular vesicles seem to be present both in peripheral and central monoamine neurons. Furthermore, since so far small granular vesicles seem to be present only in mono-amine neurons these may be used for identification of these neurons. Using

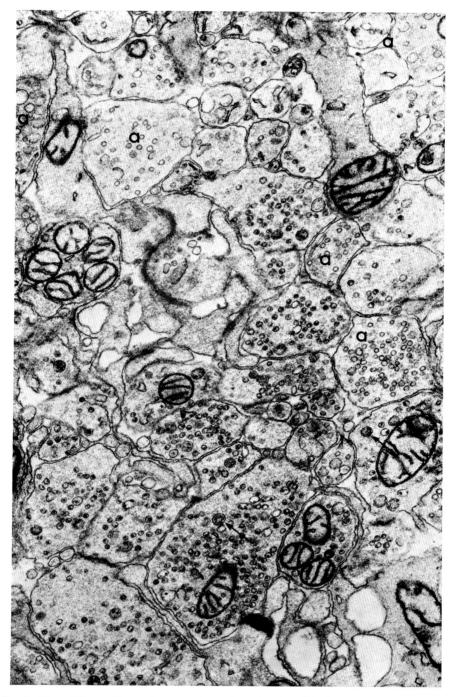

Fig. 3. Slice of the median eminence, untreated rat, incubated in buffer solution containing
α-methyl-noradrenaline (10 μg/ml). The micrograph is taken from the external layer just above
the zone adjacent to the portal vessels. A large number of boutons contains mainly small
granular vesicles and belongs probably to tubero-infundibular dopamine neurons (see FUXE
and HÖKFELT, this symposium). Also large vesicles ( ↗ ) with a more or less dense core are seen.
Some boutons (a) contain only agranular vesicles. ×35,000

pharmacological tools, such as specific blockers of membrane-uptake of the different monoamine neurons, possibilities exist to identify specifically NA, DA and 5-HT neurons.

The fact that monoamine boutons can be identified at the ultrastructural level makes it possible to estimate the monoaminergic input to various brain regions quantitatively. Thus, in the caudate nucleus about 15%, in the hypothalamic periventricular region about 3—4% and in the hypothalamic suprachiasmatic nucleus 4—5% of all boutons belong to monoaminergic neurons. These regions are according to fluorescence microscopic studies considered to be very densely innervated by monoamine nerve terminals (FUXE, 1965) which indicates that fluorescence microscopical pictures may give a somewhat exaggerated view on the relative amounts of monoamine nerve terminals. Thus, the percentage of monoamine boutons is certainly considerably lower in other brain regions, e.g. in cortical areas of cerebrum and cerebellum, where fluorescence microscopy indicates a sparse innervation (FUXE et al., 1968; HÖKFELT and FUXE, 1969). With the present technique it has also been possible to identify DA nerve endings in the median eminence (Fig. 3) (HÖKFELT, 1967c, 1968b). These nerve endings belong to tubero-infundibular DA neurons, which probably are involved in the regulation of gonadotrophin secretion from the anterior pituitary (see FUXE and HÖKFELT, 1969; see also FUXE and HÖKFELT, this symposium), probably via an axo-axonic influence in the median eminence (HÖKFELT, 1967c, 1968b).

Of great interest is to elucidate the synaptic relations between monoamine boutons and other nervous structures. These studies have, however, so far been hampered by the fact that the incubation procedure causes certain distorsions in morphology such as glial and extracellular swelling. Thus, the interpretation of the findings should be given with caution. In the hypothalamic areas probable NA and expecially 5-HT boutons are to a certain extent associated with synapses of type 1 (GRAY, 1961). However, clearcut synapses of type 1 are only very rarely seen in connexion with DA boutons in the caudate nucleus, in spite of the fact that this type of synapses are very often seen in connexion with non-monoaminergic boutons in the same section. Thus, the incubation procedure does not seem to destroy the synaptic complexes which also according to recent studies e.g. by PFENNINGER (personal communication) are very resistent to various types of rough treatment, e.g. hypertonic solutions. If synapses of type 1 indeed are considered as the site of synaptic transmission—a question which is by no means fully elucidated (see e.g. AKERT et al., 1969)—then the question arises whether a very limited percentage of all DA boutons are "functionally active" or whether the synaptic junctions may be transient structures present only at the time of transmission. On the other hand, a number of other possibilities have to be kept in mind, e.g. DA boutons may have morphologically different synapses, DA boutons may make axo-axonic contacts or DA may be released from the boutons at any place regardless the presence of structurally distinct synapses. This question is now under study using an incubation medium containing 10% Dextran T 70 (Pharmacia, Sweden), a polysaccharide with a molecular weight of about 70,000, which almost completely prevents extracellular swelling (Fig. 4).

Serial sectioning of 75 DA boutons in the caudate nucleus have revealed that in about 50% of these boutons no mitochondria are present. These findings are of a

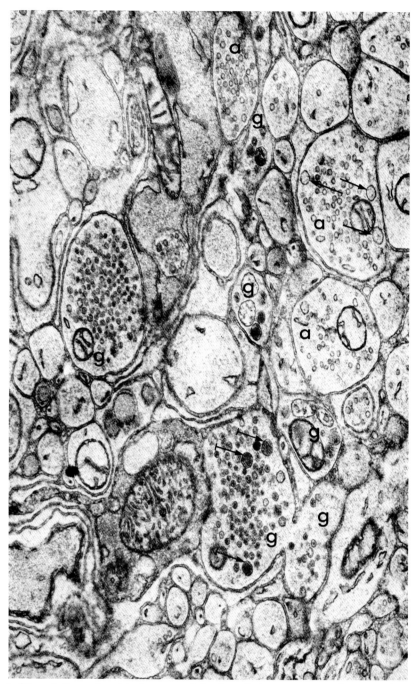

Fig. 4. Slice of the periventricular zone of the hypothalamus, untreated rat, incubated in Tyrode buffer solution containing 10% Dextran T70 (an anhydrous glucose polymer, MW 70,000, Pharmacia, Sweden) and α-methyl-noradrenaline (10 μg/ml). A number of boutons (*g*) containing granular vesicles, probably belonging to noradrenaline or 5-hydroxytryptamine nerve terminals, are seen together with boutons (*a*) containing only agranular vesicles. Note the absence of extracellular swelling usually observed in brain slices after the incubation procedure (*cf.* HÖKFELT, 1968a). ×35,000

certain interest since it is generally assumed that the enzyme monoamine oxidase (MAO), which inactivates the intracellular monoamines, is localized within the mitochondria. This finding would implicate either that MAO may, in addition, have also an extramitochondrial localization (cf. Stjärne, 1966) or that in certain boutons DA can be localized extragranularly without being inactivated. Since the number of DA boutons in the caudate nucleus has roughly been estimated to $3 \times 10^9$ (Andén et al., 1966) 50% of these boutons constitute a considerable part of the afferent input containing high amounts of DA, which then would not be controlled by MAO. This could be of physiological significance and should be kept in mind when studying drug effects on the caudate nucleus, especially when using rats treated with MAO-inhibitors.

## D. Small and Large Granular Vesicles

Measurements of the diameter of granular vesicles on sections from adrenergic nerves in the dilator muscle of rat iris have revealed that there seem to exist concomitantly two populations of granular vesicles within the same neuron; one population with a peak diameter at about 500 Å (small granular vesicles) and a second one with a peak at about 1,000 Å (large granular vesicles). The small granular vesicles occur in considerably higher amounts as compared to the large ones. Thus, about 98% of all vesicles in the adrenergic nerve endings in the dilator muscle of rat iris are of the small type.

Recent studies indicate that not only the size and number but also the chemical composition is different in the two types of vesicles. This assumption is mainly based on results obtained using various fixatives and "staining" procedures which will be discussed below and are summarized in the table.

1. After *glutaraldehyde-OsO₄ fixation* large granular vesicles can be found in both adrenergic and non-adrenergic neurons. The dense core in these vesicles does not seem to be dependent, at least not only, on the presence of an amine, since

Table. *Small and large vesicles in monoamine and non-monoamine neurons as revealed after various fixation and/or impregnation procedures*

The present table summarizes results from studies based on various fixation and/or impregnation procedures. The presence or the absence of an electron dense precipitate ("dense core") within the two types of vesicles have been recorded as "+" and "−", respectively.

|  | Vesicles in monoamine neurons | | Vesicles in certain non-monoamine neurons | |
|---|---|---|---|---|
|  | small | large | small | large |
| Glutaraldehyde-OsO₄ | (+)[a] | +[b] | − | + |
| Zinc-iodide-OsO₄ (Akert and Sandri, 1968) | + | − | + | − |
| Bismuth-iodide (Pfenninger et al., 1969) | − | + | − | + |
| E-PTA (Bloom and Aghajanian, 1968b) | − | + | − | + |
| KMnO₄ (Hökfelt, 1968a, 1969) | + | + | − | − |

[a] Only in certain peripheral adrenergic neurons and never in central adrenergic neurons.

[b] It should be pointed out that the degree of the density of the large vesicles may vary considerably (see Bloom and Aghajanian, 1968a). Thus, the present division into two groups ("+" or "−") only gives a schematic picture.

drugs which change amine levels do not seem to affect the large granular vesicles to any marked extent (FUXE *et al.*, 1965, 1966; TAXI, 1965; HÖKFELT, 1966; BLOOM and AGHAJANIAN, 1968). Since, in addition, glutaraldehyde is known to preserve proteins in tissues to a high extent it may be assumed that the dense core of the large granular vesicles as revealed after glutaraldehyde-OsO$_4$ fixation at least partly is correlated to the vesicular matrix, *i.e.* mainly proteins and especially perhaps enzymes. In agreement with this the dense core of the storage granules in neurosecretory neurons as revealed after glutaraldehyde-OsO$_4$ fixation does not seem to be related to the hormone content but rather to the carrier matrix (BARER and LEDERIS, 1966; BARGMANN and v. GAUDECKER, 1969).

Small granular vesicles can be demonstrated in certain peripheral adrenergic neurons after glutaraldehyde-OsO$_4$ fixation. In this case the presence of a dense core is closely correlated to the presence of amines. In the CNS, on the other hand, the same fixation procedure never reveals small granular vesicles (see *e.g.* FUXE *et al.*, 1965).

2. Using the *zinc-iodide-osmic acid (ZIO) impregnation* technique (CHAMPY, 1913; MAILLET, 1962) AKERT and SANDRI (1968) have been able to demonstrate small granular vesicles in both adrenergic and non-adrenergic (*e.g.* cholinergic) neurons. It has, however, so far not been possible to elucidate the nature of the dense core of these small granular vesicles. According to PELLEGRINO DE IRALDI and GUEUDET (1968) the dense core in vesicles in adrenergic neurons in the pineal gland is not caused by the NA or 5-HT present in these nerves. Of great interest is the finding that with this technique the large vesicles—also those in adrenergic neurons—do not contain a dense core.

3. In recent studies two new techniques have been applied to the study of nervous tissues. Thus, using *bismuth-iodide block impregnation* (PFENNINGER *et al.*, 1969) or *ethanolic phosphotungstic acid staining* (E-PTA) (BLOOM and AGHAJANIAN, 1968; JAIM-ETCHEVERRY and ZIEHER, 1969b) of ultrathin sections of glutaraldehyde fixed tissues it could be demonstrated that *only large vesicles* contained a dense interior, probably both in monoaminergic and non-monoaminergic neurons. Small vesicles, on the other hand, never were of the granular type. Of great interest was also the finding that in addition to the interior of the large vesicles also the so called dense projections at the presynaptic membrane are stained by these techniques.

4. The results discussed above (1—3) all favour the view that small and large granular vesicles are quite different types of vesicles. However, using $KMnO_4$ *fixation* (HÖKFELT, 1967b, 1968a, b, 1969) or *glutaraldehyde-dichromate-OsO$_4$ fixation* (TRANZER and THOENEN, 1968) or *formaldehyde-glutaraldehyde-dichromate fixation* (JAIM-ETCHEVERRY and ZIEHER, 1969a), procedures, which may more specifically stain the monoamine present in the vesicles, large vesicles contain a dense core in monoaminergic neurons. In agreement with this large vesicles seem to be able to take up exogenously administered amines (TRANZER and THOENEN, 1967b; HÖKFELT, 1968a; JAIM-ETCHEVERRY and ZIEHER, 1969).

The conclusions drawn from the data discussed above are that two types of intraneuronal vesicles exist both in monoaminergic and certain non-monoaminergic neurons. These vesicles are distinguished by size, number and chemical composition. *In monoaminergic neurons both types contain an electron dense core if certain fixatives such as KMnO₄ are used.* Under these circumstances the dense core probably reflects the presence of an amine, in all probability the amine that acts as the transmitter in the very neuron. Thus, two types of vesicles may be involved in the amine metabolism (synthesis, uptake, storage and/or release) of mono-aminergic neurons.

Little information is available on possible functional differences between the two types of vesicles. Due to the large number of small granular vesicles in the axon terminals, it is reasonable to assume that the bulk of transmitter is stored in the small vesicles. Furthermore, since the small vesicles are the ones localized closely to the synaptic cleft (see AKERT *et al.*, 1969; HÖKFELT, 1968a), the small ones may be associated with the quantal release of the transmitter substance. The large granular vesicles, on the other hand, seem to contain a protein matrix in addition to the amine and may have a more complex function, not only confined to pure storage of the amine. It is a tempting hypothesis that a more specific function, *e.g.* the synthesis of the amines may be localized in the large granular vesicles whereas the small granular vesicles mainly serve as pure storage vesicles.

The site of formation of the vesicles has been discussed extensively. Recent histochemical and biochemical data by DAHLSTRÖM (1966) and DAHLSTRÖM and HÄGGENDAHL (1966) have been interpreted to show that the "amine storage granules" are produced in the Golgi apparatus and transported along the axon to the nerve terminals. The demonstration of increased numbers of granular vesicles proximal to a constriction of an axon (KAPELLER and MAYOR, 1967, 1969) has been considered as evidence for this view.

This view is, however, complicated by the findings related above, that there seem to exist two types of vesicles involved in monoamine metabolism. As to the *large granular vesicles*, they are definitely present in the immediate neighbourhood of the Golgi apparatus, in the cytoplasm of the cell body, in the axon and in the terminal parts of the axon (FUXE *et al.*, 1966; HÖKFELT, 1969). Since the large granular vesicles proportionally are more frequent than the small ones in the axons (HÖKFELT, 1969) and since the granular vesicles "accumulated" proximal to a constriction seem to be mainly of the large type (KAPELLER and MAYOR, 1969) it may be that the large granular vesicles indeed emanate from the Golgi apparatus and then are transported down to the axon terminals. Their comparatively complex structure with a certain resemblance to the granular vesicles in adrenal medullary cells would further support the view that they are produced in the cell body. Also the *small granular vesicles* seem to be present in all parts of the neuron, although so far no certain evidence has been presented for their presence in the immediate neighbourhood of the Golgi apparatus. Furthermore, since the pro-portions of large to small granular vesicles is different in different parts of the neuron it may be speculated that the two types have different sites of formation, *e.g.* the small vesicles may be formed locally in all parts of the neuron. Whether this formation takes place from neurotubules (see *e.g.* DE ROBERTIS, 1964), mito-chondria (SPRIGGS *et al.*, 1967), from axonal endoplasmic reticulum or the nerve cell membrane (*e.g.* CHALAZONITIS, 1968), from so called complex (GRAY, 1961a) vesicles (see LEONHARDT, 1967) or from large granular vesicles (see Fig. 2) remains to be seen. In the latter case small and large granular vesicles would represent different stages of a cycle in which large granular vesicles are transformed into small ones.

# E. General Conclusions

Electron microscopic studies on $KMnO_4$ fixed nervous tissue have revealed that both peripheral and central monoamine neurons are characterized by dense core or granular vesicles. Two types of granular vesicles are present, so called small (diameter about 500 Å) and large (diameter about 1,000 Å) granular vesicles. Both of them are probably involved in monoamine metabolism but they differ not only in size, number and chemical composition but also presumably in function. Both types occur in all parts of the neuron, *i.e.* in the cell body, in the axon and in the nerve terminals. They are most frequent in terminal axonal enlargements and most sparse in the axons. However, the proportions between the two types seem to differ in the various parts of the neuron. Thus, the large granular vesicles seem to be proportionally more frequent in the axons than in the terminal axonal enlargements. This difference in the proportion of small and large granules in the various parts of the neuron may indicate a different site of formation for the two types of vesicles. Thus, large granular vesicles may be formed in the cell body, whereas small granular vesicles could be formed in all parts of the neuron either from large granular vesicles or from quite different structures.

## References

AGHAJANIAN, G. K., BLOOM, F. E.: Electron-microscopic autoradiography of rat hypothalamus after intraventricular H³-norepinephrine. Science **153**, 308–310 (1966a).
— — Localization of tritiated serotonin in rat brain by electronmicroscopic autoradiography. J. Pharmacol. exp. Ther. **156**, 23–30 (1966b).
— — Electron-microscopic localization of tritiated norepinephrine in rat brain. Effect of drugs. J. Pharmacol. exp. Ther. **156**, 407–416 (1967).
— — The formation of synaptic junctions in developing rat brain: a quantitative electron microscopic study. Brain Res. **6**, 716–727 (1968).
AKERT, K., MOOR, H., PFENNINGER, K., SANDRI, C.: Contributions of new impregnation methods and freeze etching to the problems of synaptic fine structure. In: Progress in brain research (K. AKERT and P. G. WASER, eds.), vol. 31, p. 223–240. Amsterdam-London-New York: Elsevier Publishing Company 1969.
ANDÉN, N.-E., FUXE, K., HAMBERGER, B., HÖKFELT, T.: A quantitative study on the nigro-neostriatal dopamine neuron system in rat. Acta physiol. scand. **67**, 306–312 (1966).
BARER, R., LEDERIS, K.: Ultrastructure of the rabbit neurohypophysis with special reference to the release of hormones. Z. Zellforsch. **75**, 201–239 (1966).
BARGMANN, W., GAUDECKER, BR. v.: Über die Ultrastruktur neurosekretorischer Elementargranula. Z. Zellforsch. **96**, 495–504 (1969).
BLOOM, F. E., AGHAJANIAN, G. K.: An electron microscopic analysis of large granular synaptic vesicles of the brain in relation to monoamine content. J. Pharmacol. exp. Ther. **159**, 261–273 (1968a).
— — Fine structural and cytochemical analysis of the staining of synaptic junctions with phosphotungstic acid. J. Ultrastruct. Res. **22**, 361–375 (1968b).
— BARRNETT, R. J.: Fine structural localization of noradrenaline in vesicles of autonomic nerve endings. Nature (Lond.) **210**, 599–601 (1966).
BONDAREFF, W.: Localization of α-methyl-norepinephrine in sympathetic nerve fibers of the pineal body. Exp. Neurol. **16**, 131–135 (1966).
BUDD, G. C., SALPETER, M. M.: The distribution of labelled norepinephrine within sympathetic nerve terminals studied with electron microscope radioautography. J. Cell Biol. **41**, 21–32 (1969).
CARLSSON, A.: Drugs, which block the storage of 5-hydroxytryptamine and related amines. In: Handbuch der experimentellen Pharmakologie (V. ERSPAMER, ed.), Ergänzungswerk, Bd. XIX, S. 529–592. Berlin-Heidelberg-New York: Springer 1966.

Carlsson, A., Hillarp, N.-Å., Waldeck, B.: Analysis of the Mg$^{++}$-ATP dependent storage mechanism in the amine granules of the adrenal medulla. Acta physiol. scand. **59**, Suppl. 215, 1–38 (1963).

Chalazonitis, N.: Formation et lyse des vésicules synaptiques dans le neuropile d'*Helix pomatia*. C. R. Acad. Sci. (Paris) **266**, 1743–1746 (1968).

Champy, C.: Granules et substances réduisant l'iodure d'osmium. J. Anat. (Paris) **49**, 323–343 (1913).

Coupland, R. E., Pyper, A. S., Hopwood, D.: A method for differentiating between noradrenaline—and adrenaline—storing cells in the light and electron microscope. Nature (Lond.) **201**, 1240–1242 (1964).

Dahlström, A.: The intraneuronal distribution of noradrenaline and the transport and life-span of amine storage granules in the sympathetic adrenergic neuron. M. D. Thesis, Stockholm (1966).

— Häggendahl, J.: Studies on the transport and life-span of amine storage granules in a peripheral adrenergic neuron system. Acta physiol. scand. **67**, 278–288 (1966).

De Robertis, E.: Histophysiology of synapses. Oxford-London-Edinburgh-New York-Paris-Frankfurt: Pergamon Press 1964.

— Pellegrino de Iraldi, A.: Plurivesicular secretory processes and nerve endings in the pineal gland. J. biophys. biochem. Cytol. **10**, 361–372 (1961 a).

— — A plurivesicular component in adrenergic nerve endings. Anat. Rec. **139**, 299 (1961 b).

Descarries, L., Droz, B.: Incorporation de noradrenaline-$^3$H (NA-$^3$H) dans le système nerveux central du rat adulte. Etude radio-autographique en microscopie électronique. C. R. Acad. Sci. (Paris) **266**, 2480–2482 (1968).

Devine, C. E.: Electron microscope autoradiography of rat arteriolar axons after noradrenaline infusion. Proc. Univ. Otago med. Sch. **45**, 7–8 (1967).

Euler, U. S. von, Lishajko, F.: Catecholamine release and uptake in isolated adrenergic nerve granules. Acta physiol. scand. **57**, 468–480 (1963 a).

— — Effect of adenine nucleotides on catecholamine release and uptake in isolated adrenergic nerve granules. Acta physiol. scand. **59**, 454–461 (1963 b).

Farrell, K. E.: Fine structure of nerve fibres in smooth muscle of the vas deferens in normal and reserpinized rats. Nature (Lond.) **217**, 279–281 (1968).

Fuxe, K.: Evidence for the existence of monoamine neurons in the central nervous system. IV. The distribution of monoamine nerve terminals in the central nervous system. Acta physiol. scand. **64**, Suppl. 247, 39–85 (1965).

— Hamberger, B., Hökfelt, T.: Distribution of noradrenaline nerve terminals in cortical areas of the rat. Brain Res. **8**, 125–131 (1968).

— Hökfelt, T.: Catecholamines in the hypothalamus and the pituitary gland. In: Frontiers in neuroendocrinology (W. F. Ganong and L. Martini, eds.), p. 47–96. New York-London-Toronto: Oxford University Press 1969.

— — Nilsson, O.: A fluorescence and electronmicroscopic study on certain brain regions rich in monoamine terminals. Amer. J. Anat. **117**, 33–45 (1965).

— — Reinius, S., Nilsson, O.: A fluorescence and electron microscopic study on central monoamine nerve cells. Anat. Rec. **155**, 33–40 (1966).

Gray, E. G.: The granule cells, mossy synapses and Purkinje spine synapses of the cerebellum: light and electron microscopic investigations. J. Anat. (Lond.) **95**, 345–356 (1961 a).

— Ultrastructure of synapses of the cerebral cortex and of certain specializations of the neuroglial membranes. In: Electron microscopy in anatomy (J. D. Boyd, F. R. Johnson, and J. D. Lever, eds.), p. 54–73. London: Edward Arnold 1961 b.

Grillo, M., Palay, S. L.: Granule-containing vesicles in the autonomic nervous system. In: Electron microscopy (S. S. Breese, Jr., ed.), vol. 2, p. U–1. New York: Academic Press 1962.

Hökfelt, T.: The effect of reserpine on the intraneuronal vesicles of the rat vas deferens. Experientia (Basel) **22**, 56–57 (1966).

— Ultrastructural studies on adrenergic nerve terminals in the albino rat iris after pharmacological and experimental treatment. Acta physiol. scand. **69**, 125–126 (1967 a).

— On the ultrastructural localization of noradrenaline in the central nervous system of the rat. Z. Zellforsch. **79**, 110–117 (1967 b).

HÖKFELT, T.: The possible ultrastructural identification of tubero-infundibular dopamine-containing nerve endings in the median eminence of the rat. Brain Res. **5**, 121–123 (1967 c).
— In vitro studies on central and peripheral monoamine neurons at the ultrastructural level. Z. Zellforsch. **91**, 1–74 (1968 a).
— Electron microscopic studies on peripheral and central monoamine neurons. M. D. Thesis, Stockholm 1968 b.
— Distribution of noradrenaline storing particles in peripheral adrenergic neurons as revealed by electron microscopy. Acta physiol. scand. **76**, 427–440 (1969).
— FUXE, K.: Cerebellar monoamine nerve terminals, a new type of afferent fibers to the cortex cerebelli. Exp. Brain Res. **9**, 63–72 (1969).
— JONSSON, G.: Studies on reaction and binding of monoamines after fixation and processing for electron microscopy with special reference to fixation with potassium permanganate. Histochemie **16**, 45–67 (1968).
— UNGERSTEDT, U.: Electron and fluorescence microscopic studies on the nucleus caudatus putamen of the rat after unilateral lesions of ascending nigro-neostriatal dopamine neurons. Acta physiol. scand. **76**, 415–426 (1969).
IVERSEN, L. L.: The uptake and storage of noradrenaline in sympathetic nerves. Cambridge: Cambridge University Press 1967.
JAIM-ETCHEVERRY, G., ZIEHER, L. M.: Cytochemistry of 5-hydroxytryptamine at the electron microscope level. II. Localization in the autonomic nerves of the rat pineal gland. Z. Zellforsch. **86**, 393–400 (1968).
— — Ultrastructural cytochemistry and pharmacology of 5-hydroxytryptamine in adrenergic nerve endings. I. Localization of exogenous 5-hydroxytryptamine in the autonomic nerves of the rat vas deferens. J. Pharmacol. exp. Ther. **166**, 264–271 (1969 a).
— — Selective demonstration of a type of synaptic vesicle with phosphotungstic acid staining. J. Cell Biol., in press (1969 b).
JONSSON, G.: Microfluorometric studies on the formaldehyde-induced fluorescence of noradrenaline in adrenergic nerves of rat iris. J. Histochem. Cytochem. **17**, 714–723 (1969).
KAPELLER, K., MAYOR, D.: The accumulation of noradrenaline in constricted sympathetic nerves as studied by fluorescence and electron microscopy. Proc. roy. Soc. B **167**, 282–292 (1967).
— — An electron microscopic study of the early changes proximal to constriction in sympathetic nerves. Proc. roy. Soc. B **172**, 39–51 (1969).
LUNDBORG, P.: Studies on the uptake and subcellular distribution of catecholamines and their α-methylated analogues. Acta physiol. scand., Suppl. **302**, 1–34 (1967).
MAILLET, M.: La technique de Champy à l'osmium iodure de potassium et la modification de Maillet à l'osmium iodure de zinc. Trab. Inst. Cajal Invest. biol. **54**, 1–36 (1962).
NORBERG, K.-A., HAMBERGER, B.: The sympathetic adrenergic neuron. Some characteristics revealed by histochemical studies on the intraneuronal distribution of the transmitter. Acta physiol. scand. **63**, Suppl. 238, 1–42 (1964).
ORDEN, L. S. VAN, BENSCH, K. G., GIARMAN, N. J.: Histochemical and functional relationships of catecholamines in adrenergic nerve endings. II. Extravesicular norepinephrine. J. Pharmacol. exp. Ther. **155**, 428–439 (1967).
— BLOOM, F. E., BARRNETT, R. J., GIARMAN, N. J.: Histochemical and functional relationships of catecholamines in adrenergic nerve endings. I. Participation of granular vesicles. J. Pharmacol. exp. Ther. **154**, 185–199 (1966).
PELLEGRINO DE IRALDI, A., GUEUDET, R.: Action of reserpine on the osmium tetroxide zinc iodide reactive site of synaptic vesicles in the pineal nerves of the rat. Z. Zellforsch. **91**, 178–185 (1968).
PFENNINGER, K., SANDRI, C., AKERT, K., EUGSTER, C. H.: Contribution to the problem of structural organization of the presynaptic area. Brain Res. **12**, 10–18 (1969).
RICHARDSON, K. C.: The fine structure of autonomic nerve endings in smooth muscle of the rat vas deferens. J. Anat. (Lond.) **96**, 427–442 (1962).
— The fine structure of the albino rabbit iris with special reference to the identification of adrenergic and cholinergic nerves and nerve endings in its intrinsic muscles. Amer. J. Anat. **114**, 173–206 (1964).
— Electron microscopic identification of autonomic nerve endings. Nature (Lond.) **210**, 756 (1966).

STJÄRNE, L.: Studies on noradrenaline biosynthesis in nerve tissue. Acta physiol. scand. **67**, 441–454 (1966).

TAXI, J.: Étude de l'ultrastructure des zones synaptiques dans les ganglions sympathétiques de la Grenouille. C. R. Acad. Sci. (Paris) **252**, 174–176 (1961 a).

— Sur l'innervation des fibres musculaires lisses de l'intestin de souris. C. R. Acad. Sci. (Paris) **252**, 331–333 (1961 b).

— Contribution à l'étude des connexions des neurons moteurs du système nerveux autonome. Ann. Sci. Nat. **7**, 413–674 (1965).

— Sur la fixation et la signification du contenu dense des vésicules des fibres adrénergiques étudiées au microscope électronique. C. R. Acad. bulgare Sci. **21**, 1229–1231 (1968).

— DROZ, B.: Étude de l'incorporation de noradrenaline-³H (NA-³H) et des 5-hydroxytrypto-phane-³H (5-HTP-³H) dans les fibres nerveuses du canal déferent et de l'intestin. C. R. Acad. Sci. (Paris) **263**, 1237–1240 (1966 a).

— — Étude de l'incorporation de noradrenaline-³H (NA-³H) et de 5-hydroxytryptophane-³H (5-HTP-³H) dans l'épiphyse et le ganglion cervical supérieur. C. R. Acad. Sci. (Paris) **263**, 1326–1329 (1966 b).

TRAMEZZANI, J., CHIOCCHIO, S., WASSERMANN, G. F.: A technique for light and electron microscopic identification of adrenalin- and noradrenalin-storing cells. J. Histochem. Cytochem. **12**, 890–899 (1964).

TRANZER, J. P., THOENEN, H.: Significance of empty vesicles in postganglionic sympathetic nerve terminals. Experientia (Basel) **23**, 123–124 (1967 a).

— — Electronmicroscopic localization of 5-hydroxydopamine (3,4,5-trihydroxy-phenyl-ethylamine), a new "false" sympathetic transmitter. Experientia (Basel) **23**, 743 (1967 b).

— — Various types of amine-storing vesicles in peripheral adrenergic nerve terminals. Experientia (Basel) **209**, 484–486 (1968).

WOLFE, D. E., AXELROD, J., POTTER, L. T., RICHARDSON, K. C.: Localizing tritiated norepinephrine in sympathetic axons by electron microscope autoradiography. Science **138**, 440–442 (1962).

WOOD, J. G.: Electron microscopic localization of amines in central nervous tissue. Nature (Lond.) **209**, 1131–1133 (1966).

— BARRNETT, R.: Histochemical demonstration of norepinephrine at a fine structural level. J. Histochem. Cytochem. **12**, 197–209 (1964).

# The Adrenergic Supply within the Avian Hypothalamus*

P. J. Sharp** and B. K. Follett**

Department of Zoology, The University of Leeds (England)

Key words: Hypothalamus — Aves — Adrenergic supply.

It is now well established that the mammalian median eminence contains abundant adrenergic terminals lying in close contact with the primary capillary plexus of the hypophysial blood vascular system (e.g. Fuxe, 1964; Fuxe and Hökfelt, 1967; Lichtensteiger and Langemann, 1966). Such an arrangement makes it likely that the neuronal system(s) which give rise to these terminals can be regarded as "neurosecretory" within the wider definition of the term proposed by Bern and Knowles (1966). Currently there is much interest in the relationship between hypothalamic monoamines and the control of the anterior pituitary which is easily equal to a similar interest shown in the pituitary regulating functions of the "Gomori positive" neurosecretions. The morphology of the "Gomori positive" hypothalamo-hypophysial system is well known throughout the vertebrates but, as yet, information about the monoamine-containing hypothalamo-pituitary systems is fragmentary, especially in sub-mammalian species.

Hypothalamic monoamines have been demonstrated in a number of birds including the pigeon (Fuxe and Ljunggren, 1965; Björklund, Falck and Ljunggren, 1968), the quail (Sharp and Follett, 1968), the house sparrow (Oehmke, Priedkalns, Vaupel-von Harnack and Oksche, 1969; Björklund et al., 1968), the chicken (Björklund et al., 1968; Enemar and Ljunggren, 1968), and the white-crowned sparrow (Warren, 1968) using the histochemical fluorescent technique of Falck and Owman (1965).

## The Median Eminence

When compared with mammals, the distribution of fluorescent terminals in the external layer of the avian median eminence is rather sparse although there is considerable variation between species. Björklund et al. (1968) found that there was a stronger fluorescence in the median eminence of the chicken (Fig. 1a) and gull than in the sparrow, goose or pigeon (Fig. 1b). Sharp and Follett (1968) were also able to show fluorescent terminals distributed evenly throughout both the anterior and posterior divisions of the quail median eminence (Fig. 1c) which appeared to be comparable in intensity with those described by Björklund et al. (1968) in the sparrow and goose. Similar observations have also been reported in the white-crowned sparrow (Warren, 1968) and house sparrow (Oehmke et al.,

* Supported by a grant from The Agricultural Research Council (AG 24/36).
** Present address: Department of Zoology, University College, Bangor, N. Wales (U.K..)

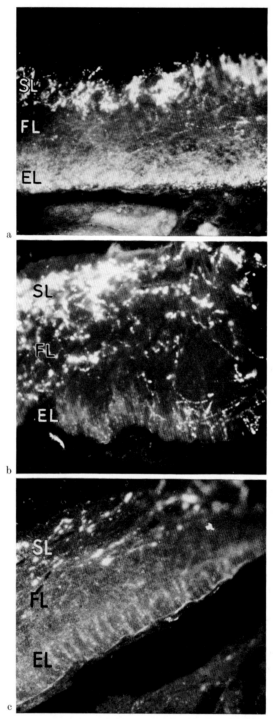

Fig. 1a–c. Sagittal section through the median eminence of a, the chicken X 190 b, the pigeon
X 300 c, the quail X 320. *EL* external layer (palisade layer), *FL* fibre layer, *SL* subependymal
layer. a, b from BJÖRKLUND and LJUNGGREN, Z. Zellforsch. **89**, 193–200 (1968); c from SHARP
and FOLLETT, Z. Zellforsch. **90**, 245–262 (1968)

1969). The terminals contain fine fluorescent granules and are orientated at right angles to the surface of the palisade layer by the many processes of the glial and ependymal cells which terminate on the primary capillary plexus. Neither the *pars tuberalis* nor the portal vessels contain any fluorescent fibres.

Above the palisade layer in the reticular zone, fluorescent structures are relatively infrequent although in all the species examined a few coarse beaded

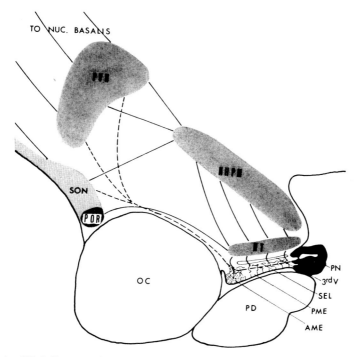

Fig. 2. A simplified diagram of a sagittal section to show the regions containing monoamines and the connections between them in the hypothalamus of the quail. The Gomori positive tracts are shown as broken lines while the monoamine-containing fibre tracts are shown by continuous lines. The density of the grey areas is proportional to the intensity of fluorescence. *AME* anterior median eminence, *NHPM* nucleus hypothalamicus posterior medialis, *NT* nucleus tuberis, *OC* optic chiasma, *PME* posterior median eminence, *PN* pars nervosa, *POR* preoptic recess, *PVN* paraventricular nucleus, *SEL* subependymal layer, *SON* supraoptic nucleus, *3rd V* third ventricle

fibres running in a rostro-caudal direction could frequently be traced for considerable distances in sagittal sections. These fluorescent fibres have been observed to enter the neural lobe in the chicken (Enemar and Ljunggren, 1968) and the starling (unpublished observation) but not in other species so far examined.

The fluorescent terminals in the palisade layer are probably derived from the monoamine-containing axons running in the sub-ependymal layer (Fig. 3). However, no photographs have yet been published which clearly show fluorescent fibres dropping through the "Gomori positive" fibre layer although logically, such an arrangement must be present (Fig. 2).

## The Posterior Hypothalamus

Fluorescent nerve terminals were found in two regions (Fig. 2) in both the quail (Sharp and Follett, 1968) and the white-crowned sparrow (Warren, 1968). In the quail these were described as the *nucleus tuberis* and the *nucleus hypothalamicus posterior medialis*; they probably correspond respectively to the ventral and extreme dorsal divisions of the *nucleus infundibularis* in the white-crowned sparrow (Oehmke, 1968). Posteriorly the two regions tend to come closer together and finally merge. Catecholamine-containing nerves run from the *nucleus tuberis* around the base of the third ventricle into the subependymal layer (Fig. 3) and thus form part of the tubero-hypophysial tract. It is not clear whether all these fibres arise from the *nucleus tuberis* or if part of the innervation comes directly from the region of the *nucleus hypothalamicus posterior medialis*.

So far it has not been possible to locate fluorescent cell bodies in the avian hypothalamus (other than in the paraventricular organ) which might give rise to the monoamine containing terminals in the median eminence. This may be a reflection of inadequate technique since even in mammals the fluorescent intensity of catecholamine-containing cell bodies in the *nucleus tuberis* is very low and best seen in pregnant or lactating animals (e.g. Fuxe and Hökfelt, 1967) or after the injection of certain drugs (e.g. Lichtensteiger and Langeman, 1966; Fuxe and Hökfelt, 1966). In the original publication on the localization of quail hypothalamic catecholamines (Sharp and Follett, 1968) it was stated that fluorescent cell bodies had been identified in the *nucleus tuberis* but this has not been confirmed in subsequent observations. Warren (1968) also points out the inconsistent appearance of structures which could be catecholamine containing cell bodies in the hypothalamus of the white-crowned sparrow. She presents photographic evidence of a group of fluorescent cell bodies lying lateral to the paraventricular organ which may be identical with those described in the pigeon (Fuxe and Ljunggren, 1965) as, *"lying in a row just caudal and parallel to the 'modified ependyma'* [paraventricular organ]".

Oehmke et al. (1969), basing their observations on the assumption that dense-core vesicles of $\sim$500 Å and $\sim$1,000 Å may represent monoamines, reported that these occur both in the perikarya and neuropile of the *nucleus tuberis* in the house sparrow. This suggests the presence of monoaminergic cell bodies in this region.

It has been shown that fluorescent cell bodies are present in the *nucleus diffusus tuberis* of the lizard (Baumgarten and Braak, 1968), thus making it clear that hypothalamic catecholamine-containing cell bodies are not a uniquely mammalian feature. However, the dopaminergic tubero-hypophysial system could be peculiar to mammals especially since dopamine does not seem to be present to any great extent in the avian neurohypophysis (Juorio and Vogt, 1967; Enemar and Ljunggren, 1968).

Recently, a noradrenergic hypothalamo-hypophysial system has been described in the rat (Björklund, Falck, Hromek, Owman and West, 1970) which appears to originate outside the basal hypothalamus. Could this noradrenaline-containing system be homologous with the one found in birds?

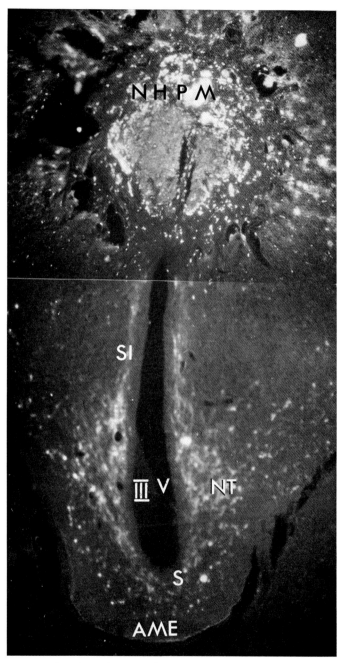

Fig. 3. Transverse section through a quail hypothalamus at the level of the anterior median eminence showing a lesion in the nucleus hypothalamicus posterior medialis. The adrenergic fibre tracts in the stratum cellulare internum are intact. X 160 *AME* anterior median eminence, *NHPM* nucleus hypothalamicus posterior medialis, *NT* nucleus tuberis, *S* subependymal layer, *SI* stratum cellulare internum, *III V* third ventricle

7*

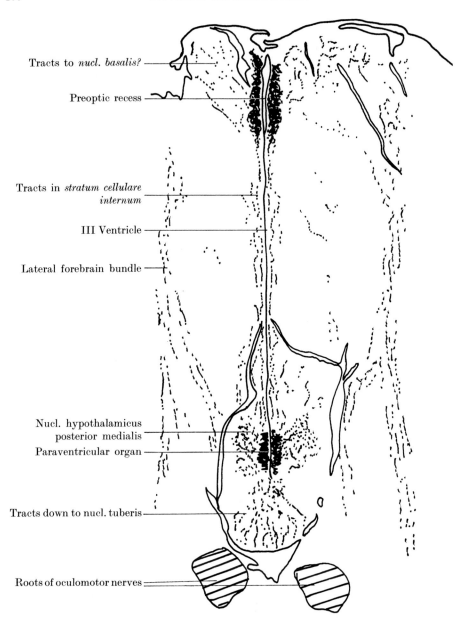

Tracts to *nucl. basalis?*

Preoptic recess

Tracts in *stratum cellulare internum*

III Ventricle

Lateral forebrain bundle

Nucl. hypothalamicus posterior medialis

Paraventricular organ

Tracts down to nucl. tuberis

Roots of oculomotor nerves

Fig. 4. Sketch of a horizontal section through the quail hypothalamus above the level of the optic chiasma, taken from a composite photograph, to show the connecting adrenergic pathways

In *Xenopus laevis*, Goos and van Oordt (1969) have shown that the hypophysial monoaminergic terminals originate in a pair of adrenergic nuclei which lie in a region corresponding to the *nucleus hypothalamicus posterior medialis*. The possibility that a similar distribution may be found in birds is not supported by lesion experiments in the quail, for when this zone was destroyed the fluorescent tracts running down into the *nucleus tuberis* were unaffected (see Fig. 3).

Since the *nucleus tuberis* and *nucleus hypothalamicus posterior medialis* both contain many cell bodies embedded in fluorescent fibres it is likely that the activities of these two areas are dependent upon adrenergic mechanisms. It is therefore of interest to note that if either or both of these areas are lesioned out in the quail the gonadotrophic functions of the anterior pituitary are completely blocked (SHARP and FOLLETT, 1969). The two nuclei are connected by two sets of monoaminergic tracts (SHARP and FOLLETT, 1968; WARREN, 1968): one set runs in the *stratum cellulare internum* close to the wall of the third ventricle (Fig. 3) and the other curves round through the lateral regions of the hypothalamus.

The *nucleus hypothalamicus posterior medialis* seems to be centrally placed to receive, modulate or transmit information conveyed in adrenergic pathways between the anterior hypothalamus, "higher brain" centres or lower brain stem and the *nucleus tuberis* or median eminence. This is illustrated in Fig. 4 in which fluorescent tracts can be seen running in the *stratum cellulare internum* connecting with the anterior hypothalamus whilst lateral pathways join the forebrain bundle.

## The Anterior Hypothalamus

This region is characterized by the magnocellular neurosecretory paraventricular and supraoptic nuclei which are embedded in monoaminergic nerve fibres (SHARP and FOLLETT, 1968; WARREN, 1968; OEHMKE et al., 1969) similar to those described in mammals (e.g. FUXE and HÖKFELT, 1967; ZAMBRANO, 1968). Ultrastructural studies on the house sparrow (OEHMKE et al., 1969; PRIEDKALNS and OKSCHE, 1969) have shown that these adrenergic fibres are in synaptic contact with the neurosecretory cells.

The lateral divisions of the supraoptic nucleus of the quail do not seem to be so richly innervated with adrenergic fibres as in the white-crowned sparrow but in all the birds studied the medial division is characterized by a well developed plexus of monoaminergic terminals (Fig. 2) lying just beneath the wall of the third ventricle in the preoptic recess.

The origin of the adrenergic terminals surrounding the magnocellular cells is still unknown but it could be extrahypothalamic. In mammals it has been established that these nerve terminals contain noradrenaline and are derived from fibres in the lateral forebrain bundle originating in the pons and medulla (see FUXE and HÖKFELT, 1967). A similar distribution has been suggested in the pigeon (FUXE and LJUNGGREN, 1965) and may well occur in the quail (see Fig. 4).

In both the pigeon and the quail a further portion of the fluorescent tract in the forebrain bundle continues anteriorly to the *nucleus basalis* and the forebrain. This may correspond to the dopaminergic neuronal system originating in the hindbrain and terminating in the forebrain described in mammals (see ANDÉN, DAHLSTRÖM, FUXE and LARSSON, 1966). In support of an avian dopaminergic mesencephalo-forebrain system is the presence of high concentrations of dopamine in the avian *nucleus basalis* (JUORIO and VOGT, 1966).

## The Monoaminergic Supraoptico-Hypophysial System

Monoamine-containing fibres have been clearly shown associated with the classical " Gomori positive" axons coursing down the posterior border of the optic chiasma towards the median eminence (see Fig. 2) in the quail (Sharp and Follett, 1968), the white-crowned sparrow (Warren, 1968) and the house sparrow (Oehmke et al., 1969). This tract can be traced to the intensely fluorescent area previously described in the medial division of the supraoptic nucleus. Ultrastructural observations on the supraoptico-hypophysial tract in the house sparrow (Oehmke et al., 1969) would seem to support the presence of an adrenergic component since both presumptive monoaminergic and neurosecretory granules were identified. The fluorescent fibres of this system become lost in the general fluorescence of the anterior portion of the *nucleus tuberis* but it cannot be excluded that they may pass directly to the median eminence.

In conclusion, it appears that there are a number of different adrenergic pathways in the avian hypothalamus which could play a part in the integrative aspects of the hypothalamic control of the anterior pituitary. Much work remains to be done to identify both the sources and the types of monoamine contained in these systems.

### References

Andén, N.-E., Dahlström, A., Fuxe, K., Larsson, K., Olson, L., Ungerstedt, U.: Ascending monoamine neuron systems to the telencephalon and diencephalon. Acta physiol. scand. **67**, 313–326 (1966).

Baumgarten, H. G., Braak, H.: Catecholamine im Gehirn der Eidechse (*Lacerta viridis* und *Lacerta muralis*). Z. Zellforsch. **86**, 574–602 (1968).

Bern, H. A., Knowles, F. G. W.: Neurosecretion. In: Neuroendocrinology, vol. 1 (ed. Martini, L., and W. F. Ganong), p. 139–186. New York and London: Academic Press 1966.

Björklund, A., Falck, B., Ljunggren, L.: Monoamines in the bird median eminence. Failure of cocaine to block the accumulation of exogenous amines. Z. Zellforsch. **89**, 193–200 (1968).

— — Hromek, F., Owman, Ch., West, K.: Distribution and identification of the monoamine fibre systems in the rat neurohypophysis by means of stereotaxic and microspectrofluorimetric techniques. Brain Res. **17**, 1–23 (1970).

Enemar, A., Ljunggren, L.: The appearance of monoamines in the adult and developing neurohypophysis of *Gallus gallus*. Z. Zellforsch. **91**, 496–506 (1968).

Falck, B., Owman, Ch.: A detailed methodological description of the fluorescence method for the cellular demonstration of biogenic monoamines. Acta Univ. Lund., Sectio II, No 7 (1965).

Fuxe, K.: Cellular localization of monoamines in the median eminence and infundibular stem of some mammals. Z. Zellforsch. **61**, 710–724 (1964).

— Hokfelt, T.: Further evidence for the existence of tubero-infundibular dopamine neurons. Acta physiol. scand. **66**, 243–244 (1966).

— — The influence of central catecholamine neurons on the hormone secretion from the anterior and posterior pituitary. In: Neurosecretion (ed. Stutinsky, F.). IV. Intern. Symp. of Neurosec., p. 165–177. Berlin-Heidelberg-New York: Springer 1967.

— Ljunggren, L.: Cellular localization of monoamines in the upper brain stem of the pigeon. J. comp. Neurol. **125**, 355–382 (1965).

Goos, H. J. Th., Oordt, P. G. W. J. van: Aminergic control of the pars intermedia in *Xenopus laevis* tadpoles. Fifth Conf. of European Comparative Endocrinologists, Utrecht 24–29 Aug. Abstr. (1969).

Juorio, A. V., Vogt, M.: Monoamines and their metabolites in the avian brain. J. Physiol. (Lond.) **189**, 489–518 (1967).

LICHTENSTEIGER, W., LANGEMANN, H.: Uptake of exogenous catecholamines by monoamine-containing neurons of the central nervous system: Uptake of catecholamine by arcuato-infundibular neurons. J. Pharm. exp. Ther. **151**, 400–408 (1966).

OEHMKE, H.-J.: Regionale Strukturunterschiede im Nucleus infundibularis der Vögel (Passeriformes). Z. Zellforsch. **92**, 406–421 (1968).

— PRIEDKALNS, J., VAUPEL-VON HARNACK, M., OKSCHE, A.: Fluoreszenz- und elektronen-mikroskopische Untersuchungen am Zwischenhirn-Hypophysensystem von *Passer domesticus*. Z. Zellforsch. **95**, 109–133 (1969).

PRIEDKALNS, J., OKSCHE, A.: Ultrastructure of synaptic terminals in Nucleus infundibularis and Nucleus supraopticus of *Passer domesticus*. Z. Zellforsch. **98**, 135–147 (1969).

SHARP, P. J., FOLLETT, B. K.: The distribution of monoamines in the hypothalamus of the Japanese quail, *Coturnix coturnix japonica*. Z. Zellforsch. **90**, 245–262 (1968).

— — The effect of hypothalamic lesions on gonadotrophin release in Japanese Quail (*Coturnix coturnix japonica*). Neuroendocrinology **5**, 205–218 (1969).

WARREN, S. P.: Primary catecholamine fibres in the ventral hypothalamus of the white-crowned sparrow, *Zonotrichia leucophrys gambelii*. Master's Thesis, University of Washington (1968).

ZAMBRANO, D.: The effect of nialamide and L-dopa on the synaptic endings of the neurosecretory neurons of the supraoptic nucleus of the rat. Neuroendocrinology **3**, 99–106 (1968).

# Adrenergic Neurons in the Lower Spinal Cord of the Pike (Esox lucius) and their Relation to the Neurosecretory System of the Neurophysis spinalis caudalis* ** ***

H. G. Baumgarten and H. Wartenberg

Department of Anatomy and Neuroanatomy, University of Hamburg (West-Germany)
(Head: Prof. Dr. Dr. E. Horstmann)

**Key words:** Spinal cord — Neurophysis spinalis caudalis — Teleosts — Adrenergic neurons — Neurosecretion.

Recent investigations carried out on the neural lobe and median eminence of different vertebrate species by means of fluorescence microscopy have demonstrated adrenergic neuron systems which most probably contact neurosecretory fibres. Furthermore the nuclei of origin of the neurohypophysial tracts have been found to be profusely innervated by noradrenergic nerve terminals. Corresponding electron microscopical investigations gave evidence for the presence of axonal enlargements containing a mixed population of empty small vesicles and small and large granular vesicles which are known to be typical constituents of synaptic varicosities of monoamine storing neurons. Thus there is morphological evidence for a direct adrenergic influence upon storage and release of neurosecretions. Since the caudal neurosecretory organ of teleosts in many respects resembles the hypothalamic neurosecretory system it seemed reasonable to assume that the urophysis might possess an adrenergic modulatory system. This possibility was tested on the spinal cord of the pike.

## Light-, Fluorescence- and Electronmicroscopical Findings

Semi-thin sections through the lower spinal cord corresponding to the largest circumference of the urophysis reveal that the central canal is situated dorsally and surrounded by a multistratified epithelium. At the lateral and ventral aspects of the central canal large and irregularly shaped cells with multilobed nuclei occur; their cytoplasm contains huge amounts of a fine to coarse granular material which stains intensely with toluidine-blue. Such cells correspond to neurosecretory perikarya which are easily identified in the electron microscope. The spinal cord is embraced by the urophysis which is characterized by accumulations of the same basophilic substance, concentrated around numerous capillaries.

* Supported by grants from the Deutsche Forschungsgemeinschaft.
** A more detailed description will be published separately in the Zeitschrift für Zellforschung.
*** For generous supply of 5-OH-dopa and 5-OH-dopamine we are indebted to Dr. H. Thoenen, Hoffmann-La Roche, and to Prof. Dr. G. Kroneberg, Bayer.

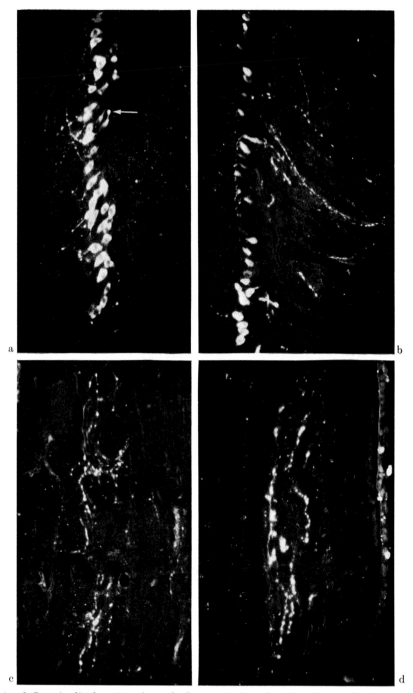

Fig. 1 a–d. Longitudinal sections from the lower spinal cord of the pike at a level just above the urophysis. Technique according to FALCK and HILLARP. a Ventrolateral circumference of the central canal. Numerous green fluorescent nerve cell bodies most of which issue a faintly fluorescent basal neurite. Arrow points to an apical dendrite terminating inside the ventricle with a bulbous enlargement. ca. ×230. b Paramedian-sagittal section showing axonal processes coursing in the glial septum. Note extremely small varicosities along the axon. ca. ×230. c Adrenergic preterminal fibre portions approaching neurosecretory nerve cell bodies and their processes. ca. ×230. d Anterior funiculus: droplet fibres descending in the median longitudinal fascicle together with neurosecretory axons. ca. ×230

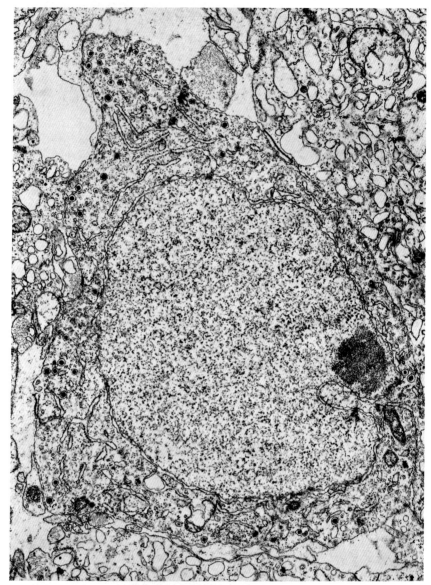

Fig. 2. Perikaryon of an adrenergic nerve cell located just below the ependymal lining of the central canal at a level of the spinal cord just above the urophysis. Control specimen. × 15,000

Electronmicroscopically these accumulations correspond to densely packed terminals of axonal processes from neurosecretory perikarya. In between both parts a weakly stained border zone is mainly composed of unmyelinated nerve fibres of different origin which form a dense neuropil.

The ependyma consists of spindle-shaped cells the nuclei of which stain weakly with toluidine blue; their cytoplasm appears light. Basally in the ependymal lining, at the ventrolateral edge of the central canal, small cells with a faintly blue stained cytoplasm can be distinguished; they are a little larger and more ovoid in shape than the ependymal cells. In sections processed for fluorescence microscopy small nerve cells are detected which exhibit a formaldehyde-induced green fluorescence and which have the same position, arrangement and frequency as the small cells located in the basal ependymal layer (Fig. 1 a, b). They are most numerous in the spinal cord corresponding to the upper part of the urophysis and the spinal cord cranial to it; a decreasing amount of such cells is seen in the ependyma facing the lower parts of the urophysis. The fluorescence of the small cells is confined to the cytoplasm, appears diffuse and shows a remarkably high intensity. Each cell is seen to issue a basal axonal process, whereas only some cells are provided with a thin weakly green fluorescent apical dendrite which extends into the ventricle. Already in its proximal portion the neurite contains beaded varicosities; the more distal portion, however, looks smooth and extremely thin. Axonal processes are seen to course in three different direction: 1) most of them traverse glial septa in a ventral or ventro-lateral direction and descend together with fibre bundles of the median longitudinal bundle; here they join neurosecretory axons and transform into beaded fibres again; small and large varicosities resembling droplets (Fig. 1 d) are met in one and the same axonal profile; 2) short neurites are found to ascend and descend in the sub-ependymal tissue layer; they intermingle with processes from neighbouring adren-ergic perikarya running alongside the central canal. Owing to their low fluorescence intensity and smallness such fibres are difficult to follow, 3) at the cranial level of the urophysis some axons turn laterally to contact processes and perikarya of neurosecretory axons (Fig. 1 c).

According to microspectrographical findings and according to the results of chemical determinations the green fluorescent substance may be noradrenaline.

## Electronmicroscopical Findings

Both cell types bordering the ventricle of the central canal can be easily refound in the electron microscope. The epithelium of the central canal is composed of small slender ependymal cells provided with kinocilia and small nerve cells charac-terized by numerous electron dense vesicles scattered in the cytoplasm (Figs. 2, 3). The size of the vesicles varies in between 900 and 1,500 Å and the diameter of the dense core—which is of medium to high electron density—ranges between 600 and 1,000 Å. To make sure that these vesicles really can take up and store monoamines of the catecholamine group and thus can be truely recognized as the natural storage sites of the endogenous noradrenaline detected in the green fluorescent perikarya, most animals were pretreated with 5-hydroxydopa and 5-hydroxydopamine which has been found to increase the electron density of the storage sites from peripheral sympathetic nerve endings in lower vertebrates as well as those from noradrenaline storing short paraependymal neurons in the hypothalamus of *Lacerta* and *Lampetra*. Using the dense core vesicles as means of identification, the axonal enlargements of the green fluorescent perikarya were easily detected in the subependymal neuropil, the anterior funiculus and in the border zone of the upper part of the urophysis (Fig. 3, inset; Fig. 4). Bouton-like enlargements contain in addition to the large granular vesicles also small empty vesicles (about 350 Å) and are repeatedly observed in close proximity to neuro-

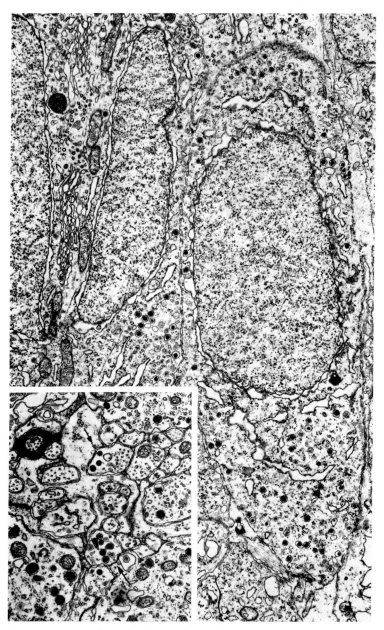

Fig. 3. Transverse section through the spinal cord just above the urophysis: ventrolateral edge of the central canal. Adrenergic nerve cell bodies containing numerous dense core vesicles. Pretreatment with 5-OH-dopa. ×14,000. Inset: transverse section through the anterior funiculus where it enters the urophysis. Arrow points to intervaricose sections of adrenergic axons, running alongside neurosecretory axons. The adrenergic fibres contain large dense core vesicles similar to those in the perikaryon. Pretreatment with 5-OH-dopamine. ×14,000

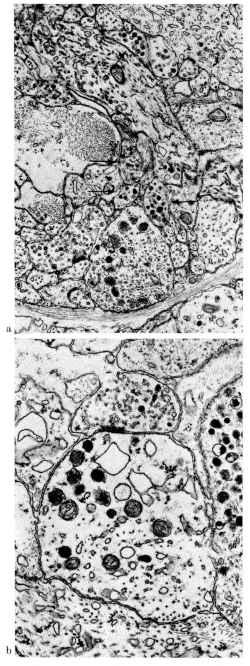

Fig. 4. a Small adrenergic boutons approaching neurosecretory fibres. The adrenergic varicosities (arrows) contain mainly large granular vesicles. Pretreatment with 5-OH-dopamine.
× 15,300. b Synaptic contact between a bouton containing small empty vesicles and a neurosecretory axon in the border zone of the urophysis. ca. × 18,300

secretory axons and to axonal beads containing mainly small empty vesicles supposed to be cholinergic in nature. Whereas the varicose enlargements of cholinergic axons are provided with membrane thickenings at synaptic contact-points no such membrane specializations are detected at points of close contacts between adrenergic varicosities and neurosecretory neurons.

Neurosecretory cell bodies, axonal processes and terminal enlargements are characterized by their content of elementary granules. Two types may be distinguished: medium sized and large granules (1,000—2,000 Å) with a strongly osmiophilic core (800—1,800 Å) and exhibiting a dense granular substructure; and large but less electron dense granules (1,500—2,600 Å) with a similar substructure of the inner core (1,000—2,500 Å) and a sometimes poorly contrasted membrane covering. The elementary granules are associated with a great number of small empty vesicles ("synaptoids") (cf. Scharrer and Kater, 1969) inside the neurosecretory terminals where they contact the perivascular space.

Unexpectedly, in untreated specimens from spring-time animals and more frequently in untreated and pretreated specimens from animals processed during autumn-time dense core vesicles resembling elementary granules were observed within the cytoplasm of endothelial cells.

## Discussion

The results of this combined fluorescence microscopical and electronmicro-scopical study on the lower spinal cord and urophysis suggest that at least part of the small periventricularly located adrenergic perikarya and their axonal processes establish contacts to some of the neurosecretory processes along their course to the neurohemal region. The adrenergic neurons show some remarkable features which distinguish them from ordinary adrenergic neurons: 1) an intense fluorescence, displayed by the perikaryon, which indicates unusually high amine concentrations; 2) the occurrence of axonal beads in the most proximal part of the neurite, 3) the presence of sometimes extraordinarily big axonal enlargements in the distal portion of the axon very much resembling the so called droplets of dopamine-containing fibres seen in the neurohypophysis and median eminence of mammals (cf. Björklund, Enemar and Falck, 1968; Björklund, 1968) and fishes (cf. Baumgarten, 1970), and finally the occurrence of an apical fluorescent dendrite terminating inside the ventricle with a bulbous enlargement. Therefore these specialized adrenergic neurons in many respects resemble the bipolar mono-amine storing short neurons of the nucleus ependymalis hypothalami (the so called organon vasculosum) which have been discovered in most submammalian vertebrates including teleosts (cf. Baumgarten and Braak, 1967, 1968). The adrenergic neurons do not only exhibit peculiar light microscopical but as well ultrastructural features which distinguish them from ordinary peripheral or central adrenergic neurons: The perikaryon and axonal swellings as well as the inter-varicose sections contain a population of mainly large granular vesicles which—in contrast to the large granular vesicles of most adrenergic neurons—do take up and concentrate catecholamine like substances and precursors to an easily detect-able extent. For the time being we conclude that there might exist several types of functionally different populations of so called large granular vesicles in different types of noradrenaline storing neurons. It may be worth while to mention that in the periventricular hypothalamus of the rat HÖKFELT (1968) discovered noradrenaline boutons with a remarkable amount of large dense core vesicles which turned out to react to amine depleting or accumulating agents in a way similar to the small granular ones.

We do not hesitate to ascribe to such bouton-like enlargements of adrenergic axons—closely approaching neurosecretory processes and being equipped with large granular vesicles and small empty ones—the function of true synapses despite the lack of any membrane specializations. Membrane thickenings do not seem to be a prerequisite for transmission in monoaminergic neurons. The final question is: what are the presumed functions of an adrenergic innervation to the neurosecretory system? In the absence of any direct hint or proof supported by the results of pharmacological or physiological experiments the answer is a matter of speculation. But in analogy to ENEMAR's and FALCK's (1965) findings on the significance of the adrenergic innervation to the hormone producing intermedia cells in *Rana temporaria* it might be assumed that the short local adrenergic neurons in the lower spinal cord of teleosts antagonize the hormone releasing effects of the cholinergic excitatory influence, i.e. inhibit the release of neurosecretory material.

## References

BAUMGARTEN, H. G.: Die Verteilung von Dopamin, Noradrenalin und 5-Hydroxytryptamin im Zentralnervensystem von *Lampetra fluviatilis*. (To be published 1970.)
— BRAAK, H.: Catecholamine im Hypothalamus vom Goldfisch (*Carassius auratus*). Z. Zellforsch. **80**, 246–263 (1967).
— — Catecholamine im Gehirn der Eidechse (*Lacerta viridis* und *Lacerta muralis*). Z. Zellforsch. **86**, 574–602 (1968).
BJÖRKLUND, A.: Monoamine-containing fibres in the pituitary neurointermediate lobe of the pig and rat. Z. Zellforsch. **89**, 573–589 (1968).
— ENEMAR, A., FALCK, B.: Monoamines in the hypothalamo-hypophysial system of the mouse with special reference to the ontogenetic aspects. Z. Zellforsch. **89**, 590–607 (1968).
ENEMAR, A., FALCK, B.: On the presence of adrenergic nerves in the pars intermedia of the frog, *Rana temporaria*. Gen. comp. Endocr. **5**, 577–580 (1965).
SCHARRER, B., KATER, S. B.: Neurosecretion. XV. An electron microscopic study of the corpora cardiaca of *Periplaneta americana* after experimentally induced hormone release. Z. Zellforsch. **95**, 177–186 (1969).

# Biogenic Amines in the Tuber Cinereum of *Xenopus laevis* Tadpoles. Electron and Fluorescence Microscopical Observations

J. Peute* and H. J. Th. Goos

Zoological Laboratory, State University of Utrecht (The Netherlands)

**Key words:** Tuber cinereum — *Xenopus laevis* tadpoles — Biogenic amines.

## Introduction

It is generally accepted that in Amphibia the activity of the adenohypophysis is regulated by the neurosecretory centres of the hypothalamus (Jørgensen, 1968). Evidence that this also accounts for the activity of the pars intermedia was obtained by Kastin and Ross (1965). They observed that lesions in the hypothalamus of *Rana pipiens* caused a darkening of the skin and a depletion of the intermediate lobe. Likewise, lesions in the caudal hypothalamus were seen to result in darkening of the skin in *Rana temporaria* (Goos and Peute, unpublished results). These data indicate that the main hypothalamic factor regulating the pars intermedia activity has an inhibitory effect and is thus correctly named "melanotrope inhibiting factor" (MIF).

According to Dierickx (1965, 1967) the MIF is not produced by peptidergic neurosecretory cells of the preoptic nucleus, for extirpation of the nucleus does not affect the skin melanophores of *Rana temporaria*. In *Rana pipiens* Dierst and Ralph (1962) succeeded in localizing a MIF centre in the hypothalamus caudal to the optic chiasm.

Using fluorescence and electron microscopical techniques respectively, Goos and van Halewijn (1968) and Peute (1968) observed a nucleus of monoamine-containing neurons in the caudal hypothalamus of *Xenopus laevis*. Goos (1969) obtained some evidence that this nucleus might be the actual source of the MIF. Indeed Enemar and Falck (1965) and Enemar and Iturriza (1967) could demonstrate the presence of monoamines in the intermediate lobe of *Rana temporaria* and *Bufo arenarum* respectively, and Iturriza (1966, 1969), Dierst-Davis *et al.* (1966) and Goos (1969) found possible evidence of the MIF being a monoamine.

The present experiments were serving two purposes: first it was tried to verify the hypothesis that the aminergic nucleus in the caudal hypothalamus of *Xenopus laevis* produces the MIF and secondly it was tried to identify the granules that store monoamines in the rostral tip of the nucleus, i.e. the paraventricular organ.

* The authors are indebted to Prof. Dr. P. G. W. J. van Oordt for critically reading the manuscript, and his stimulating enthusiasm. Thanks are due to Miss M. Kolhorn Visser and Mr. H. van Kooten for technical and photographical assistance.

# Material and Methods

Tadpoles of *Xenopus laevis* were used that had reached stage 49/50 of Nieuwkoop and Faber's normal table (1956). They were adapted to a dark background for 24 hours and subsequently divided into three groups. The first remained in normal tapwater on a dark background for 21 hours. In the tapwater of the second group 1.2 mg/l reserpine was dissolved. The animals were kept in this solution on a dark background for six hours. The tadpoles of the third group were first placed in a solution of 50 mg/l iproniazide in water for 18 hours, and immediately thereafter for another three hours in a D. L. DOPA solution of 50 mg/l tapwater. The third group was also kept on a dark background.

## Fluorescence Microscopy

From each group five animals were fixed in liquid nitrogen for the histological demonstration of bioamines in the caudal hypothalamus with the aid of Falck's method (1965). This technique was applied to serial sagittal sections of the head region of 7 µ.

## Electron Microscopy

From each group the brains of three tadpoles were immersed for one hour in a fixation fluid containing one part of Karnovsky's mixture (1965) and one part osmium tetroxide 2%, both in cacodylic buffer pH 7.2 at a temperature of 3°C. Dehydration was performed in acetone and propylen oxide. The tissue was embedded in a mixture of DDSA, Araldite and Epon (3:1:1). Thin sections were contrasted with uranyl acetate in methanol 70% followed by lead citrate (Reynolds, 1963). Electron microscope: Zeiss EM 9 A.

In order to determine whether or not the number of certain vesicles in the cells studied was affected by the drugs, 50 median cell sections of each group were photographed at a magnification of 27,000. From each cell the apical half was measured by means of a planimeter. The area obtained in this way was further reduced by the area of mitochondria, lysosomes, Golgi area and endoplasmic cisternae. The remaining cytoplasmic areas of the 50 cells were added up and divided by 50, resulting in an average cytoplasmic area. In these cytoplasmic areas the total number of each class of vesicles was counted and divided by 50. Thus the average number of vesicles per cytoplasmic area was obtained. From these data the average number of granules per surface unit was calculated. The results have been plotted in a diagram giving the number of each class of vesicles per 100 cm².

## Observations

### Melanophores

Because of the adaptation to a dark background the melanophores of the control animals remained between stage 4 and 5 of the Hogben and Slome (1931) index throughout the experiment. As described by Goos (1969) reserpine caused an initial aggregation of the melanophores within one hour. However, after four hours this was followed by a renewed dispersion, so that at the end of the experiment the original stage was retained. At the end of the consecutive treatment with iproniazide and DOPA the melanophores had aggregated down to stage 1.5.

### Fluorescence Microscopy

In the caudal hypothalamus of the control animals a pair of fluorescent nuclei was observed, situated along the third ventricle. The effect of reserpine on these nuclei was most distinct after a six hour treatment. At that time the cells of these nuclei appeared to be completely devoid of fluorescent material. This situation lasted to the end of the experiment. After treatment with iproniazide, followed by DOPA, the amount of fluorescent material in the cells of these nuclei had increased. Moreover, a fluorescent tract was observed, connecting these nuclei with the pars intermedia via the median eminence. An identical fluorescence was present in the intermediate lobe.

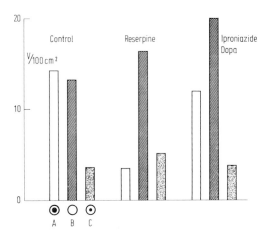

Fig. 1. Three classes of vesicles (A, B, C) can be observed in the type I cells of the paraventricular organ of *Xenopus laevis* tadpoles. The diagram shows the number of vesicles per square unit in control, reserpine treated, and iproniazide/DOPA treated tadpoles

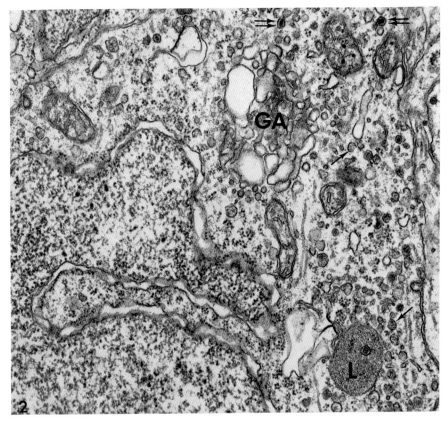

Fig. 2. The apical part of a type I neuron of the paraventricular organ in an iproniazide/DOPA treated tadpole. ⇉ class A vesicles; → class B vesicles; *GA* Golgi area; *L* Lysosome

*Electron Microscopy*

In a previous ultrastructural study of the paraventricular organ, two types of nerve cells were observed (PEUTE, 1969). The type I cells contained dense-core vesicles of about 1,000 Å in diameter, whereas the dense-core vesicles of the type II cells measured about 1,350 Å in diameter. Both cell types were characterized by intraventricular protrusions, forming a dense intraventricular network. In the present material only few type II cells were observed. This made it impossible to conclude about any effects of reserpine or iproniazide/DOPA treatment on the granulation of this cell type. In the type I cells three classes of vesicles could be observed: class A) dense-core vesicles, the core being 600–700 Å in diameter, the vesicle measuring about 1,000 Å; class B) vesicles with a grey content and a more or less irregular outline or even with a broken membrane, measuring about 1,100 Å; class C) vesicles of approximately 1,000 Å in diameter with a grey content, and in addition a small dense core, 200–400 Å in diameter.

The average cytoplasmic area in control, reserpine treated and iproniazide/DOPA treated animals was respectively 494, 541, 523 cm$^2$. After treatment with reserpine the number of class A vesicles per surface unit had considerably decreased (Fig. 1), whereas the number of class B vesicles remained more or less constant. The number of class C vesicles had also increased to a certain extent. Following the iproniazide/DOPA treatment the number of class A and class C vesicles per square unit had remained near the control level, whereas the number of class B vesicles had distinctly increased (Figs. 1 and 2).

# Discussion

A treatment with reserpine for six hours ended in a complete disappearance of fluorescent monoamines from the caudal hypothalamus of *Xenopus laevis* tadpoles, including the paraventricular organ. In the latter the number of class A vesicles strongly decreased. This relationship seems to indicate that it is the class A vesicles that are storing monoamines in the paraventricular organ. Reserpine caused an augmentation of the class C vesicles, which can be explained by assuming that the class C vesicles are class A vesicles that are extruding monoamines. So it may be assumed that in the present material and under these conditions, monoamines are released from dense-core vesicles with a mean diameter of 1,000 Å. Such a hypothesis would be in accordance with the opinion of several authors including CLEMENTI *et al.* (1966); BAK and HASSLER (1967); MATSUI (1967); ZAMBRANO (1968). However, others have described a correlation between the monoamine content and the number of vesicles with a mean diameter of about 400 Å, a.o. AGHAJANIAN and BLOOM (1967); BONDAREFF (1965); FUXE *et al.* (1965); TAXI and DROZ (1967). A possible explanation for this discrepancy may be the difference between the species and the tissues studied as well as between the fixation methods used.

In the iproniazide/DOPA experiment an aggregation of the melanophores was observed, which means that secretion of the MIF had increased. At the same time the aminergic nuclei in the caudal hypothalamus had stored large amounts of fluorescent material. Moreover, contrary to the situation in the controls such material could also be observed in a fibre tract running towards the pars intermedia of iproniazide/DOPA treated animals. These results add to the conclusion of Goos (1969) that the MIF is a bioamine and one of the secretory products of the caudal hypothalamus.

In the type I cells of the paraventricular organ iproniazide/DOPA caused an increase in the amount of class B vesicles. It may well be that it is these vesicles that contain the large amounts of monoamines produced under the experimental conditions. This being true, there are two possibilities. First, the class B vesicles contain monoamines insensitive to reserpine and different from those present in the class A and C vesicles. Secondly, it may be that class B vesicles represent newly formed aminergic vesicles in which the monoamines are not stored for a longer period. The latter would then take place only when class B vesicles are transformed into class A vesicles. Experiments are carried out to verify the above hypotheses.

## Summary

The effects of reserpine and iproniazide/DOPA treatment on the paired aminergic nucleus in the caudal hypothalamus of *Xenopus laevis* tadpoles was studied by fluorescence microscopy. In addition, the most rostral tip of this nucleus, the paraventricular organ, was studied ultrastructurally. New evidence has come forward that the MIF is a bioamine synthesized in this nucleus. In the type I cells of the paraventricular organ three classes of vesicles with a mean diameter of 1,000 Å were observed. It is argued that these vesicles are involved in the synthesis, the storage and the release of monoamines.

## References

Aghajanian, G. K., Bloom, F. E.: Electron-microscopic localization of tritiated norepinephrine in rat brain: Effect of drugs. J. Pharmacol. exp. Ther. **156**, 407–416 (1967).

Bak, I. J., Hassler, R.: Wirkung von Iproniazid und 1-DOPA auf die dense-core vesicles in der Substantia nigra bei der Maus. Naturwissenschaften **54**, 47 (1967).

Bondareff, W.: Submicroscopic morphology of granular vesicles in sympathetic nerves of rat pineal body. Z. Zellforsch. **67**, 211–219 (1965).

Clementi, F., Mantegazza, P., Botturi, M.: A pharmacologic and morphologic study on the nature of the dense-core granules present in the presynaptic endings of sympathetic ganglia. Int. J. Neuropharmacol. **5**, 281–285 (1966).

Dierickx, K.: On the neurosecretory control of the pars intermedia of the hypophysis in the frog. Naturwissenschaften **52**, 109–110 (1965).

— The function of the hypophysis without preoptic neurosecretory control. Z. Zellforsch. **78**, 114–130 (1967).

Dierst-Davis, K., Ralph, C. L., Pechersky, J.: Effects of pharmacological amines on the hypothalamus of *Rana pipiens* in relation to the control of skin melanophores. Gen. comp. Endocr. **6**, 409–419 (1966).

Enemar, A., Falck, B.: On the presence of adrenergic nerves in the pars intermedia of the frog, *Rana temporaria*. Gen. comp. Endocr. **5**, 577–583 (1965).

— Iturriza, F. C.: Adrenergic nerves in the pars intermedia of the pituitary in the toad, *Bufo arenarum*. Z. Zellforsch. **77**, 325–330 (1967).

Falck, B., Owman, Ch.: A detailed description of the fluorescence method for the cellular localization of biogenic amines. Acta Univ. Lund, Sect. II, **7**, 1–24 (1965).

Fuxe, K., Hökfelt, T., Nilsson, O.: A fluorescence and electronmicroscopic study on certain brain regions rich in monoamine terminals. Amer. J. Anat. **117**, 33–46 (1965).

Goos, H. J. Th.: Hypothalamic control of the pars intermedia in *Xenopus laevis* tadpoles. Z. Zellforsch. **97**, 118–124 (1969).

— Halewijn, R. van: Biogenic amines in the hypothalamus of *Xenopus laevis* tadpoles. Naturwissenschaften **55**, 393–394 (1968).

Hogben, L., Slome, D.: The pigmentary effector system. VI. The dual character of endocrine co-ordination in amphibian colour change. Proc. roy. Soc. B **108**, 10–53 (1931).

Iturriza, F. C.: Monoamines and control of the pars intermedia of the toad pituitary. Gen. comp. Endocr. **6**, 19–25 (1966).

— Further evidences for the blocking effect of catecholamines on the secretion of melanocyte-stimulating hormone in toads. Gen. comp. Endocr. **12**, 417–426 (1969).

JØRGENSEN, C. B.: Central nervous control of adenohypophysial functions. In: Perspectives in endocrinology. Hormones in the lives of lower vertebrates, ed. by E. J. W. BARRINGTON and C. B. JØRGENSEN, p. 469–541. London and New York: Academic Press 1968.

KARNOVSKY, M. J.: A formaldehyde-glutaraldehyde-fixative of high osmolality for use in electron microscopy. J. Cell Biol. **27**, 137 A–138 A (1965).

KASTIN, A. J., ROSS, G. T.: Melanocyte-stimulating hormone activity in pituitaries of frogs with hypothalamic lesion. Endocrinology **77**, 45–48 (1965).

MATSUI, T.: Effect of reserpine on the distribution of granulated vesicles in the mouse median eminence. Neuroendocrinology **2**, 99–106 (1967).

NIEUWKOOP, P. D., FABER, J.: Normal table for *Xenopus laevis* Daudin. Amsterdam: North-Holland Publ. Co. 1956.

PEUTE, J.: Granulierte Nervenzellen im Tuber cinereum von *Xenopus laevis*. Naturwissenschaften **55**, 393–394 (1968).

— Fine structure of the paraventricular organ of *Xenopus laevis* tadpoles. Z. Zellforsch. **97**, 564–575 (1969).

REYNOLDS, E. J.: The use of lead citrate at high pH as an electron opaque stain in electron microscopy. J. Cell Biol. **17**, 203–212 (1963).

TAXI, J., DROZ, B.: Localisation d'amines biogènes dans le système neurovégétatif périphérique. In: Neurosecretion, ed. by FR. STUTINSKY, p. 191–203. Berlin-Heidelberg-New York: Springer 1967.

ZAMBRANO, D.: On the presence of neurons with granulated vesicles in the median eminence of rat and dog. Neuroendocrinology **3**, 141–155 (1968).

# The Effects of Antiandrogens on the Hypothalamus

T. H. Schiebler and D. W. Meinhardt

Department of Anatomy, University of Würzburg (West-Germany)

**Key words:** Antiandrogens — Hypothalamus — Catecholamines.

Antiandrogens are substances which competitively inhibit the action of male sex hormones on their target organs (Neumann *et al.*, 1965). Neumann's idea (Neumann and Elger, 1966) that these substances act via the hypothalamus is deduced from the observation that cyproterone induces an increase in the level of gonadotropin. Since the action of testosterone on the hypothalamic receptors is inhibited competitively, an increase in hypothalamic activity is observed, which results in an increase of gonadotropin production in the anterior lobe of the pituitary. Neumann's concept was the starting point for our studies and we investigated by histochemical means in which way antiandrogens affect the hypothalamus.

Young rats received a daily injection of 1 mg of cyproterone acetate, starting on the first postnatal day at the latest; these injections were given for up to 44 days. On the day following the last injection the animals—as well as a group of control animals—were killed. The presence of catecholamines was determined in freeze-dried cryostat sections by means of formalin-induced fluorescence; for the demonstration of neurosecretion paraffin-embedded material was stained using Bock's modification of the chrome-alum-haematoxylin method. — Furthermore, animals castrated immediately after birth and kept alive for up to 50 days as well as untreated male rats served as controls.

If cyproterone acetate is administered from the first postnatal day onwards, the fluorescence of the hypothalamus is greatly affected (Fig. 1). Beginning on the 20th postnatal day a distinct increase in intensity is observed in all regions known to show fluorescence in the normal animal. In the nuclei supraopticus and paraventricularis the fluorescence is bound only to the interneuronal neuropil particularly in the immediate vicinity of the nerve cells. It appears to be of special importance that the surface of the altogether non-fluorescent perikarya shows a number of extremely fine nodules which contain fluorescent material (Fig. 1b). These nodules may represent synapses. This finding does not apply to all nerve cells of the hypothalamus. In the nucleus periventricularis, nucleus arcuatus and others we find nerve cells, which, after treatment, show a strong cytoplasmic fluorescence. Also the nerve fibres lying between the different nuclei show a general increase in fluorescence and an obvious increase in the number of varicosities. Following treatment the changes in the region of the median eminence are particularly striking (Fig. 2). Apart from the characteristic increase in intensity in the whole system, the treatment also causes a widening of the zona externa, in which catecholamine-containing fibres are observed. The widening takes place in the direction of the zona interna, where the fibres approach the portal vessels;

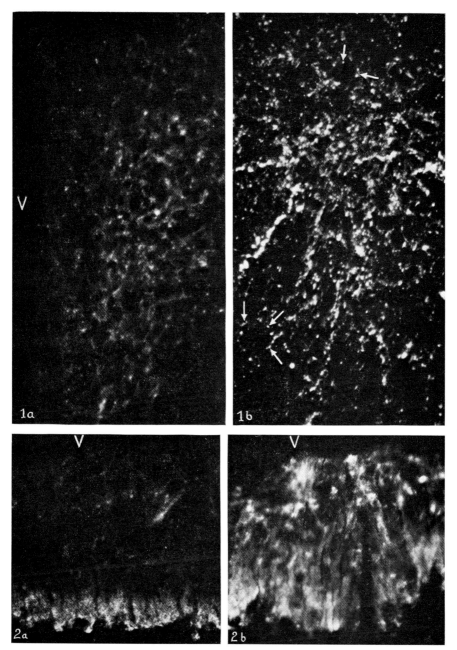

Fig. 1. a Nucleus paraventricularis of an untreated rat from the 31st postnatal day. b Nucleu. paraventricularis ofa rat from the 42nd postnatal day after cyproterone acetate treatment Note the distinct increase of the fluorescence intensity. The surface of the non-fluorescent perikarya shows extremely fine nodules with fluorescent material (arrow). *V* III. Ventricle.
× 150

Fig. 2. a Median eminence of an untreated rat from the 42nd postnatal day. b Median eminence of a rat on the 40th postnatal day after cyproterone acetate treatment. A strong increase of the fluorescence intensity and a widening of the catecholamine containing external zone in the direction of the internal zone. *V* III. Ventricle. × 150 furthermore an increased number of fluorescent fibres are seen to be in contact with the vessels of the portal system.

Of special interest is the reaction of the classical neurosecretory system following antiandrogen treatment. We observe a distinct increase in the amount of neurosecretory material in the nuclei supraopticus and paraventricularis and the median eminence after approximately 24 days of treatment. — Castration has exactly the same effect as has cyproterone acetate, as far as the intensity of fluorescence and neurosecretion are concerned.

The problem is now, how to interpret these observations. We would like to start from the fact that cyproterone treatment and castration have a dual effect on the hypothalamus: they both stimulate the aminergic as well as the peptidergic system. — As far as the *aminergic system* is concerned, the results are particularly interesting since the existing school of thinking postulates that this system regulates the sexual system (Spatz, 1951; Flerkó, 1954; Szentágothai, 1964). It seems feasible that cyproterone and castration interrupt the feed- backmechanism so that the hypothalamo-infundibular system is put into a state of increased activity. Although it is known that the catecholamines are not identical with the releasing factors, we think that nevertheless a similar type of action can be considered. This would mean that antiandrogens and castration lead to an increased production of releasing factors, which in turn stimulate the production of gonadotropin in the anterior lobe of the hypophysis.

Another point is the simultaneous effect of antiandrogens on the *peptidergic neurosecretory system*. The following hypothesis can be put forward which is based on the observation that a higher intensity of fluorescence is observed in the nodular thickenings found on the surface of the perikarya of the nuclei supraopticus and paraventricularis. Since it is known that the hypothalamus plays an important role in the sexual directive action, we assume that the interference has above all an effect on the neurones of the anterior hypothalamus. This is the region where the hypothalamo-infundibular or aminergic system originates. We think that in a sort of "short-circuit" nerve fibres from the anterior hypothalamus run to the cells of the nuclei supraopticus and paraventricularis, and indeed there have been a number of recent publications about the innervation of neurosecretory cells (Falck, 1964; Bargmann, 1965; Polenov and Senchik, 1966). However, there have been no suggestions as to the site where these nerve fibres originate. We, too, are not in the position to prove morphologically beyond any doubt the existence of these assumed direct fiber connections between small-celled nuclei and the classical neurosecretory areas. Nevertheless, our results, which show an increase in total fluorescence in the anterior hypothalamus, in the various nerve fibres, and in the neuropil of the nuclei supraopticus and paraventricularis, seem to indicate that these hypothetical connections do indeed exist. This would mean that the classical neurosecretory cells in the rat are part of the regulatory system of sexual functions.

## References

Bargmann, W.: Über Synapsen im endokrinen System. Nova Acta Leopoldina, N.F. **30**, 199–206 (1965).
Falck, B.: Cellular localization of monoamines. Prop. Brain Res. **8**, 28–44 (1964).

FLERKÓ, B.: Zur hypothalamischen Steuerung der gonadotropen Funktion der Hypophyse. Acta morph. Acad. Sci. hung. **4**, 475–492 (1954).

NEUMANN, F., RICHTER, K. D., GÜNZEL, P.: Wirkungen von Antiandrogenen. Zbl. Vet.-Med. **12**, 171–188 (1965).

— ELGER, W.: Permanent changes in gonadal function and sexual behaviour as a result of early feminization of male rats by treatment with an antiandrogenic steroid. Endokrinologie **50**, 209–225 (1966).

POLENOV, A. L., SENCHIK, J. I.: Synapses on neurosecretory cells of the supraoptic nucleus in white mice. Nature (Lond.) **211**, 1423 (1966).

SPATZ, H.: Neues über die Verknüpfung von Hypophyse und Hypothalamus. Acta neuroveg. (Wien) **3**, 5–49 (1951).

SZENTÁGOTHAI, J.: The parvicellular neurosecretory system. In: Progress in brain research, vol. 5, Lectures on the diencephalon (ed. W. BARGMANN and J. P. SCHADÉ), p. 135–146. Amsterdam-London-New York: Elsevier Publ. Co. 1964.

# Ultrastructure of the Median Eminence of the Toad, *Bufo bufo*, Following Transections of the Hypothalamus at Different Levels*

P. E. BUDTZ

Zoophysiological Laboratory A, Juliane Mariesvej 32, Copenhagen Ø (Denmark)

**Key words:** Median eminence — *Bufo bufo* — Transections of the hypothalamus — Ultrastructure.

In the zona externa of the toad median eminence 5 different types of neurons can be differentiated, mainly based on the appearance of vesicles and granules (BUDTZ, 1967; RODRÍGUEZ, 1969). Little is known, however, about the origin of these neurons. The presence of two nerve tracts to the median eminence, originating at different hypothalamic cell groups of *Bufo arenarum* has been demonstrated by RODRÍGUEZ et al. (1967).

In order to throw light on the origin of the ultrastructurally different nerve tracts to the median eminence the hypothalamus was transectioned at 4 different levels, namely: just behind the optic chiasma (denervation III, 20 animals), in the rostral part of the optic chiasma (denervation IV b, 7 animals), just rostrally to the optic chiasma (denervation IV a) and in front of the preoptic nucleus (denervation VI, 3 animals); 13 toads served as unoperated controls. Animals were sacrificed at intervals between 3 h und 4 months.

The effects on the ultrastructure of the zona externa were similar following denervation III and IV b, namely an initial degeneration of neurons after 3 h, which continued during the first week and was completed after 3 weeks but was followed by degenerative changes in the capillaries. Only few type I fibres (with granules of 1,000–1,300 Å diameter) were normal. Denervation IV a and denervation VI had the same effect, but different from that following denervations at the lower levels. The result was a temporary aggregation of granules of type I and a high number of myelin or dense bodies, temporary since no significant difference could be observed after 6 weeks when compared with normals.

From the experiments it was therefore concluded, that in *Bufo bufo* all types of neurons terminating in the zona externa of the median eminence originate in an area caudal to the bulk of the preoptic nucleus, but dorsally or rostrally to the optic chiasma. Some of the type I-fibres (1,000–1,300 Å granules) appear to originate at a level below the optic chiasma as indicated by the survival of some of these fibres after denervation III.

---

* The full extent of this work is to be published in Z. Zellforsch., 1970.

# References

BUDTZ, P. E.: Ultrastructure of the median eminence of the toad, *Bufo bufo,* under normal and experimental conditions. Gen. comp. Endocr. **9,** 436–437 (1967).

RODRÍGUEZ, E. M.: Ultrastructure of the neurohemal region of the toad median eminence. Z. Zellforsch. **93,** 182–212 (1969).

— VEGA, J. A., LA MALFA, J. A.: The different origins of the hypothalamohypophysial tracts of the toad, *Bufo arenarum* H. Gen. comp. Endocr. **9,** 487 (1967).

# Investigations on the Hypothalamo-Neurohypophysial Neurosecretory System of the Grass Frog (*Rana pipiens*) after Transection of the Proximal Neurohypophysis. III. Ultrastructure and Hormone Content of the Distal Stump*

H.-D. Dellmann and E. M. Rodríguez**

Department of Veterinary Anatomy, University of Missouri, Columbia Mo. 65201 (U.S.A.)

Key words: Ultrastructure — Pressor activity — Neurohypophysis — Transection — *Rana pipiens*.

Various structural and physiological changes are known to occur in the proximal as well as in the distal stumps of transected axons in the central and peripheral nervous system (Hild, 1951; Christ, 1962; Etkin, 1962; Kreutzberg, 1963; Lubinska, 1964; Schlote, 1964, 1966a, b; Christ and Nemetscheck-Gansler, 1965; Blümcke, Niedorf and Rode, 1966; Dellmann and Dale, 1966; Dellmann, Dale, Eldridge and Owsley, 1967; Iturizza and Restelli, 1967; and others). In the distal stump of interrupted neurosecretory axons Hild (1951), Christ (1962), Etkin (1962), Dellmann and Dale (1966), Iturriza and Restelli (1967), and Dellmann and Owsley (1968) observed an increased amount of chromalum-hematoxylin-phloxin positive (CHP +) and/or paraldehyde-fuchsin-positive (PAF +) substance in the first few days following the lesion; based upon this particular staining affinity it was generally assumed that this substance represented neurosecretory material.

Although electron-microscopic studies (Christ and Nemetscheck-Gansler, 1965; Dellmann, Dale, Owsley and Eldridge, 1968) have shown the existence of an increased number of neurosecretory granules in the vicinity of the transection site, further own investigations in the distal portion of the transected hypothalamo-hypophysial neurosecretory system indicated that other structural components may possibly be responsible for the positive Go and/or PAF reaction.

Consequently the present studies were carried out to characterize at the fine structural level the changes in the distal stump of transected neurosecretory nerve fibers in the immediate vicinity of the lesion; the observation period covered the

* This work was supported by grants 5RO1 NB 06641 NEUA and 5RO1 07492 NEUA from the National Institutes of Health and by the Space Sciences Research Center of the University of Missouri. The technical assistance of Mrs. Gladys Clark is gratefully acknowledged. We thank Mr. Ray Faup for maintaining the electron microscope in excellent operating condition and Mr. Jorge Ribas for valuable help in the photography laboratory.

** Fellow of the Consejo Nacional de Investigaciones Científicas y Técnicas de la República Argentina.

first nine days after the transection during which, in previous light microscopic studies (DELLMANN and OWSLEY, 1968), the most spectacular changes were observed in the distal stump. To make the functional interpretation of the morphological findings more meaningful and more reliable the vasopressor activity of the median eminence (distal stump; see Fig. 1) was determined by bioassay procedures.

## Material and Methods

The investigations were carried out on grass frogs, *Rana pipiens*, kept under constant temperature ($18 \pm 2°$ C), light (dark:light $= 12:12$) and humidity conditions (animals immersed in water up to the head).

After transection of the proximal neurohypophysis according to the technique previously described using a 0.1% MS 222 (Sandoz) solution for anaesthesia (DELLMANN and OWSLEY, 1968), three animals were sacrificed for morphological studies at each of the following time periods after the operation: 6, 12, 24, 36, 48 hours, 6 and 9 days; 7 sham operated animals served as controls. The animals were of the southern, non-hibernating variety and were sacrificed between January 31 and February 18, 1969.

After decapitation the fixative (threefold aldehyde mixture) according to RODRÍGUEZ (1969) was immediately brought into contact with the operated area by application through the operation opening in the skull and infusion into the preoptic recess and the lateral ventricles, then the entire brain was quickly exposed and fixed by immersion for 30 minutes; after careful dissection of the areas adjacent to the lesion, the tissue remained in the fixative for another $1^1/_2$ hours. After 2 hours postfixation in a 1% osmium tetroxide solution (pH 7.2) and *en bloc* staining with uranyl acetate according to KARNOVSKY (1967) the tissue was embedded in araldite 502, the sections were stained with lead citrate according to VENABLE and COGGESHALL (1965) and examined with an RCA EMU 3 electron microscope at 50 kV.

For the bioassay procedures one group of 6 animals was sacrificed at 6 hours, 2 groups of 7 and 6 animals at 1 day, two groups of 8 and 6 animals at 2 days, on group of 6 animals at 9 days and 1 group of 3 animals at 15 days after the transection; two groups of 6 and one group of 4 animals served as controls. The animals were of the northern, hibernating variety; they were fed ad libidum with tadpoles from the beginning of April and sacrificed between April 24 and June 5, 1969.

After decapitation of the animals the median eminences were carefully dissected, pooled and homogenized in 0.25% acetic acid at $0°$ C; the homogenates were obtained with a teflon pestle turning for two minutes at equal speeds for all extracts. The homogenates were then placed into boiling water for 3 minutes and subsequently centrifuged at 3,000 RPM for 10 minutes.

The pressor activity of the extracts was measured by the method of DEKANSKY (1952) with some modifications. After anaesthesia with 12% ethanol, a carotid artery and a jugular vein were cannulated and tracheotomy was performed. Dibenzyline, 300 µg/100 g was given intravenously to block sympathetic activity.

Generally a $(2+2)$ assay design was used and when the pressor activity of the sample was very low $(2+1)$ assays were performed.

Pitressin (Parke, Davis & Co.) was used as standard preparation.

## Results

### I. Morphological Findings

The postoperative ultrastructural changes can be subdivided into two phases, a first phase covering approximately the period between the operation and 2 days, and a second phase which starts at around $1^1/_2$ days. The overlapping of the two phases within the same animal is due to the different speed at which the changes develop in individual axons.

**First Phase**

Throughout this phase the axonal structures observed at the site of transection or in its immediate vicinity undergo the following quantitative and/or qualitative changes:

### a) Neurosecretory Granules

One of the main features which distinguishes most of the axons at 6 hours with regard to the controls is the increase in the number of neurosecretory granules (1,300–1,700 Å); this increase is particularly obvious at the proximal end of the transected axons, but not restricted to it. It can also be observed to a lesser degree in more distal portions of the axon (Fig. 1). Sometimes these are the only parts where an increase can be observed, the very proximal end of the axon remaining essentially devoid of neurosecretory granules.

Subsequently no essential changes in the number of granules can be observed at the transection site in those axons that are filled with granules; in the axons which contain no or only a few neurosecretory granules the number of granules increases. In more distal portions of the axon the number of granules continues also to increase, often within axonal dilatations (Fig. 2), till around 48 hours after the transection.

Connections between neurosecretory granules and tubular formations are frequently observed (see below, Fig. 2); transitional forms between tubular dilatations and dense granules are also common (Fig. 2).

### b) Vesicles Containing Moderately Electron Dense Material

At 6 hours these vesicles (1,500–4,000 Å) are often found in a considerable number intermingled with other axonal organelles (Fig. 1). A slight but constant increase in their number can be observed during the first phase, but becomes particularly obvious toward its end.

Most of these vesicles are round or oval (Fig. 1); often pear-shaped vesicles or vesicles with very irregular outlines are observed. Furthermore they are characterized by their granular, moderately electron dense content and the fact that a considerable number of them are surrounded by more than one membrane (Fig. 1). Occasionally transitional forms are observed between dense granules and these vesicles as well as between them and large dense lamellar bodies.

### c) Large Dense Lamellar Bodies

These lamellar bodies occur either together with other axonal organelles or are found to occupy almost the entire axon, with only a few tubules, filaments and/or small dense lamellar bodies among them (Fig. 1). At 6 hours the large dense lamellar bodies are the most striking and, at least in some axons, one of the most abundant organelles. A slight increase in the number of large dense lamellar bodies

Fig. 1. a Schematic drawing of a midline longitudinal section through the investigated area; *inf* infundibulum, *me* median eminence, *nl* neural lobe, *oc* optic chiasm, *tr* transection. The rectangle indicates the area represented in Fig. 1a and the hatched median eminence area the tissue used for bioassay procedures. b Represents approximately the area within the rectangle of Fig. 1a. The rectangle indicates the area which was generally sectioned for ultrastructural investigations; the enlarged dark proximal ends of the disconnected axons are clearly visible underneath the ependymal lining e. Semithin araldite section, toluidin blue, ×420. c Axons in the distal stump, 6 hours after the transection. Note the ultrastructural

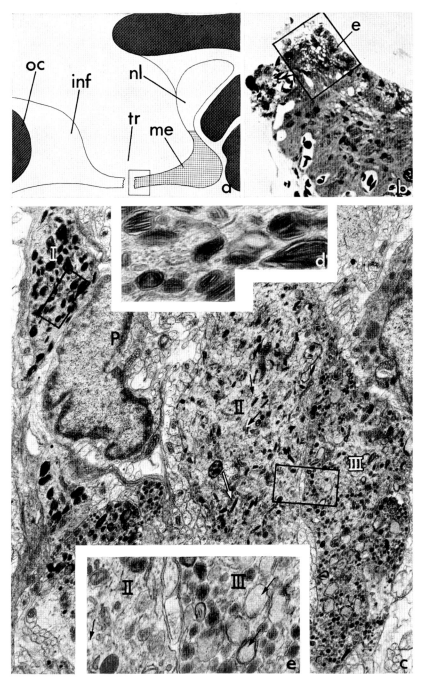

differences in axons I, II, and III. Axon I, close to a pituicyte (*p*) contains almost exclusively large, dense lamellar bodies, axon II a larger number of small dense lamellar bodies (arrows) and axon III neurosecretory granules and vesicles filled with moderately electron dense material. ×8,785. d Represents the area outlined in axon I in Fig. 1c with large and small dense lamellar bodies. ×37,250. e Represents the area outlined in axons II and III in Fig. 1c with microtubules and tubular formations (arrow) in axon II and neurosecretory granules and vesicles filled with moderately electron dense material (arrow) in axon III. ×20,500 can be observed during the first 36 hours and is followed by a more pronounced one at 2 days.

The large dense lamellar bodies (1,400–6,000 Å long; 1,100–2,600 Å wide) are predominantly oval, elongated structures which may also occur, however, in almost any other shape (Fig. 1). The internal structure of these bodies, roughly parallel lamellae separated by empty spaces or electron dense material, is obvious in most of them (Fig. 1). Quite frequently the lamellae are so densely packed, that the entire body appears as a black, structureless organelle. In some of the dense lamellar bodies portions of these bodies are non lamellated and filled with moderately electron dense material (Fig. 1). The smaller ones of these large dense lamellar bodies are frequently seen to be surrounded by a very clearly visible membrane separated from the internal lamellae by a space filled with moderately electron dense material (Fig. 1).

### d) Small Dense Lamellar Bodies

These lamellar bodies are generally found to be scattered over the axon together with the various other structures found during this phase (Fig. 1). Because of their size (1,500–4,800 Å long, up to 600 Å wide) they are generally much less prominent than the large dense lamellar bodies. The number of small dense lamellar bodies present at 6 hours does not seem to change during the first 36 hours, but a noticeable increase can be observed at 48 hours.

The small dense lamellar bodies are rodlike structures, which contain parallel lamellae in their center, whereas the ends of the rod are either filled with moderately electron dense structureless material or structures similar to mitochondrial cristae; indeed, numerous transitional forms can be observed between slender elongated mitochondria and small dense lamellar bodies.

### e) Mitochondria

The mitochondrial population during the first phase is subject to great quantitative and qualitative variations. Those parts of the axon that are densely packed with dense granules contain only a few or even no mitochondria. In those portions, however, where tubular formations (see below) are found either alone or associated with other structures (Fig. 1), the number of mitochondria is considerably higher. It is quite interesting to notice that at 6 hours after the transection frequently those parts of the axon that contain small dense lamellar bodies do not contain any or only very few mitochondria, although we would like to emphasize that the presence of small dense lamellar bodies does not exclude the presence of mitochondria in this part of the axon. Subsequently the number of mitochondria increases between 12 and 36 hours and is found to have considerably decreased at 48 hours.

The dimensions of the mitochondria vary within rather wide limits (330 to 3,300 Å in width, up to 2 microns in length). The thin mitochondria are more frequently associated with the tubular formations than the thicker ones. Furthermore they are characterized by the presence of relatively few cristae and the fact that two ends of the mitochondria are often linked by a considerably smaller intermediate portion. A thickening of the mitochondria is indicative for the beginning transformation of these organelles into small dense lamellar bodies.

## f) Tubular Formations

At 6 hours a considerable number of those neurosecretory axons which do not contain a great amount of neurosecretory granules are characterized by the presence of a frequently very elaborate system of tubular formations (Fig. 1) which is very poorly developed in the normal axon. But even in those parts of the axon, especially at the site of transection, which contain only a moderate amount of or a few neurosecretory granules, tubular formations, sometimes very sparse, often very densely packed, can be observed. With increasing time intervals between transection and sacrifice of the animal the density and the width of the tubular formations increase also reaching a maximum development at around 24 hours which appears to be maintained over a period of at least 24 hours.

The fact that the tubular formations are membrane bound (appr. 50 Å) makes it very easy to differentiate them from the neurotubules. At 6 hours the tubular formations (110–330 Å thick) are generally empty or filled occasionally with slightly electron dense material and possess dilatations up to 440 Å in width. At 12 hours the tubular formations have increased in width (130–450 Å) and the larger dilatations (750 Å) of these tubular formations are filled with moderately electron dense material; at this period neurosecretory granules are observed to be connected with the tubular formations. At 24 hours (Fig. 2) a still further increase in size can be observed (130–550 Å), a considerable number of dilatations (750 Å) filled with moderately electron dense material is present (Fig. 2) and likewise numerous neurosecretory granules are connected to the tubular formations. At 36 hours, while the density of the tubular formations is still maintained at 24 hours' level, their width has decreased (110–360 Å); the maximum size of the tubular dilatations is 550 Å. At 48 hours, with still approximately the same density as at 24 hours, a further decrease in the width of the tubular formations can be observed (110–270 Å) the size of the dilatations remaining the same as at 36 hours.

## g) Neurofilaments

While neurofilaments are generally inconspicuous at 6 hours after the transection, they become very prominent structures in the subsequent stages of the first phase (Fig. 2). They are found to run in bundles which fill a considerable part of the nondilated part of the axon and which then curve through the axonal dilatations in often whorl-like arrangements which in most instances occupy the center of these dilatations.

## Second Phase

This phase begins at around 36 hours after the transection. At this time only a few fibers undergo changes which become more pronounced and more frequent with increasing time after the operation. As many of the changes in the distal stump are identical with the changes in the disconnected neural lobe (DELLMANN and OWSLEY, 1969a; STERBA and BRÜCKNER, 1969), the description will be restricted to the events at the very proximal end of the interrupted axons and in its immediate vicinity.

At the beginning of this phase the degenerative changes occur in nerve fibers in their normal, interpituicytic position. At and especially after two days pituicytic phagocytic activity becomes very pronounced (Fig. 3). At this time changes also

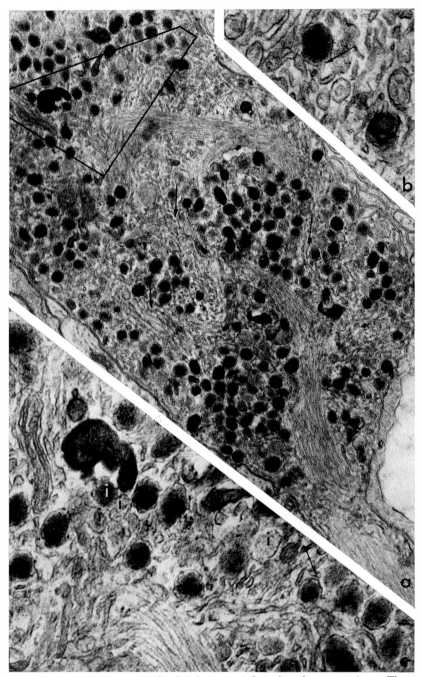

Fig. 2a–c. Neurosecretory axon in the distal stump, 1 day after the transection. a The axon is filled with dense granules, bundles of filaments and a multitude of tubular formations (arrows). ×23,400. b Note the connection between tubular formations and neurosecretory granules, the tubular formations lined by a unit membrane filled with moderately electron dense material and the vesicles intermediate between tubular formations and neurosecretory granules. ×72,000. c Represents the area outlined in Fig. 2a; neurosecretory granules, filaments, tubular formations, tubular dilatations filled with electron dense material (arrow) as well as some intermediate forms (i) between tubular dilatations and neurosecretory granules are present. ×78,390

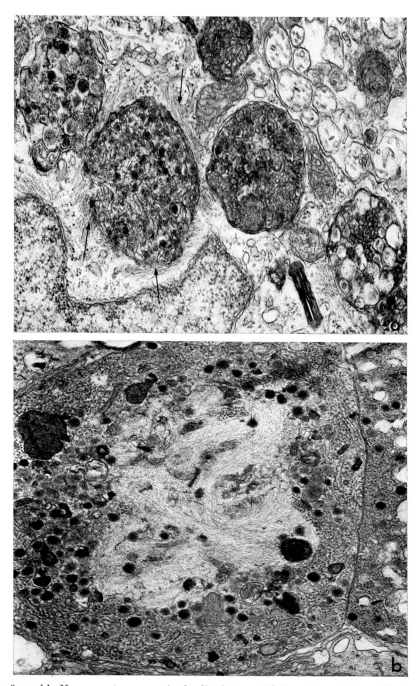

Fig. 3a and b. Neurosecretory axons in the distal stump $1^1/_2$ days (a) and 6 days (b) after the transection. a Neurosecretory axons are found in intrapituicytic position and characterized by the first signs of degeneration (for further information see text); note the presence of numerous filaments (arrows) around the largest axon. ×32,513. b Whorls of filaments, a few neurosecretory granules and well developed peripheral but apparently inactive (see text) tubular formations characterize this axon at 6 days. ×17,613 occur in axons or axon fragments in intrapituicytic position. The following changes are observed in the nerve fibers before they are engulfed by pituicytes:

### a) Neurosecretory Granules

An increase in size, in the width of the space between bounding membrane and granule, a loss of electron density, a loss of the membrane and/or fusion of the membrane of several granules are the characteristic changes of the neurosecretory granules at the beginning of degeneration (Fig. 3). These changes eventually lead to the formation of very large multilamellate bodies.

### b) Vesicles Filled with Moderately Electron Dense Material and Various Other Vesicles

The vesicles filled with moderately electron dense material disappear during this period and are only occasionally found at 6 days. At this time empty vesicles (Fig. 3) besides vesicles containing some moderately electron dense material in the periphery surrounded by one or more frequently by several layers of membranes predominate. Some of these vesicles are found to be up to 6,000 Å in diameter.

### c) Large and Small Dense Lamellar Bodies

At the beginning of this phase these two types of dense lamellar bodies are easily discernible. Subsequently they increase in number and in the later phases of degeneration they become undistinguishable from other lamellar formations within the axon.

### d) Mitochondria

A direct transformation of the slender elongated mitochondria into small dense lamellar bodies or swelling and subsequent incorporation into the lamellar systems of the degenerating axon are the changes that are observed in the mitochondria during this phase.

### e) Tubular Formations

After 48 hours the tubular formations seem to have lost their importance. Although they still occur at 6 (Fig. 3) and even 9 days after the transection and sometimes even in a considerable number, a general decrease in their number is observed. They closely resemble the tubular formations during the initial phase, with only very few dilatations.

### f) Neurotubules and Neurofilaments

While neurotubules decrease in number rather rapidly after 36 hours and are practically absent at 6 days, the neurofilaments are characterized by a high increase in number. They have a tendency to occupy the center of the proximal end of the transected axon (Fig. 3) in a complicated, interwoven, whorl-like arrangement.

Ultimately all axons, regardless of their appearance before degeneration, will have similar morphological appearance.

### g) Pituicytes and Other Cells

During the entire phase the pituicytes have a high phagocytic activity (Fig. 3) and the observed changes are similar to the ones described previously (Dellmann and OWSLEY, 1969a; STERBA and BRÜCKNER, 1969). Together with the intra-pituicytic lysis of axon fragments an increase in the number of intracellular fila-ments often particularly concentrated around the engulfed axons is frequently observed (Fig. 3).

## II. Pharmacological Findings

The results of the rat blood pressor assay are represented in Fig. 4; a rise in hormonal activity in the distal stump area (including the entire median eminence; Fig. 1) is observed 1 day after the transection followed by a subsequent decrease in activity.

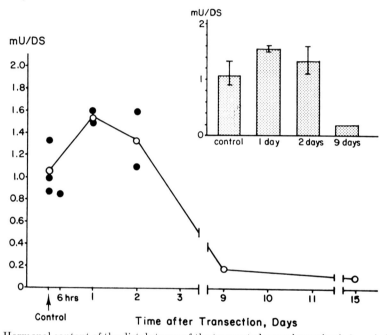

Fig. 4. Hormonal content of the distal stump of the transected neurohypophysis (area indicated in Fig. 1b). The black dots represent the individual values in mU per distal stump (*DS*), the white dots the mean values, which coincide with individual values at days 9 and 15 after the transection. In the histogram the means and highest and lowest values are represented

## Discussion

The study of the distal stump of transected neurosecretory nerve fibers reveals a far more complicated ultrastructural organization of this area than expected from previous preliminary studies (CHRIST and NEMETSCHECK-GANSLER, 1965; DELLMANN, DALE, OWSLEY and ELDRIDGE, 1968). Furthermore, the determination of the vasopressor activity of the distal stump and the adjacent median eminence yields a hormone increase 24 hours after the interruption of the neurosecretory pathway. Based upon these results it can be attempted to correlate light micro-scopic and ultrastructural findings, to determine the possible origin and signi-ficance of the structures found in the distal stump and to establish the relationship between pharmacological and fine structural observations and thus find a reasonable explanation for the possible origin of the increased hormone content of the distal stump.

### Correlation between Light Microscopic and Ultrastructural Findings

An increase in the amount of chromalum-hematoxylin-phloxin (CHP) + and/ or paraldehyde fuchsine (PAF) + substance is observed in the distal stump of the transected hypothalamo-neurohypophysial tract as early as 15 minutes after the operation. A further increase is found during the next 24 or 48 hours until, at around 4 days, small Herring bodies occur which represent disintegrating neuro-secretory nerve fibers (Dellmann and Owsley, 1968). Based upon the assumption that the CHP+ and/or PAF + substance represents neurosecretory material, the positive reaction furnished an argument in favor of the local origin of this material (Christ, 1962; Dellmann and Owsley, 1968, literature references). Neuro-secretory granules have indeed been observed in the distal stump under the electron microscope (Christ and Nemetscheck-Gansler, 1965; Dellmann, Dale, Ows-ley and Eldridge, 1968); the present study confirms these reports and does not leave any doubt as to the presence of an increased number of neurosecretory granules at the very proximal ends of a considerable number of the disconnected axons as well as in their immediate vicinity. However, in comparing the PAF reaction with the number of dense granules it becomes difficult to correlate the results, i.e. the PAF reaction is more intense than expected from the number of neurosecretory granules present at the ultrastructural level.

Are there any other organelles which could possibly be made responsible for a positive PAF reaction? Throughout the entire observation period, but especially at its very beginning, large and small dense lamellar bodies were observed to be one of the most striking and prominent intraaxonal organelles. They frequently occupied axonal dilatations entirely (Fig. 1) or were a major part of them; often these lamellar bodies were within the range of the resolution of the light micro-scope. We have been able to show in the neurohypophysis of cattle (Dellmann and Owsley, 1969b) and of dehydrated rats (unpublished observations) that dense lamellar bodies give a positive PAF reaction; thus we can reasonably assume that the large elongated PAF + granules observed under the light microscope in the axons and axonal dilatations of the distal stump represent dense lamellar bodies rather than neurosecretory granules. These dense lamellar bodies are considered to be the expression of a degenerative process (see below), which con-firms Scharrer's (1962) earlier opinion that the positive CHP reaction in the distal stump may be due to degenerating neurosecretory nerve fibers.

During the second phase, fragmentation of the neurosecretory nerve fibers and phagocytosis of these fragments by the pituicytes occur. The huge dense lamellar bodies resulting from this phagocytic activity appear as PAF+ complexes in the light microscope (Dellmann and Owsley, 1969a) and are primarily responsible for the Gomori positive reaction in the stump at this time.

The tubular formations whose greatest development in the transected axons is observed during the first 48 hours after the transection are presumably function-ing in hormone transport and concentration (see below). As aldehyde fuchsin has been shown to give a positive reaction with oxytocin and lysine-vasopressin (Gutierrez and Sloper, 1969) we further hypothesize that part of the PAF+

and/or CHP+ reaction is due to the presence of these hormone containing tubular formations.

### Origin and Significance of the Distal Stump Structures

The question as to the possible origin of some of the structures observed in the distal stump is sometimes rather difficult to answer because of their absence in the control animals and their presence at 6 hours, the earliest observation time after transection. Further information needs to be obtained through additional studies which are on their way.

It is very likely that some of the organelles in the distal stump originate in situ. A backflow from more distal parts of the axon and a local formation may be realized for others.

On the basis of our present findings the sometimes relatively high increase in the number of neurosecretory granules, especially at the very proximal end of the interrupted fibers within the first 12 hours after the transection, can only be accounted for by the existence of a lesion directed backflow of granules from more distal parts of the axon; a bidirectional flow of axoplasm seems to be an established fact (LUBINSKA, 1964; BANKS, MANGNALL and MAYOR, 1969), however, the extent of the axoplasmic movement remains to be determined (ZELENA, LUBINSKA and GUTMANN, 1968). An observation in favor of a backflow predominating in the neighborhood of the transection is the whorl-like arrangement of the neurofilament bundles which suggests localized axoplasmic streaming (SCHLOTE, 1966a; JOHNSON et al., 1969). This arrangement of filaments is lacking in the proximal stump where a backflow is very unlikely to occur. At a later time after transection the observation of connections between neurosecretory granules and tubular formations and the presence of intermediate forms between these granules and tubular dilatations filled with moderately electron dense material make the tubular origin of some of the neurosecretory granules, especially at around 24 hours, very probable.

Vesicles filled with moderately electron dense material are present in the distal stump at 6 hours and there again the investigation of the events earlier after the transection will possibly yield more information as to their origin. A comparison with the changes occuring in the neural lobe seems to indicate that these vesicles may represent enlarged dense granules or may be the result of the fusion of several dense granules. As these vesicles are often surrounded by several membranes it seems reasonable to assume that they will eventually form dense lamellar bodies; in fact some of the dense lamellar bodies may represent peripheral sections through these vesicles. The vesicles filled with moderately electron dense material are considered to be one of the first indications of degenerative changes within the axon; the fact that during the first phase after the transection considerably less vesicles were present than during the second phase when a definite degeneration of the neurosecretory axons occurs is in favor of this interpretation.

More than one origin seems to be possible for the large dense lamellar bodies. Because of their size and the fact that transitional forms are not observed we think that it is rather unlikely that the large dense lamellar bodies represent degenerating mitochondria. The observation of several layers of lamellae around the vesicles filled with moderate electron dense material makes a vesicular origin of these bodies very likely. On the other hand it appears that localized intraaxonal degeneration may also result in the formation of large dense lamellar bodies (Blümcke et al. 1966). This opinion is further supported by the occurence of similar but larger dense lamellar bodies which are known to be the result of axonal degeneration.

It is rather difficult if not impossible to draw a clear line of demarcation between large and small dense lamellar bodies; however, we do not have any doubt as to the mitochondrial origin of the small ones. Numerous transitional forms, such as thickening of the mitochondrial cristae and an increase in their electron density and the persistence of the outer compartment in some of the dense lamellar bodies indicate that this interpretation is correct; this confirms Schlote's (1966) earlier hypothesis. It is quite interesting to notice that there exists an inverse numerical relationship between mitochondria and small dense lamellar bodies. At 6 hours dense lamellar bodies are generally far more numerous than mitochondria (although both may coexist in almost equal numbers), during the next 24 hours, the relationship changes in favor of the mitochondria until, at 48 hours, an increase in the number of small dense lamellar bodies is observed. This fact seems to indicate that the small dense lamellar bodies have to be considered as degenerating mitochondria rather than a special form of mitochondria as proposed by Schlote (1966).

The increase in the number of mitochondria between 12 and 36 hours is particularly obvious in those parts of the axons where tubular formations predominate. In the portions of the axon where neurosecretory granules prevail, the number of mitochondria remains essentially unchanged.

One of the most interesting and probably functionally most significant axonal structures are the tubular formations; because of their very extensive development at our earliest observation time, it is extremely difficult to hypothesize on their possible origin. Based upon the fact that tubular formations occur in the normal axon (although only to a very limited extent) and that they are limited by a unit membrane, which distinguishes them very clearly from the neurotubules, we assume that the tubular formations in our experimental animals derive by proliferation from those normally present. We consider the sequence of changes through which the tubular formations go between the beginning and the end of our observation period as the morphological expression of important functional changes. The increase in extent and width of these tubular formations together with an increase in electron density of their content between 6 and 24 hours might be related to the increase in the hormonal content of the distal stump. The subsequent slendering and eventual disappearance of the tubular formations may again be related to the decrease in hormonal content. The possibility of a correlation between tubular formations and hormones is further substantiated by the observation of vesicles and neurosecretory granules connected to the tubular formations suggesting a tubular origin of these structures.

According to the above considerations, we propose three possible explanations for the increase in hormonal content observed in the distal stump area 24 hours after the transection: 1) The increase is due to a backflow of neurosecretory granules from the neural lobe, 2) the increase is caused by a backflow within tubular formations and subsequent concentration therein of extragranular hormones (GINSBURG, 1968) which are present within the more distal parts of the axons and 3) the increase is due to an axoplasmic backflow of extragranular hormones. Of these three possibilities the first two ones are by far more likely to be realized. Although there is a considerable increase in the amount of neurosecretory granules at the proximal ends of the disconnected fibers and in their immediate vicinity, the overall increase as compared to the neural lobe and to the proximal stump is so small that it seems very unlikely that this increase can account for a major part of the hormonal increase. On the other hand, the increase in the number of tubular formations, the diameter increase of these tubules, the fact that numerous tubular dilatations are observed and that transitional forms can be demonstrated between these dilatations and neurosecretory granules, are arguments in favor of the second hypothesis. A function very similar to the Golgi apparatus in the perikaryon is visualized for the tubular formations, although neurosecretory granule formation is obviously not necessary for an increase in hormone activity. A further and final argument in favor of the first two explanations for the hormonal increase is the fact, that the increase in neurosecretory granules as well as the changes in the tubular formations parallel the increase in pressor activity and that in turn a decrease in pressor activity is accompanied by definite morphological signs of decreased or even ceased neurosecretory activity and also changes in the tubular formations in the distal stump. More reliable criteria are certainly furnished by a combination of electron microscopic and pharmacological studies rather than light microscopic ones; thus, at a time when the distal stump is still CHP+ is appears that the structures responsible for this positive reaction are mostly other than neurosecretory granules and that the hormone activity has dropped to an almost nonmeasurable level.

In conclusion, we would like to emphasize that ultrastructural and functional reactive changes occur in the distal stump as a response to transection; these changes occur within the first phase between 6 hours and 2 days after the transection and represent a true beginning of regeneration. They are followed by degenerative changes during the second phase starting at 36 hours which lead to the morphological and functional death of the disconnected portion of the axon.

## Summary

During the first postoperative phase, between 6 and 48 hours, the following features characterize the disconnected neurosecretory axons: a) Neurosecretory granules are often particularly numerous at the proximal end of the disconnected axons; their number increases over the entire phase. b) Large dense lamellar bodies which are considered to occur as a consequence of localized intraaxonal degeneration; their number also increases during the entire phase. c) Small dense lamellar bodies representing transformed mitochondria, increase noticeably in number at the end of this phase. d) Vesicles containing moderately electron dense material are found to become more numerous during the entire period. e) Mitochondria increase in number between 12 and 36 hours, but decrease at 48 hours. f) Tubular formations, dilatations, and vesicles connected to them reach a maximum development in width and density at 24 hours: these tubular formations, are believed to be involved in extragranular hormone transport from more distal portions of the axons leading to an increase in hormone content of the distal stump at 24 hours. All these structures with the exception of mitochondria are considered to be responsible for the paraldehyde fuchsin-positive reaction observed under the light microscope during this phase. Based upon these observations the first phase is considered to be the beginning of a regeneration. The second phase begins at around 36 hours and is characterized by degenerative phenomena. A considerable decrease in the number of dense granules, mitochondria and tubular formations and a concommitant increase in vesicles containing a moderately electron dense material, dense lamellar bodies and filaments, fragmentation of axons and phagocytic activity of pituicytes go parallel with a decrease in the hormone activity of the distal stump.

## References

Banks, P., Magnall, D., Mayor, D.: The re-distribution of oxidase, noradrenaline and adenosine-triphosphatase in adrenergic nerves constricted at two points. J. Physiol. (Lond.) **200**, 745–762 (1969).

Blümcke, S., Niedorf, H. R., Rode, J.: Axoplasmic alterations in the proximal and distal stumps of transected nerves. Acta neuropath. **7**, 44–61 (1966).

Christ, J. F.: The early changes in the hypophysial neurosecretory fibers after coagulation. In: Neurosecretion, p. 125–147 (eds. H. Heller and R. B. Clark). New York: Academic Press 1962.

— Nemetscheck-Gansler, H.: Zur Ultramorphologie der Veränderungen im neurosekretorischen System nach Koagulation des Hypophysenstiels. Z. Naturforsch. **20**, 278–281 (1965).

Dekanski, J.: The quantitative assay of vasopressin. Brit. J. Pharmacol. **7**, 567–572 (1952)[1]

Dellmann, H.-D., Dale, H. E.: Morphology, structure and vasotocin content of the neurosecretory hypothalamo-hypophysial system of the grass frog (*Rana pipiens*) under normal and experimental conditions. Anat. Rec. **154**, 336–337 (1966).

— — Eldridge, L. F., Owsley, P. A.: Changes in the structure and function of the neurosecretory hypothalamo-neurohypophysial system in the distal stump of the transected neurohypophysis of the grass frog (*Rana pipiens*). In: Proc. XVIIIth World Vet. Congr., p. 724. Paris: Muray Print 1967.

— — Owsley, P. A., Eldridge, L. F.: Morphological and functional changes in the distal hypothalamo-neurohypophysial system of the grass frog (*Rana pipiens*) after transection of the proximal neurohypophysis. Experientia (Basel) **24**, 383–386 (1968).

— Owsley, P. A.: Investigations on the hypothalamo-neurohypophysial neurosecretory system of the grass frog (*Rana pipiens*) after transection of the proximal neurohypophysis. I. Light microscopic findings in animals kept at 18°C environmental temperature. Z. Zellforsch. **87**, 1–16 (1968).

— — Investigations on the hypothalamo-neurohypophysial neurosecretory system of the grass frog (*Rana pipiens*) after transection of the proximal neurohypophysis. II. Light and electron microscopic findings in the disconnected distal neurohypophysis with special emphasis on the pituicytes. Z. Zellforsch. **94**, 325–336 (1969a).

— — Ultrastructure of Herring bodies in the bovine neurohypophysis. Anat. Rec. **163**, 176 (1969b).

Dierickx, K.: The gonadotrophic center of the tuber cinereum hypothalami and ovulation. Z. Zellforsch. **77**, 188–203 (1967).

Etkin, W.: Neurosecretory control of the pars intermedia. Gen. comp. Neurol. **2**, 161–169 (1962).

Ginsburg, M.: Molecular aspects of neurohypophysial hormone release. Proc. roy. Soc. B **170**, 27–36 (1968).

Gutierrez, M., Sloper, J. C.: Reaction in vitro of synthetic oxytocin and lysine-vasopressin with the pseudoisocyaninchloride technique used for the demonstration of neurohypophysial neurosecretory material. Histochemie **17**, 73–77 (1969).

HILD, W.: Untersuchungen über das Verhalten der „neurosekretorischen Bahn" nach Hypophysenstieldurchtrennungen, Eingriffen in den Wasserhaushalt und Belastung der Osmoregulation. Virchows Arch. path. Anat. **319**, 526–546 (1951).

ITURRIZA, F. C., RESTELLI, M. A.: Neurosecretion in the distal stump of the sectioned hypothalamic-hypophyseal tract in the toad. Z. Zellforsch. **81**, 297–302 (1967).

JOHNSON, S., SMITH, R. S., LOCK, S. S. H.: Accumulation of material at severed ends of myelinated nerve fibers. Amer. J. Physiol. **217**, 188–191 (1969).

KARNOVSKY, M. J.: The ultrastructural basis of capillary permeability studied with peroxidase as a tracer. J. Cell Biol. **35**, 213–236 (1967).

KREUTZBERG, G.: Enzymhistochemische Veränderungen in Axonen des Rückenmarks nach Durchtrennung der langen Bahnen. Dtsch. Z. Nervenheilk. **185**, 308–318 (1963).

LUBINSKA, L.: Axoplasmic streaming in regenerating and normal nerve fibers. In: Progress in brain research, vol. 13, Mechanisms of neural regeneration, p. 1–66 (eds. M. SINGER and J. P. SCHADE). Amsterdam-London-New York: Elsevier 1964.

RODRÍGUEZ, E. M.: Fixation of the central nervous system by perfusion of the cerebral ventricles by a threefold aldehyde mixture. Brain Res. **15**, 395—412 (1969).

SCHARRER, B.: Discussion of CHRIST's paper. In: Neurosecretion, p. 144 (eds. H. HELLER and R. B. CLARK). New York: Academic Press 1962.

SCHLOTE, W.: Die läsionsbedingten primär retrograden Veränderungen der Axone zentraler Nervenfasern im elektronenmikroskopischen Bild. Acta neuropath. (Berl.) **4**, 138–157 (1964).

— Zur Abgrenzung reaktiver von regenerativen Vorgängen im Axoplasma zentraler Nervenfasern. Verh. Dtsch. Ges. Path. 50. Tagg, p. 277–280. Stuttgart: Gustav Fischer 1966a.

— Der Aufbau von Schichtenkörpern im Axoplasma durchtrennter Opticusfasern distal der Läsion. J. Ultrastruct. Res. **16**, 548–568 (1966b).

VENABLE, J., COGGESHALL, R.: The use of a simple lead citrate stain in electron microscopy. J. Cell Biol. **25**, 407–408 (1965).

ZELENA, J., LUBINSKA, L., GUTMANN, E.: Accumulation of organelles at the ends of interrupted axons. Z. Zellforsch. **91**, 200–219 (1968).

# Mechanism of Release of Neurohypophyseal Materials

## Mechanism of Release of Neurohypophyseal Hormones

Niels A. Thorn

Institute of Medical Physiology C, University of Copenhagen (Denmark)

**Key words:** Neurohypophysis — Hormones — Mechanism of release.

The hypothalamo-neurohypophyseal system of course fulfils the criteria for a neurosecretory system, since this concept has been formulated on the basis of the function of that system.

a) The nerve cells can receive stimuli from other neurons and conduct these stimuli.

b) They elaborate secretory material demonstrable by histological technique.

c) They store and release under a strict control physiologically active substances (vasopressin and oxytocin), which affect organs lying distant from the central nervous system.

We have for some time in our laboratory been interested in the mechanism of release of these hormones.

Let us discuss some of the problems involved as I see them:

### 1. Does Release Only Take Place at Nerve Endings?

It has long been assumed that the stimuli for release of vasopressin do not act on the peripheral nerve endings but affect structures more proximally.

This concept has been strengthened recently by the finding that agents which cause release of hormone in intact animals (e.g. nicotine and amyl nitrite) do not affect the release from isolated neural lobes (see Thorn, 1966). Also, it seems that stimuli which can cause a release from neural lobes in vitro do not do so from isolated hypothalamus preparations containing the supraoptic and paraventricular nuclei which were demonstrated to contain hormone (Bie and Thorn, 1967). In these experiments it was impossible to be sure that the possibilities for access of the stimulating substances to the perikarya was ideal, but a long time of incubation and strong stimuli were applied. Usually hormone in only a fraction of the total contents in the neurohypophysis can be extracted from the hypothalamus. That release apparently does not take place from the hypothalamus might be due to several causes: One could be that the depolarization processes do not change the perikaryal membrane in the same way as the axonal membrane. Other possibilities are that the brain-blood barrier in this region is tight, or that the chemical state of the hormone is such that it is not freely releasable. The latter 2 facts might explain the probable lack of release in the proximal part of the axon.

## 2. Possible Role of Acetylcholin in Release Processes

It has earlier been suggested that acetylcholin functions as a transmitter substance at the nerve endings in the release of vasopressin and oxytocin from the neurohypophysis. However, recent studies by LEDERIS and LIVINGSTON (1969) and LA BELLA (1968) have shown that acetylcholin is localized to specific nerve endings and probably specific granules in the neurohypophysis and that it seems to function exclusively in vascular regulations in this region. Its function relevant to the release of vasopressin and oxytocin thus seems to be to transmit afferent nerve impulses to the supraoptic and paraventricular nuclei and not to mediate the release of hormones by a direct action on the nerve endings in the neural lobe. It might be added that a suggestion by LEVEQUE and SMALL (1959) that pituicytes secrete a substance that stimulates secretion of hormone by an action directly on the nerves has not found much support.

## 3. Do Nerve Endings Located Elsewhere in the System than in the Neurohypophysis Take Part in Release?

It has been suggested that the continued secretion of vasopressin after stalk section might be due to a release from intact nerve endings in the eminentia mediana. The function of this region is still not well examined. FUXE (1964) showed a high concentration of monoamines in the median eminence. MATSUI and KOBAYASHI (1965) found a high concentration of monoamine oxydase in the same region (see also FOLLETT et al., 1966). MONROE (1967) in electron-micrographic studies found a group of small calibered axons, which terminate around the infundibular capillaries of the portal system. Their function is unknown. The studies of BIE and THORN (1967) previously quoted, might be taken as support for the hypothesis that there seem to be no vasopressinergic nerve endings in the eminentia, which release hormone to the blood.

The question whether there is any penetration of vasopressin through the blood brain barrier has been studied by two groups recently. HELLER et al. (1968) found that vasopressin injected into the plasma of rabbits moved into the cerebro-spinal fluid. VORHERR et al. (1968) did not find any passage of vasopressin into the cerebro-spinal fluid of dogs. Both groups found an increase in the content of cerebro-spinal fluid vasopressin under circumstances of anesthesia or hemorrhage. It is uncertain whether it may be inferred from these experiments that vasopressin may be released directly to the cerebro-spinal fluid somewhere on the ventricular wall.

## 4. Hormone Pools in the Nerve Endings, Presence of a Pool of Easily Releasable Hormone

Vasopressin and its "carrier protein", neurophysin, are present in the nerve endings in two anatomically different loci. The major part is found in the granules, but some vasopressin and neurophysin seems to be present free in the axoplasm (GINSBURG, 1968).

Recent studies by HOPE and his coworkers have demonstrated that the chemical properties of neurophysin, a "specific" protein isolated from neural lobes, may vary with the preparation technique. The feature about neurophysin that has been considered unique, has been its capacity to bind vasopressin and oxytocin. Thus it has been considered to function as a carrier protein. The binding capacity has been found by different groups to differ pretty much. Other substances in the neurohypophysis can bind vasopressin and oxytocin (Wu and Saffran, 1969).

Functionally, there seems to be an easily releasable pool, which comprises only about 5–10% of the totally extractable hormone. This has been demonstrated in in vitro experiments on rat neural hemilobes (Thorn, 1966). About 5% af the vasopressin extractable was released during stimulation with a high concentration of potassium in the medium. No more than this percentage could be mobilized during such a stimulation, even after further subdivision of the neural hemilobes, prolongation of the stimulation period, or after increasing the calcium concentration in the medium fivefold. Daniel and Lederis (1967) also using hemilobes of rats, showed that the amount released decreases with the time of stimulation, too.

Sachs et al. (1967) showed that pituitaries taken from bled dogs released much less vasopressin in vitro in response to electrical or potassium stimulation than pituitaries from non-bled animals.

The same phenomenon was found concerning release in vivo. The release was not a simple function of the total hormone content of the gland. What would seem to be a direct evidence for the metabolic heterogeneity of the pool of neurohypophyseal vasopressin was given by Sachs and Haller (1968). The pool of neurohypophyseal vasopressin was labelled with $^{35}$S. The specific activity of the hormone secreted in response to excess potassium in vitro or to bleeding in vivo, was several times greater than that of the hormone remaining in the gland.

The limited release capacity was not due to anoxia of the tissue or a negative feedback from secreted vasopressin. The phenomenon was also found using electrical stimulation of guinea pig neural lobes. Nothing is known about the anatomical basis for the easily releasable pool. One might speculate on different possibilities. One would be that the easily releasable pool is extragranular hormone or hormone in granules of a special maturity or closeness to the axonal membrane. Another possibility is that the neurons go through cycles of activity (Zambrano and de Robertis, 1966) or that the hormone is within a special population of neurons.

Acetylcholine output from a stimulated ganglion shows conditions similar to those just described. Also noradrenaline in splenic nerve endings is found in two stores, only one of which is easily available (Gillespie and Kirkepar, 1966). Apparently here is another point where the function of the neurons in this neuroendocrine system resembles that of ordinary nerve cells.

How hormone "precursor" is transferred into the easily releasable pool is unknown. One way it might happen is by breakage of secretory granules or leakage from them, possibly during exocytosis. The way the pool is regulated is unknown.

A variety of stimuli can cause a rapid depletion of stainable material from the neurohypophysis. However, there is no correlation between this change and the release of biologically active material (hormone) (Barer and Lederis, 1966). The biochemical mechanisms involved in the changes in the neurosecretory material are still obscure. It might be that some of it is due to release of an unknown substance (Sloper, 1966).

## 5. Barriers that Hormone Must Pass During Secretion

The hormone must pass a number of barriers before being secreted. It would seem that if secretion occurs by exocytosis the passing of the barriers after the axonal membrane would present serious problems. These barriers are represented by two layers of basement membrane, a layer of interstitial tissue and the fenestrated capillary wall.

## 6. Electrical Phenomena Associated with Hormone Release

As summarized by GINSBURG (1968) there seems to be good evidence that the cells in the hypothalamo-neurohypophyseal system function as neurons as concerns their electrical activity. Recently DYBALL and KOIZUMI (1969) have further supported this by demonstrating that stimuli which are known to release vasopressin and oxytocin also excite electrically units in the supraoptic and paraventricular system.

The electrical activity of the nerve endings after stimulation subsides much earlier than the secretory response (DYBALL, 1969).

## 7. Role of Calcium in the Release Process

That calcium is an essential factor in excitation secretion coupling was shown by DOUGLAS and his co-workers in studies of the release of hormone from isolated neural lobes (see DOUGLAS, 1968).

Biochemical studies have shown that small concentrations of calcium ions detach arginine and lysine-vasopressin as well as oxytocin from their loose binding to carrier protein (SMITH and THORN, 1965; THORN, 1966; GINSBURG et al., 1966). The experiments involved gel filtration in which calcium inhibited the binding of arginine-vasopressin to neurophysin and film dialysis experiments in which the same phenomenon was shown for lysine-vasopressin. There was no effect of magnesium, sodium, acetylcholin, noradrenalin or serotonin. The concentration of calcium for inhibition of binding is critical. The mechanism of the effect is unknown. It may involve interference at charged sites or an allosteric effect. The same effect has been found in relation to the binding of isoleucin[3]-leucin[8]-oxytocin to carboxymethyl-dextran, a complex considered similar to vasopressin-neurophysin (SCHÄKER, 1968). This reaction with calcium seems important in the release mechanism, but *when* it occurs is not quite clear. If no reverse pinocytosis takes place, it may be crucial in liberating neurophysin-bound-vasopressin within the nerve endings and allow the nonapeptide to be transported more freely to the blood. If reverse pinocytosis takes place, its function would be to detach vasopressin from neurophysin in the pericapillary space, thus facilitating its further transport to plasma, or it may detach it when the complex has reached the blood vessels. On the other hand, dissociation of vasopressin from neurophysin might mean something for the properties of the latter. It might be possible that such a dissociation eases the transport of neurophysin across the axon membrane. After this it might then be taken up by the pituicytes. It is also possible that during the latter part of exocytosis processes hormone dissociated from neurophysin passes the region where granules have been in contact with the cell membrane.

## 8. Role of Energy in the Release Process

Poisner and Douglas (1968a, b) have demonstrated the presence of adenosine triphosphate and adenosine triphosphatase activity in neurosecretory granules from the neurohypophysis. Addition of ATP to suspensions of granules stimulated

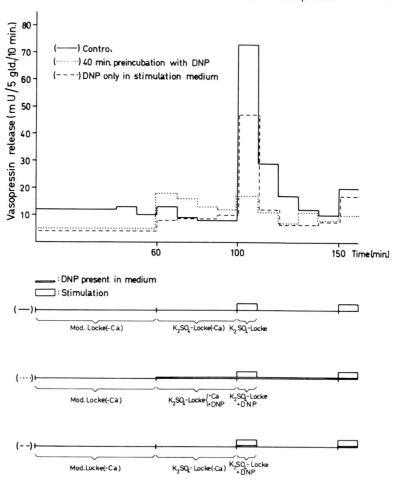

Fig. 1. Effect of DNP (0.5 mM) on calcium induced release of vasopressin. The incubation procedure is indicated in the lower part of the figure. (From Warberg and Thorn, 1969)

erlease of vasopressin weakly. This suggested to them that ATP and ATPase participate in the storage and release of vasopressin. Such a process might be linked with complex dissociation from the axoplasm. However, it might also be so that the process is part of a contractile step in exocytosis. Poisner and Trifaro (1969) have demonstrated various phenomena in the action of ATP on catechol-amine granules which might support such a concept. The fact that calcium was not essential for this process would seem to mean that calcium, if it is essential for exocytosis, might act by producing a contact between granules and the axon membrane in the nerve endings (or calcium might cause a break-down intracellularly of granules). DOUGLAS and coworkers (1965) have shown that the metabolic inhibitors DNP, IAC, cyanide and others had no effect on the baseline rate of release, but seriously hampered the release on stimulation by potassium or calcium.

DOUGLAS et al. interpreted their experiments to show that an energy dependent link is essential for the release of the hormone, or, alternatively that the inhibitor might act by blocking production of some intermediate required to prime the hormone extrusion mechanism.

However, the experiments forming the basis for DOUGLAS and POISNER's concept were few. So we decided to repeat DOUGLAS and POISNER's experiments on the effect of metabolic inhibitors on the in vitro release of vasopressin. We have used two inhibitors: Dinitrophenol and iodoacetate in a concentration of 0.5 and 3 mM, respectively. We have two different sorts of stimulation, one is stimulating the neurohypophysis in vitro by adding potassium to a regular Locke medium, and the other way is to add calcium to a calcium-free potassium sulphate Locke medium. The essential finding is seen in Fig. 1. It is seen that if calcium is introduced to a potassium sulphate Locke medium in which five sets of hemilobes have been incubated for some time, there is a release of hormone. This release is only a small fraction of the total contents. It is about 5% of the total contents. A second stimulation causes release of a smaller amount of hormone. Now, if we incubate the glands in a medium containing dinitrophenol only during stimulation, this is the broken curve you see, there is some inhibition of the release. If we incubate the hemilobes for a longer period (the dotted line) there is a stronger inhibition of the release. Here it has nearly been abolished. We have made similar experiments with iodoacetate, and found essentially similar results concerning the inhibition. However, the inhibition was smaller. Now, if we should try to interpret these findings, of course one of the possibilities is that energy is really necessary for the release process itself, and that what has been done by adding metabolic inhibitors is inhibiting a reverse pinocytosis. However, there is one other possibility at least. It we look at the baseline rate of secretion during the period when the gland was incubated with dinitrophenol we see that there was an increased baseline rate of release of hormone during the preincubation with inhibitors. This may then have caused a depletion of the easily releasable store of the hormone. If no repletion has taken place, that means that even if we have calcium available for the secretion there can occur no release of hormone. An increased baseline rate of release during lack of glucose and oxygen was noted by SACHS and HALLER (1968). They did not try to study the effect of either factor alone.

To obtain a reliable effect of the metabolic inhibitors they have to be allowed to act for some time. In this way, however, several of the many partial functions of the cells may be effected such as:

a) maintenance of membrane integrity,

b) maintenance of sequestration of calcium by actively accumulating processes,

c) possible maintenance of easily releasable hormone.

Even if ATP causes a release of vasopressin from isolated granules and if metabolic inhibitors inhibit the release these findings do not prove that energy is involved in the processes most directly involved in the release of the hormone, and in the author's opinion do not support the existence of exocytosis as the normal secretory process.

### 9. Hypotheses for Cellular Mechanism of Release of Vasopressin

Two hypotheses have been advanced for the nature of the cellular mechanisms involved in the release of vasopressin which occurs when impulses reach the nerve

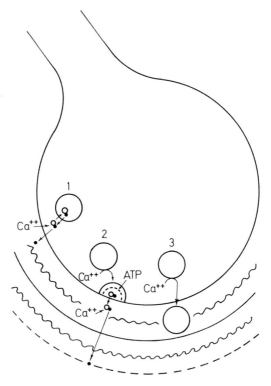

Fig. 2. Main possibilities for the mechanism of release of vasopressin: 1) Complex dissociation; 2) Exocytosis; 3) Extrusion of granule + membrane. (This possibility is not very likely)

endings in the neurohypophysis. Douglas and coworkers (Douglas and Poisner, 1964; Douglas, 1968) suggested that "reverse pinocytosis" involving the contents of neurosecretory granules was the most likely explanation.

Although very recently electron micrographs have been published which seem to demonstrate exocytosis in the pars distalis of amphibia (Bunt, 1969; Masur, 1969) no such findings seem to exist in mammals in a physiological state and certainly no findings demonstrating correlation between frequency of exocytosis and intensity of secretion.

One biochemical support of exocytosis would be the demonstration that vasopressin and neurophysin are always released in a fixed ratio reflecting the ratio in the granules.

The question whether vasopressin and neurophysin under physiological conditions leave the neuron as a complex cannot be answered at present. FAWCETT *et al.* (1968) labelled neurophysin in a few dogs by $^{35}$S cystein. When vasopressin release in such animals was stimulated violently by hemorrhage, labelled neurophysin and vasopressin were released, but with a much smaller proportion of neurophysin than was found in the neural lobe. Stimulation in vitro of neural lobes from such animals showed a higher proportion of neurophysin release. In experiments using an indirect method for detection of possible release of binding protein from isolated neural hemilobes of rats THORN (1966) could not find any such release. GINSBURG and IRELAND (1966) stimulated release of vasopressin from isolated neurosecretory granules by changes in pH of the medium. No demonstrable increase in supernatant protein was found. *A tentative conclusion seems to be that neurophysin may be released, but that there is no fixed ratio between vasopressin and neurophysin released.*

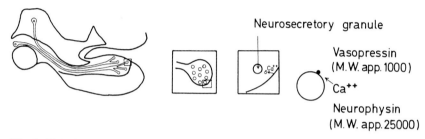

Fig. 3. Main features of the complex dissociation hypothesis for release of vasopressin

It seems probable that under certain circumstances hormone may pass the barriers between the storage location and the blood vessels independently of carrier protein. However, the pH and ionic composition (especially concentration of calcium) in the fluids outside the neurons are such that a dissociation would immediately occur in case the hormone should leave the axons bound to neurophysin.

Little attention has so far been paid to a possible release of the non-neurophysin-protein material in the granules.

*It seems to the present reviewer that there is as yet no proof that reverse pinocytosis takes place under physiological circumstances in the mammalian neurohypophysis. In many of the systems where exocytosis has been observed structually or suggested from biochemical studies, very strong stimulation has been used. It might be that there is a spectrum of release mechanisms ranging from release of vasopressin alone over "partial" to "total" reverse pinocytosis, depending on the strength of stimulation and the maturity of the material stored in the neurohypophysis.*

Whether reverse pinocytosis takes place or not it is necessary to explain the fate of the granule membranes, since the general consensus of opinion seems to be that they stay in the cells. The evidence for this being the case in monoaminergic cells has recently been summarized by DOUGLAS (1968).

A different hypothesis, the "complex dissociation" hypothesis, in the secretion mechanism has been put forward by SMITH and THORN (1965), THORN (1966), and supported by GINSBURG *et al.* (1966). According to this hypothesis, calcium detaches nonapeptide from its binding to the carrier protein in a pool of "easily releasable" hormone located within the nerve endings. The free nonapeptide then passes through the barriers to the blood. There must be a steep concentration gradient over these barriers, and there is a fairly high blood flow in the region. The two hypotheses may be compared with similar hypotheses for noradrenaline release from sympathetic nerve endings (HEDQUIST et al., 1968; FOLKOW et al., 1967). A crucial point in this hypothesis is the problem whether the stimulated nerve endings allow a reasonably free passage of vasopressin (and oxytocin). Some preliminary studies done in our laboratory, using $H^3$-lysine-vasopressin and ox neurohypophyses seem to support that this is the case (PLISKA, VILHARDT and THORN, in preparation).

## 10. Possible Role of Enzymic Break-Down of Vasopressin in the Secretion

An interesting recent development has been the demonstration of the presence in neurohypophyseal tissue of enzymes which destroy vasopressin (PLISKA, VILHARDT and THORN, 1970). Such enzymes have previously been demonstrated to be present in the hypothalamus. When tritiated lysine-vasopressin was added to tissue pieces from the neurohypophysis of oxen, a considerable break-down of hormone occurred. Split products were identified by thin layer chromatography in the tissue. It is possible that a considerable part of the hormone produced is broken down without ever reaching the blood stream. Such a condition would be in agreement with the suggestion by SMITH and FARQUHAR (1966) for anterior pituitary cells. Possibly, the findings of MASUR and HOLTZMAN (1969) could support such a notion. The localization of the enzymes in the neural lobe tissue is unknown, but it is known that hormone in granules is protected against enzymatic breakdown (WEINSTEIN et al., 1961). The enzymes might be localized to the axoplasm. LEBLOVA and RYCHLIK (1960) found oxytocin-destroying enzymes located there. It is possible that the "vasopressinase" can only attack hormone which has been liberated from binding to neurophysin. No information is available as yet on the possible control of the activity of the inactivating enzyme systems. If exocytosis is the normal process, the enzymes might take care of hormone that was spilt over from disintegrated or releasing granules.

## 11. Relation of Release to Synthesis

One can divide the pool of hormone in the whole system into two: That in the perikaryal part of the system, and that in the nerve endings (neurohypophysis). It is then possible to study the reactions of hormone in these two pools to different procedures. This was done by VILHARDT (1969) in our laboratory who studied the effect of dehydration and overhydration on vasopressin content and neurosecretory material in the system of rats as well as on the amount of hormone released after stimulation.

The result of these studies was that heavy overhydration for 4 hours causes more than doubling of the vasopressin content of the neurohypophysis with no change in the amount released on one stimulation by high potassium in vitro, or in the amount found in the hypothalamus (Table). The effect of overhydration seemed well documented since it was demonstrated also after 48 hours and 5 days (see also FENDLER *et al.*, 1968).

Table. *Effect of overhydration and dehydration on vasopressin content in neurohypophysis and hypothalamus and on amount of hormone released in vitro after stimulation by a high potassium concentration in the medium.* (From VILHARDT, 1969)

| | No. of expts. | Neurohypophysis | | Hypothalamus | |
|---|---|---|---|---|---|
| | | A | B | A | B |
| Normal | 5 | 776± 80 | 52±11 | 146±36 | 5±1 |
| Overhydrated 48 hours[a] | 3 | 1,128± 95[c] | 26± 1 | 35± 4[c] | 2±1[c] |
| Overhydrated 5 days[a] | 5 | 1,245±104[d] | 47± 3 | 45±19 | 2±1 |
| Dehydrated 48 hours | 6 | 412± 49[d] | 20± 6[c] | 111±40 | 10±5 |
| Dehydrated 10 days | 2 | 23± 5[d] | 3± 1[c] | 26± 7 | 2±1 |
| Overhydrated 4 hours[b] | 5 | 1,906±158[d] | 59±26 | 71±16 | 2±1[c] |

A = Vasopressin content in mU/1,000 g rat.
B = Amount of vasopressin (mU/1,000 g rat) released on a single stimulation with high K Locke solution.
[a] 10 ml of water per rat 4 times per 24 hrs.
[b] 10 ml of water per rat per hour.
[c] Statistically significant difference from normal group, $p < 0.05$.
[d] Statistically significant difference from normal group, $p < 0.005$.

The amount of stainable neurosecretory material varied in parallel with the changes in hormone content.

If this increase in neural lobe content is an expression of an unchanged rate of production in spite of a stop of the release, this may have several interesting consequences. One could then estimate the rate of production. This would be about 250 mU/1,000 g rat per hour. Using a method employed by SLOPER (1966) the approximate secretion rate per 1,000 g rat would be equivalent to 45 mU/ 1,000 g/hour. This means that during antidiuresis only 15–20% of the synthesized vasopressin is secreted. The rest would probably be destroyed enzymatically in the neurohypophysis by enzymes of the type found in preliminary experiments by PLISKA, VILHARDT and THORN.

If this calculation has any relation to the conditions in the gland, it has an important bearing on a problem mentioned by SACHS (1960). Studying the uptake of $^{35}$S labelled cystine after infusion into the 3rd ventricle of dogs he found a ratio of the specific activity of vasopressin from the hypothalamus over that in the neurohypophysis of 2–5. SACHS points out that considering the total amount of neurohypophyseal hormone and assuming that the secretion rate of vasopressin is 5 mU/hour (SHANNON, 1942), this ratio should be of the order of 400. He therefore concludes that it is possible that part of the hormone is synthesized in the neural lobe. However, if SLOPER's probably more realistic estimate for vasopressin secretion rate (44.5 mU/hour) is used, and if we assume that this represents less than 15% of the production rate (which consequently would be of the order of 300 mU/hour) then the ratio calculated in the same way that SACHS did would be less than 6.7. This is compatible with the findings of SACHS. The hypothesis of a synthesis of vasopressin in the neural lobe therefore seems to be unnecessary.

If the vasopressin secretion has such a small efficiency, and if neurophysin is synthesized and released with the vasopressin without any transformation to vasopressin anywhere, this means that the function besides production of granule membranes involves production of a considerable amount of hormone and of protein which is not used in the action of the system. This would seem to be a rather extravagant, uneconomic way of function, but probably necessary for the execution of the refined function[1]. It appears from Vilhardt's experiments that the rate of synthesis does not seem to be very intimately coupled to the rate of release, since depletion of the store in the neural lobe takes place during dehydration, and since during overhydration there is a marked accumulation of hormone.

## 12. Release of Vasopressin-Like Material from Bronchogenic Carcinoma Cells

Large amounts of vasopressin-like material are produced in certain cases of bronchogenic carcinoma. It is unknown what the mechanism of release of antidiuretic material from the tumour tissue is. It is possible that the abnormal cells constantly leak hormone, but the possibility of necrosis and consequent release of necrotic cell contents also exists.

Utiger (1968) stated that electron microscopic studies showed material in the tumour cells in his case which was similar to granules in neurohypophyseal tissue. Neurophysin has not been isolated from tumour tissue. It would seem unlikely that the cells possess the normal apparatus for the controlled release. At least the output of hormone in the urine is excessive.

### References

Barer, R., Lederis, K.: Ultrastructure of the rabbit neurohypophysis with special reference to the release of hormones. Z. Zellforsch. 75, 201–239 (1966).
Bie, P., Thorn, N. A.: In vitro studies of the release mechanism for vasopressin in rats. II. Studies of the possible release of hormone from hypothalamic tissue. Acta endocr. (Kbh.) 56, 139–145 (1967).
Bunt, A. H.: Fine structure of the pars distalis and interrenalis Taricha torosa after administration of metopirone (SU-48 85). Gen. comp. Endocr. 12, 134–147 (1969).
Daniel, A. R., Lederis, K.: Release of neurohypophysial hormones in vitro. J. Physiol. (Lond.) 190, 171–187 (1967).
Douglas, W. W., Poisner, A. M.: Stimulus-secretion coupling in a neurosecretory organ: The role of calcium in the release of vasopressin from the neurohypophysis. J. Physiol. (Lond.) 172, 1–18 (1964).
— Ishida, A., Poisner, A. M.: The effect of metabolic inhibitors on the release of vasopressin from the isolated neurohypophysis. J. Physiol. (Lond.) 181, 753–759 (1965).
— Stimulus-secretion coupling: The concept and clues from chromaffin and other cells. Brit. J. Pharmacol. 34, 451–474 (1968).
Dyball,R. E.J .: The time relation between the secretory and electrical responses of supraoptic neurones to osmotic stimuli. J. Physiol. (Lond.) 203, 67–68 P (1969).
— Koizumi, K.: Electrical activity in the supraoptic and paraventricular nuclei associated with neurohypophysial hormone release. J. Physiol. (Lond.) 201, 711–722 (1969).
Fawcett, C. P., Powell, A. E., Sachs, H.: Biosynthesis and release of neurophysin. Endocrinology 83, 1299–1310 (1968).

---

1 The enzymes present in the nerve endings and in the perikaryal region might be nonspecific proteolytic enzymes. They could have a function in transforming a precursor protein into nonapeptide in that region.

FENDLER, K., HEFCO, V., LISSÁK, K.: The effect of dehydration and repeated water loading on the supraoptic-neurohypophyseo-neurosecretory system and the ADH content of the neurohypophysis in the rat. Acta physiol. Acad. Sci. hung. **34**, 285–293 (1968).

FOLKOW, B., HÄGGENDAL, J., LISANDER, B.: Extent of release and elimination of noradrenaline at peripheral adrenergic nerve terminals. Acta physiol. scand., Suppl. **307** (1967).

FOLLETT, B. K., KOBAYASHI, H., FARNER, D. S.: The distribution of monoamine oxidase and acetylcholinesterase in the hypothalamus and its relation to the hypothalamo-hypophysial neurosecretory system in the white-crowned sparrow. Z. Zellforsch. **75**, 57–65 (1966).

FUXE, K.: Cellular localization of monoamines in the median eminence and the infundibular stem of some mammals. Z. Zellforsch. **61**, 710–724 (1964).

GILLESPIE, J. A., KIRKEPAR, S. M.: The uptake and release of radioactive noradrenaline by the splenic nerves of cat. J. Physiol. (Lond.) **187**, 51–68 (1966).

GINSBURG, M.: Production, release, transport and elimination of the neurohypophysial hormones. In: BERDE, B. (ed.), Neurohypophysial hormones and similar polypeptides. In: Handbuch der experimentellen Pharmakologie, Bd. 23, S. 286–371. Berlin-Heidelberg-New York: Springer 1968).

— IRELAND, M.: The role of neurophysin in the transport and release of neurohypophysial hormones. J. Endocr. **35**, 289–298 (1966).

— JAYASENA, K., THOMAS, P. J.: Preparation and properties of porcine neurophysin and the influence of calcium on the hormone-neurophysin complex. J. Physiol. (Lond.) **184**, 387–401 (1966).

HEDQUIST, P., LAGERCRANTZ, H., STJÄRNE, L.: Adenine nucleotides and catecholamine mobilization in adrenal medulla and in sympathetic nerves. Acta physiol. scand. **74**, 40–41 A (1968).

HELLER, H., HASAN, S. H., SAIFI, A. Q.: Antidiuretic activity in the cerebrospinal fluid. J. Endocr. **41**, 273–280 (1968).

LA BELLA, F. S.: Storage and secretion of neurohypophyseal hormones. Canad. J. Physiol. Pharmacol. **46**, 335–345 (1968).

LEBLOVA, S., RYCHLIK, I.: Inhibition of enzyme inactivation of oxytocin by amino acids. Coll. českoslov. chem. Commun. **25**, 2926–2929 (1960).

LEDERIS, K., LIVINGSTON, A.: Acetylcholine and related enzymes in the neural lobe and anterior hypothalamus of the rabbit. J. Physiol. (Lond.) **201**, 695–709 (1969).

LEVEQUE, J. E., SMALL, M.: The relationship of the pituicyte to the posterior lobe hormones. Endocrinology **65**, 909–915 (1959).

MASUR, S. K.: Fine structure of the autotransplanted pituitary in the red eft, *Notophthalmus viridescens*. Gen. comp. Endocr. **12**, 12–32 (1969).

MATSUI, T., KOBAYASHI, H.: Histochemical demonstration of monoamine oxidase in the hypothalamo-hypophysial system of the tree sparrow and the rat. Z. Zellforsch. **68**, 172–182 (1965).

MONROE, B. G.: A comparative study of the ultrastructure of the median eminence, infundibular stem and neural lobe of the hypophysis of the rat. Z. Zellforsch. **76**, 405–432 (1967).

PLISKA, V., VILHARDT, H., THORN, N. A.: In vitro uptake and breakdown of tritiated lysine-vasopressin by neurohypophyseal tissue from the ox. To be published (1970).

POISNER, A. M., DOUGLAS, W. W.: A possible mechanism of release of posterior pituitary hormones involving adenosine triphosphate and an adenosine triphosphatase in the neurosecretory granules. Mol. Pharmacol. **4**, 531–540 (1968).

— — Adenosine triphosphate and adenosine triphosphatase in hormone-containing granules of posterior pituitary gland. Science **160**, 203–204 (1968).

— TRIFARO, J. M.: The role of adenosine triphosphate and adenosine triphosphatase in the release of catecholamines from the adrenal medulla. III. Similarities between the effects of ATP on chromaffin granules and on mitochondria. Molec. Pharmacol. **5**, 294–299 (1969).

SACHS, H.: Vasopressin biosynthesis. I. In vivo studies. J. Neurochem. **5**, 297–303 (1960).

— HALLER, E. W.: Further studies on the capacity of the neurohypophysis to release vasopressin. Endocrinology **83**, 251–262 (1968).

— SHARE, L., OSINCHAK, J., CARPI, A.: Capacity of the neurohypophysis to release vasopressin. Endocrinology **81**, 755–770 (1967).

Schäker, W.: Untersuchungen über einen Oxytocin-Karboxymethyldextran-Komplex und den immunologischen Nachweis von Isoleucin³-Leucin⁸-Oxytocin nach Immunisierung mit dem Hormon-Dextran-Komplex. Acta biol. med. germ. **20**, 203–222 (1968).

Shannon, J. A.: The rate of liberation of the posterior pituitary antidiuretic hormone in the dog. J. exp. Med. **76**, 387–399 (1942).

Sloper, J. C.: Hypothalamic neurosecretion. Brit. med. Bull. **22**, 209–215 (1966).

Smith, M. W., Thorn, N. A.: The effects of calcium on protein-binding and metabolism of arginine vasopressin in rats. J. Endocr. **32**, 141–151 (1965).

Smith, R. E., Farquhar, M. G.: Lysosome function in the regulation of the secretory process in cells of the anterior pituitary gland. J. Cell Biol. **31**, 319–347 (1966).

Thorn, N. A.: In vitro studies of the release mechanism for vasopressin in rats. Acta endocr. (Kbh.) **53**, 644–654 (1966).

Utiger, R. D.: Disorders of antidiuretic hormone secretion. Med. Clin. N. Amer. **52**, 381–391 (1968).

Vilhardt, H.: Influence of prolonged overhydration and dehydration on vasopressin content and neurosecretory material in the hypothalamo-neurohypophysial system of rats. Acta physiol. scand. **76**, 30–31 A (1969).

Vorherr, M., Bradbury, M. W. B., Hoghoughi, M., Kleeman, C. R.: Antidiuretic hormone in cerebrospinal fluid during endogenous and exogenous changes in its blood level. Endocrinology **83**, 246–250 (1968).

Weinstein, H., Malamed, S., Sachs, H.: Isolation of vasopressin containing granules from the neurohypophysis of the dog. Biochim. biophys. Acta (Amst.) **50**, 386–389 (1961).

Wuu, T. C., Saffran, M.: Isolation and characterization of a hormone-binding polypeptide from pig posterior pituitary powder. J. biol. Chem. **25**, 482–490 (1969).

Zambrano, D., de Robertis, E.: The secretory cycle of supraoptic neurons in the rat. A structural-functional correlation. Z. Zellforsch. **73**, 414–431 (1966).

# The Role of the Neurophysins in Storage and Release of Hormones

D. B. Hope (Oxford)

*(Manuscript not received)*

# Electrical Discharge Patterns in Hypothalamic Neurosecretory Neurones Associated with Hormone Release*

R. E. J. Dyball

Department of Anatomy, University of Bristol (England)

**Key words:** Hypothalamus — Secretory neurones — Hormone release — Electrical discharge patterns.

There is a clearly defined nervous pathway connecting the neural lobe of the pituitary gland and the hypothalamus, and Harris (1955) showed that electrical stimulation of this hypothalamo-hypophysial tract would release oxytocin and vasopressin. It has been suggested, therefore, that an increase in the electrical activity, in the form of action potentials, of the neurones in the supraoptic and paraventricular nuclei is associated with neurohypophysial hormone release. Several attempts have been made to show that stimuli which release one or both these hormones also increase the electrical activity in the supraoptic and paraventricular nuclei (see Cross and Silver, 1966). However when recordings are made from neuronal units in the central nervous system it is difficult to be certain of the type of neurone from which the recordings are being made, even if the location of the recording electrode is known. To overcome this difficulty the technique of antidromic stimulation of the neural lobe was developed for the identification of supraoptic and paraventricular neurones in rats (Yagi, Azuma and Matsuda, 1966; Dyball, 1969b; Dyball and Koizumi, 1969). After neurosecretory units had been identified in this way their spontaneous discharge rate was monitored before and after intracarotid injections of hypertonic and isotonic NaCl solutions. The mean change in firing rate following the injections was then compared with the mean change in plasma ADH concentration at different time intervals after similar injections.

## Materials and Methods

Male Wistar rats approximately 200 g in weight, were anaesthetized with urethane (1.5 g/kg) and their right common carotid arteries were cannulated for the injection of hypertonic or isotonic sodium chloride solution. One group of animals was then prepared for blood collection by the insertion of cannulae into their right external jugular veins (to collect blood from the head). After the injection of heparin solution (1,000 iu) through the cannulated right femoral vein, 1 ml blood samples were collected into polythene centrifuge tubes, before and at varying time intervals after intracarotid injections of 0.25 ml of 1 molar NaCl solution or

* The author is much indebted to Professor B. A. Cross for his help in the preparation of the manuscript and to Miss P. Pountney for technical assistance. The work was supported by a grant from the Medical Research Council.

0.25 ml isotonic NaCl solution (at a rate of 0.6 ml/min). The blood samples were centrifuged and the resulting plasma samples were assayed as soon as possible (within $1^1/_2$ hours) for anti-diuretic activity in the ethanol-anaesthetised, water-loaded rat using the apparatus described by Dyball, Lane and Morris (1966). Rats from the other group were placed in a model H 200 Hoffman Reiter hypophysectomy instrument (H. Neuman & Co.) and a concentric stimulating electrode was introduced through the hollow ear piece of the instrument so that its tip lay just below the hypophysis (Dyball, 1969b). Using the hypophysectomy instrument as a head holder, electrical recordings were then made from single hypothalamic units using recording apparatus not essentially different from that used by Dyball and Koizumi (1969). Recordings were only made from those units from which antidromic action potentials could be elicited by single pulse stimulation of the neural lobe.

## Results

Fig. 1 A shows a photograph of a typical oscilloscope sweep which was trig-gered by a pulse delivered to the neural lobe. The first deflection is a stimulus

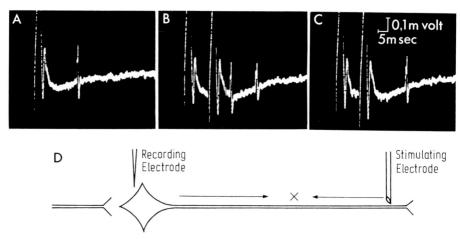

Fig. 1. Photographs of typical oscilloscope sweeps showing how neurosecretory units are identified: A Single stimulus pulse followed by an antidromic action potential; B 2 pulses and 2 action potentials; C 2 pulses but only 1 action potential since the first one had collided with a spontaneous spike; D Diagram to show the collision of spontaneous and antidromic action potentials

artefact and it is followed by an antidromic action potential. Typically the refractory period for the neurosecretory neurones was less than 5 msec so that two pulses delivered to the neural lobe with a 10 msec interval caused the appear-ance of 2 action potentials at the cell body, in the paraventricular nucleus in this case (see Fig. 1 B). To be completely certain that the action potentials recorded after the stimulus shocks are not spontaneous action potentials the collision technique illustrated in Fig. 1 D can be used. If a stimulus pulse is delivered to the neural lobe while a spontaneous action potential is travelling down the axon, no antidromic action potential will be seen at the soma since the two potentials will collide and cancel each other out. However a second pulse delivered to the neural lobe a few milliseconds later will give rise to the expected antidromic spike. This is illustrated in Fig. 1 C in which a train of 2 pulses was delivered to the neural lobe triggered by a spontaneous action potential. The first antidromic spike met the descending spontaneous spike and was cancelled out whereas the second appeared as expected.

After the identification of neurosecretory units in this way the effects of intra-carotid injection of isotonic and hypertonic solutions were tested. Fig. 2A shows the mean ± S.E. changes in firing rate caused by 30 injections of hypertonic and

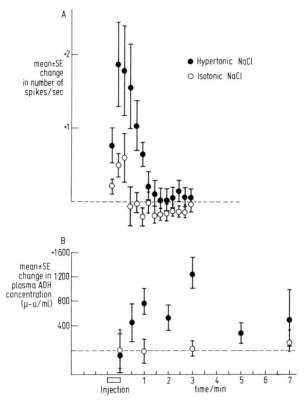

Fig. 2. A The mean ± S.E. changes in firing rate of supraoptic neurones caused by intracarotid injections of hypertonic and isotonic NaCl solution. B The mean ± S.E. changes in plasma ADH caused by similar isotonic and hypertonic injections

27 injections of isotonic NaCl on the 18 supraoptic units tested. Fig. 2B shows the mean ± S.E. changes caused by similar hypertonic and isotonic injections on the plasma concentrations of ADH (6 animals in each group). It can be seen that both firing rate and plasma ADH level were increased by the hypertonic injections but that isotonic injections had very little effect.

Fig. 3 shows the effects of 38 hypertonic and 33 isotonic injections on units of the paraventricular nucleus. It can be seen that hypertonic injections caused a considerably smaller change in discharge rate in the paraventricular nucleus than in the supraoptic nucleus.

Fig. 4 shows in the form of a block diagram the proportion of these injections which caused excitatory, inhibitory or inconclusive responses. A response was considered to have been excitatory if the number of spikes in 3 or 4 of the four

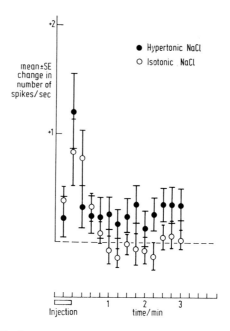

Fig. 3. The mean ± S.E. changes in firing rate of paraventricular neurones caused by intracarotid injections of hypertonic and isotonic NaCl solution

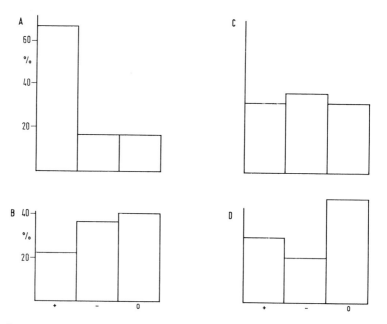

Fig. 4 A–D. The proportion of the intracarotid injections which produced excitatory (+),
inhibitory (−) or inconclusive (○) results: A Supraoptic nucleus, hypertonic injection.
B Supraoptic nucleus, isotonic injection. C Paraventricular nucleus, hypertonic injection.
D Paraventricular nucleus, isotonic injection

15 second periods starting immediately after the injection was higher than in a comparable control period, and to have been inhibitory if the number of spikes in 3 or 4 of them was less than in the control periods. Responses which fell into neither of these categories were considered as inconclusive. It can be seen that only in the case of the effects of hypertonic injections on the supraoptic nucleus was any marked excitation seen.

## Discussion

These results confirm earlier findings (CROSS, NOVIN and SUNDSTEN, 1969; DYBALL, 1969a; DYBALL and KOIZUMI, 1969; YAGI et al., 1966) that in addition to their secretory properties, the neurosecretory neurones of the neurohypophysis behave electrically in a way comparable to other neurones. Furthermore, although an increase in the firing rate of these neurosecretory neurones is associated with hormone release, the two events are not necessarily synchronous. If the maximum rate of hormone release is associated directly with the maximum rate of firing, it might be expected that the peak of electrical activity would precede the peak of plasma ADH level by a short period of time since the half life of vasopressin in blood is approximately 1 minute (GINSBURG, 1968). However the observed delay is approximately $2^1/_2$ minutes so hormone discharge probably continues after the subsidence of the electrical response. The possibility remains that when more units are tested a substantial number of longer responses will be observed.

The first part of the discussion has been concerned only with the supraoptic nucleus. But a similar investigation has been made on paraventricular neurones. Figs. 3 and 4 suggest that paraventricular units are less sensitive to hypertonic injections but it is possible that as experimental results accumulate more osmo-sensitive units will be found. The initial excitation during and immediately after the injections of hypertonic and isotonic NaCl, which is comparable to the excitation seen in the supraoptic nucleus after isotonic NaCl injection, is probably a non-specific effect. The most likely explanation is that the volume of the fluid injected causes minute movements of the tip of the recording electrode against the cell from which the recordings are being made and so excites it mechanically.

A further piece of evidence which suggests that there is a functional difference between the two nuclei is that although only 1 of the 19 supraoptic units tested was not spontaneously active, 5 out of the 18 paraventricular units were not active and would not have been detected had the neural lobe not been stimulated. This comparative lack of spontaneous activity has also been noted by CROSS et al. (1969) in the paraventricular nucleus of rabbits.

## Summary

Blood samples were taken and assayed for antidiuretic activity before and at different time intervals after intracarotid injections of isotonic and hypertonic sodium chloride solutions. In addition unit recordings were made from hypothalamic neurosecretory neurones, identified as such by antidromic stimulation of the posterior pituitary, following similar isotonic and hypertonic injections.

The peak of plasma antidiuretic activity occurred 3 minutes after the end of the injection whereas the maximum firing rate of the supraoptic units coincided with the end of the injection and the response had subsided after 1 minute. This implies a continued release of hormone after the end of the electrical response. Paraventricular units appeared to be less responsive to hypertonic injections.

## References

CROSS, B. A., NOVIN, D., SUNDSTEN, J. W.: Antidromic activation of neurones in the paraventricular nucleus by stimulation of the neural lobe of the pituitary. J. Physiol. (Lond.) **203**, 68–69 P (1969).
— SILVER, I. A.: Electrophysiological studies on the hypothalamus. Brit. med. Bull. **22**, 254–260 (1966).
DYBALL, R. E. J.: The time relation between the secretory and electrical responses of supraoptic neurones to osmotic stimuli. J. Physiol. (Lond.) **203**, 67–68 P (1969a).
— Stimulation of the neurohypophysis of the rat by a transaural approach. J. Physiol. (Lond.) **203**, 3–4 P (1969b).
— KOIZUMI, K.: Electrical activity in the supraoptic and paraventricular nuclei associated with neurohypophysial hormone release. J. Physiol. (Lond.) **201**, 711–722 (1969).
— LANE, G. J., MORRIS, R. G.: A simplified automatic device for the performance of antidiuretic assays. J. Physiol. (Lond.) **186**, 43–44 (1966).
GINSBURG, M.: Production, release, transportation and elimination of the neurohypophysial hormones. In: Handbuch der experimentellen Pharmakologie, Bd. 23, S. 286–371. Berlin-Heidelberg-New York: Springer 1968.
HARRIS, G. W.: In: Neural control of the pituitary gland. London: Edward Arnold Ltd. 1955.
YAGI, K., AZUMA, T., MATSUDA, K.: Neurosecretory cell: capable of conducting impulses in rats. Science **154**, 778–779 (1966).

# The Ultrastructure of Neurosecretory Fibre Terminals after Zinc-Iodine-Osmium Impregnation

Francis Knowles and Brian Weatherhead

Department of Anatomy, King's College, London (England)

Rainer Martin

Stazione Zoologica, Naples (Italy)

**Key words:** Neurosecretion — Fibre terminals — Ultrastructure.

The nature of the small electron-lucent vesicles present in neurosecretory neurons have been the subject of controversy for many years. Some authors have suggested that they may be synaptic vesicles containing acetylcholine since they resemble in size (c. 400–500 Å diameter) and position the synaptic vesicles in known cholinergic fibres (De Robertis and Bennett, 1954). This view has been criticised (Holmes and Knowles, 1960) because the content of these vesicles has not been positively identified.

An alternative hypothesis was proposed at the IIIrd International Symposium at Bristol in these words "That vesicles of about 300–500 Å in diameter seen in neurosecretory fibre terminations may not be true synaptic vesicles, but represent disintegration products of larger vesicles" (Knowles, 1962). Since then this idea, subsequently termed the "Fragmentation Theory" has received considerable support from observations that elementary neurosecretory vesicles fragment to form smaller, electron-lucent, vesicles (Knowles, 1963; Herlant, 1967; Normann, 1969).

This evidence for the fragmentation of elementary neurosecretory vesicles at fibre terminals supports the view that many of the small vesicles seen there might be formed as a *result* of the processes leading to neurosecretory hormone release: such evidence does not, however, exclude a possibility that some of the small vesicles might be true synaptic vesicles, containing transmitter substances which, under suitable conditions, might *cause* hormone release. If this were so it should be possible to differentiate chemically two types of small vesicle at neurosecretory fibre terminals. Thus far methods in current use in electron microscopy have distinguished only one type of small vesicle.

Akert and Sandri (1968) demonstrated that the Champy-Maillet zinc-iodine-osmium method (ZIO) previously used to reveal peripheral nerve endings with the light microscope could also be used successfully to stain the synaptic vesicles shown by the electron microscope. Clearly the application of this method to neurosecretory fibres might determine whether some, at least, of the small vesicles seen there should properly be called synaptic vesicles, with biochemical as well as morphological resemblance to synaptic vesicles present in cholinergic and adrenergic neurons.

## Materials and Methods

Small dogfish (c. 30 cm in length) of the species *Scyliorhinus stellaris* were used in the present studies. The ultrastructure of the pituitary neurointermediate lobe of this species has previously been described elsewhere in detail (Knowles, 1965).

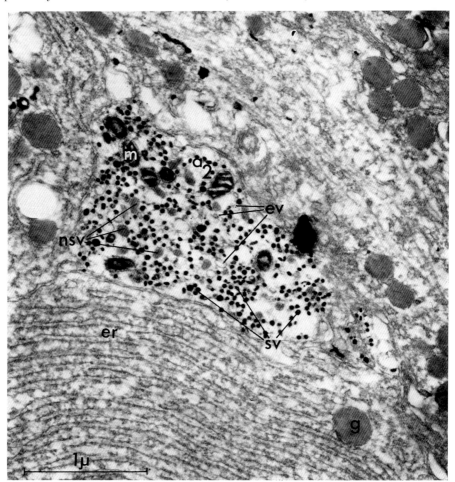

Fig. 1. *Scyliorhinus stellaris*, neurointermediate lobe impregnated by the zinc-iodine-osmium method. An $A_2$ neurosecretory fibre terminal making contact with the synthetic pole of an intrinsic intermedia cell. Note the small densely stained vesicles (*sv*), the small electron-lucent vesicles (*ev*) and the neurosecretory vesicles (*nsv*). *er* endoplasmic reticulum of the intrinsic intermedia cell; *m* mitochondrion; *g* secretory granule of the intrinsic intermedia cell

A modification of the Akert-Sandri technique was used (see Martin, Barlow and Miralto, 1969). Instead of direct immersion of the tissue in zinc, iodine and osmium tetroxide, the animals, anaesthetised with MS 222, were first perfused with glutaraldehyde (filtered sea water 80 ml; 50% glutaraldehyde 7 ml; distilled water 13 ml; pH adjusted to 7.2 with 0.1 N NaOH) at room temperature. 80 ml of the fixative was injected through the heart, the pituitary was dissected out and immersed in a further volume of fixative for one hour; it was then washed in physiological saline and incubated in the zinc-iodine-osmium mixture at 4°C for 12 hours. Subsequently it was dehydrated in acetone and embedded in Durcupan (Fluka).

Since the neurosecretory fibres to be studied, in the neurointermediate lobe, are believed to regulate MSH synthesis and release and thereby the colour of the animal, attention was paid to the state of illumination, and the background on which the animals were maintained. Comparative studies in this respect will form the subject of a later communication. Here the relationship between the fibre terminals and their state of functional activity will receive only brief mention.

## Results

The results obtained by the method described above differ from any hitherto described for the electron microscopic examination of neurosecretory tissues. In direct contrast to previous observations the elementary neurosecretory vesicles,

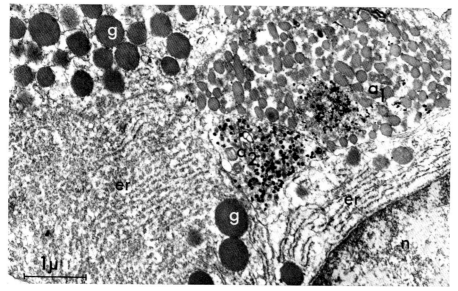

Fig. 2. Dual innervation of the synthetic pole of an intrinsic intermedia cell by both A$_1$ ($a_1$) and A$_2$ ($a_2$) neurosecretory fibres. $n$ nucleus of intrinsic intermedia cell; $er$ endoplasmic reticulum; $g$ secretory granule

diameter c. 1,800 Å, were rendered only very slightly electron-dense, but most of the smaller vesicles at the fibre terminals became intensely electron dense (Fig. 1). Tissue incubation for more than 12 hours increased the electron density of some other tissue components, e.g. mitochondria, but shorter periods of incubation resulted in a clear distinction between the "synaptic" vesicles and other components in the neurosecretory fibres.

Previous studies on the ultrastructure of the neurosecretory innervation of the pituitary intermedia cells of *Scyliorhinus* indicated a dual innervation (KNOWLES, 1965), with Type A or peptidergic fibres making direct synaptoid contacts with the synthetic poles of the intrinsic intermedia cells and Type B, or aminergic, fibres making similar contacts with the release poles. The present studies reveal an even greater complexity of innervation.

In the earlier description two classes of fibre innervating the synthetic pole were noted, distinguished by the size of their contained elementary neurosecretory vesicles, respectively 1,800 and 1,000 Å in diameter. At the time it was suggested

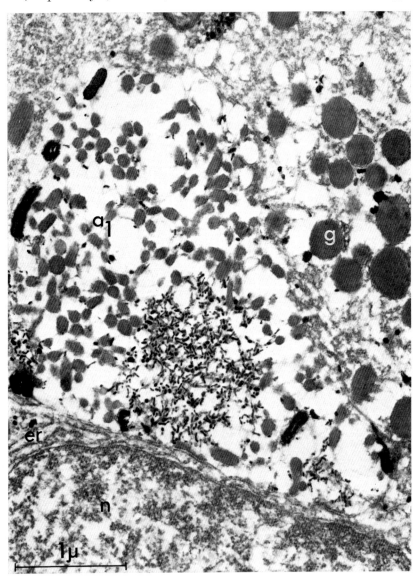

Fig. 3. Type $A_1$ neurosecretory fibre terminal in contact with the synthetic pole of an intermedia cell. Note the elongated form of the densely stained small vesicles. *er* endoplasmic reticulum; *g* secretory granule; *n* nucleus

that both might be Type A fibres ($A_1$ and $A_2$), but the precise nature and distribution of that fibre with smaller vesicles ($A_2$) was left open to question. The present investigation has shown that the intrinsic cells are commonly innervated by *both* types of fibre, at their synthetic poles (Fig. 2). Closer examination of the fibres with smaller vesicles revealed greater morphological resemblances to B than to $A_1$ fibres. Until the $A_2$ fibres have been studied in greater detail this term $A_2$ will be used here, but the possibility that they are aminergic must be envisaged. For the present it will suffice to remark that at least three types of neurosecretory fibre

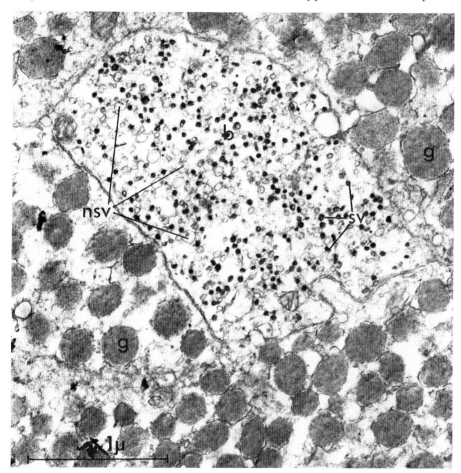

Fig. 4. Type B neurosecretory fibre terminal making contact with the release poles of inter-media cells. Note the small strongly stained vesicles (*sv*) and the large electron-lucent neurosecretory vesicles, some of which contain small dense cores (*nsv*). *g* secretory granules

make direct contact with cells of the pituitary neurointermediate lobe of *Scyliorhinus*.

In the $A_1$ fibres ZIO-positive vesicles were frequently grouped together, with or without accompanying small electron-lucent vesicles, to form small circumscribed areas, generally close to the points of contact between the $A_1$ fibres and intrinsic cells (see Fig. 2). In contrast the ZIO-positive vesicles in $A_2$ and B fibres were more evenly dispersed throughout the terminals.

In all classes of fibre terminal two states could be distinguished, as follows:

11*

(1) In some fibre terminals there were many tightly packed elementary neuro-secretory vesicles and many ZIO-positive vesicles were present.

(2) In other terminals small electron-lucent vesicles were more frequent, but there were relatively few elementary neurosecretory vesicles and many of these appeared "empty". The number of ZIO-positive vesicles also seemed less, and in many instances these vesicles were notably elongate in form (Fig. 3).

An abundance of small vesicles both ZIO-positive and -negative associated with few and "empty" neurosecretory vesicles may indicate an active fibre. Therefore it is interesting to note that B fibres in animals maintained on illuminated white backgrounds showed these features to a marked degree (Fig. 4). Under these conditions the dogfish is maximally pale and MSH secretion minimal, so the supposition that the B fibre shown is in a state of activity would accord well with the widely held view that these aminergic fibres inhibit MSH release.

A possibility that aminergic fibres might inhibit MSH synthesis should also be envisaged, and in this connection it is interesting to note that the $A_2$ (or B ?) fibres innervating the synthetic poles of intrinsic cells appeared active in animals on illuminated white backgrounds, but less active in animals in darkness. Conversely, preliminary observations indicate that the $A_1$ fibres were more active in darkness. Such correlations might indicate that the $A_1$ fibres are excitatory and the $A_2$ and B fibres inhibitory in action.

## Discussion

Precise correlation between conditions of illumination and background, states of MSH synthesis and release, and functional activity of A and B fibres and their ultrastructure must await a more detailed investigation of these parameters. Meanwhile it is worthy of note that the present results indicate that the ZIO-positive vesicles appear to be more elongated in fibres that are presumed to be active and that Pellegrino de Iraldi and Gueudet (1968) have described an elongation of ZIO-positive vesicles in adrenergic nerves after reserpine treatment.

The functional and biochemical interpretations of these findings must await a better knowledge of the specificity of the zinc-iodine-osmium method. Pellegrino de Iraldi and Gueudet (1968) have shown that the stained component is neither catecholamine nor indoleamine, but whether the method may stain acetylcholine as suggested by Akert and Sandri (1968), or part of an acetylcholine complex, is still an open question. For the present no claim that the method stains a transmitter substance in neurosecretory fibre terminals is made, but attention is drawn to the main interest of the observations, namely, that they demonstrate some chemical affinity as well as morphological affinity between the synaptic vesicles of cholinergic fibres and small vesicles at neurosecretory fibre terminals.

Whether small vesicles at neurosecretory fibre terminals may arise by fragmentation of elementary neurosecretory vesicles cannot be determined from the present studies alone. It is, however, clear from the greater electron density of the small ZIO-positive vesicles that if they arise from the larger vesicles, the contents of the surrounding membranes of the latter must undergo some marked change during this process. The presence of small electron-lucent vesicles together with small electron-dense vesicles (Fig. 1) shows that size of vesicle alone does not determine their staining affinities. Chemical identification of the contents, which evidently reduce osmium in the presence of zinc and iodine, is therefore of paramount importance.

The specificity of the zinc-iodine-osmium method is open to question, and its chemical basis is not yet known. It principal interest for students of neurosecretion is that it does, for the first time, stain some of the so-called synaptic vesicles in neurosecretory fibres and thus makes more feasible an analysis of the part they may play in hormone release.

### References

AKERT, K., SANDRI, C.: An electron-microscopic study of zinc iodide-osmium impregnation of neurons. I. Staining of synaptic vesicles at cholinergic junctions. Brain Res. **7**, 286–295 (1968).

DE ROBERTIS, E. P., BENNETT, H. S.: Submicroscopic vesicular component in synapses. Fed. Proc. **13**, 35 (Abstract) (1954).

HERLANT, M.: Mode de libération des produits de neurosécrétion. In: Neurosecretion (ed. F. STUTINSKY), p. 20–35. Berlin-Heidelberg-New York: Springer 1967.

HOLMES, R. L., KNOWLES, F. G. W.: "Synaptic vesicles" in the neurohypophysis. Nature (Lond.) **185**, 709–711 (1960).

KNOWLES, Sir F.: In discussion following paper by HELLER, H., and LEDERIS, K., Characteristics of isolated neurosecretory vesicles from mammalian neural lobes. In: Neurosecretion (eds. HELLER, H., and CLARK, R. B.). Mem. Soc. Endocr. **12**, 49–50 (1962).

— Techniques in the study of neurosecretion. In: Techniques in endocrine research (eds. ECKSTEIN, P., KNOWLES, F., p. 57–75. London-New York: Academic Press 1963.

— Evidence for a dual control, by neurosecretion, of hormone synthesis and hormone release in the pituitary of the dogfish, *Scylliorhinus stellaris*. Phil. Trans. B. **249**, 435–455 (1965).

MARTIN, R., BARLOW, J., MIRALTO, A.: Application of the zinc iodide-osmium tetroxide impregnation of synaptic vesicles in cephalopod nerves. Brain Res. **15**, 1–16 (1969).

NORMANN, T. CH.: Experimentally induced exocytosis of neurosecretory granules. Exp. Cell Res. **55**, 285–287 (1969).

PELLEGRINO DE IRALDI, A., GUEUDET, R.: Action of reserpine on the osmium tetroxide zinc iodide reactive site of synaptic vesicles in the pineal nerves of the rat. Z. Zellforsch. **91**, 178–185 (1968).

# Electron Microscopic and Autoradiographic Study on the Neurosecretory System of Albino Rats with Special Consideration of the Pituicyte Problem

J. Krsulovic, A. Ermisch and G. Sterba

Laboratory of Neurobiology, Leipzig (DDR)

**Key words:** Neurosecretion — Pituicytes.

As to the functional role of pituicytes there are two main opinions. Some workers assume they play the same role as glia cells in the central nervous system, that is a supportive, especially trophic, function (Hartmann, 1958; Fujita and Hartmann, 1961; Polenov and Belenkii, 1964). Others propose that pituicytes have a special function related to neurosecretory activity (Ortmann, 1951; Kurosumi, 1964). The fact that, after transection of the pituitary stalk, pituicytes are able to phagocytize NSM (Sterba and Brückner, 1967, 1969; Dellmann and Owsley, 1969) suggests that also in the intact animal a process of degradation may take place.

It seems to be important to obtain more information about the characteristics of the relationship between neurosecretory cells and pituicytes. With this aim the neurosecretory system of the rat, known to be involved in the regulation of water metabolism (Bargmann and Scharrer, 1951), has been further investigated in normal and dehydrated animals. The correlation of metabolic and morphologic changes, especially in those areas where pituicytes are in close contact with neurosecretory terminals, was given special attention.

## Material and Methods

Male adult albino rats weighing 150–200 g were used.

*Electron Microscopy.* Neural lobes of ten rats (4 controls and 6 deprived of water for seven days) were investigated. Prefixation with glutaraldehyde (4%) was performed in situ, and in two animals by perfusion. For postfixation a mixture of $OsO_4$ and $K_2Cr_2O_7$ was used (Wohlfarth-Bottermann, 1957). "Staining" followed according to Reynolds (1963). Electron microscopes used were KEM 1–1 and SEM of VEB Fernsehelektronik, Berlin-Oberschöneweide.

*Autoradiography.* Fourteen rats were used. Preliminary values reported here concern only four among these animals (2 controls, and 2 dehydrated for seven days). The rats were injected subcutaneously with $^{35}S$-DL-cystine (Isocomerz Dresden, specific activity 66 mCi/mM). 3–5.2 μCi per gram body weight, and killed by decapitation at different intervals (1–3–6–10–15–20 and 24 hours) after the injection. The four rats considered here belong to the ten-hour group. The hypophyses were quickly removed and, after fixation in Bouin, embedded in paraffin. In two animals (1 control and 1 dehydrated) a piece of tissue was fixed in glutaraldehyde and $OsO_4$-$K_2Cr_2O_7$ and further processed for electron microscopy.

All the counts were corrected in relation to the amount of $^{35}S$-DL-cystine injected, the exposure time, and the half-life of $^{35}S$.

## Results

In electron micrographs of the neurohypophysis of normal rats two kinds of neurosecretory nerve endings can be observed: (1) a "storage form" with closely

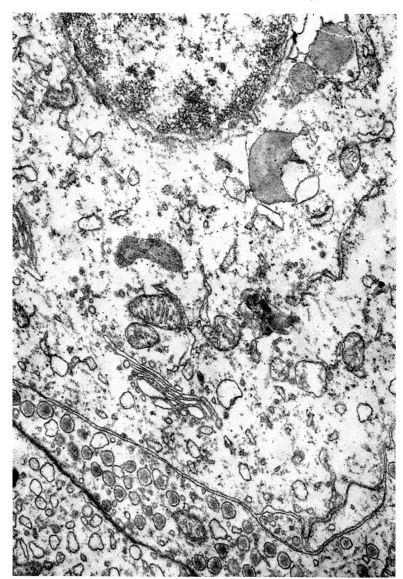

Fig. 1. Electron micrograph of neurohypophysis of a control rat. Part of a normal pituicyte and two neurosecretory nerve endings. ×35,000

packed elementary granules (EG), and (2) an "active form" containing mainly residual granules. The first appears to be more numerous. Normal pituicytes predominate and are characterized by a mean nuclear volume of $120 \mu^3$. The rough endoplasmic reticulum is poorly developed. The membranes bounding the characteristic osmiophilic granules sometimes shows continuity with those of the Golgi apparatus and the smooth endoplasmic reticulum, which often fuse with

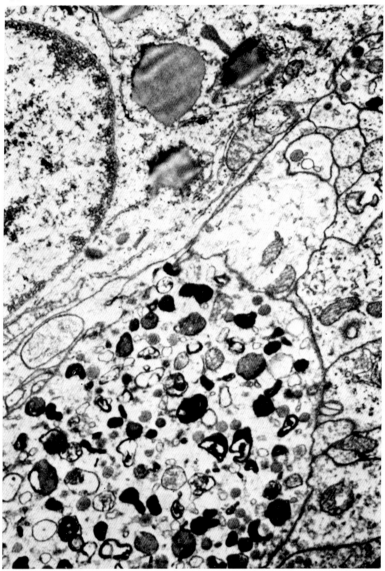

Fig. 2. Electron micrograph of neurohypophysis after seven days of dehydration. Part of an hypertrophied pituicyte surrounded by several nerve endings, the large one remarkably modified in comparison to normal types. ×30,000

the plasma membrane. These spatial relationships argue in favor of interpreting the lipid droplets as important cellular constituents or organelles (Fig. 1).

After seven days of dehydration the neurosecretory axons contain only occasional EG. Instead, their terminals show residual granules and microvesicles.

Many of these nerve endings are modified or degenerated. Hypertrophied pitui-cytes are most common. Their mean nuclear volume is 190 $\mu^3$; the perinuclear cytoplasm is abundant. The amount of rough endoplasmic reticulum is substanti-

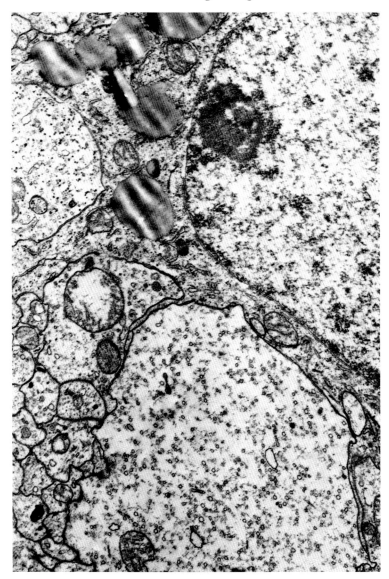

Fig. 3. Electron micrograph of hypertrophied pituicyte surrounded by several nerve endings, the large one loaded with microvesicles. $\times 20,000$

ally increased, while the Golgi apparatus appears proportionally less developed. In these pituicytes, the rough endoplasmic reticulum shows close relationships with the osmiophilic granules and extends to the periphery of the cell. The number and size of the osmiophilic granules is increased after stimulation. The ground cytoplasm is denser than in control specimens on account of increased numbers of free and membraned-bound ribosomes (Figs. 2, 3).

In autoradiographs the labelled material was found within pituicytes of normal and dehydrated rats. A precise localization of the labelled substance in the pituicyte was only possible in sections of 1 μm. In the stripping film above pituicytes of dehydrated rats more grains were found than in controls. Grain counts confirm this optical impression. This result parallels the autoradiographic observations on the hypothalamic neurosecretory nuclei (NSO and NPV). In these neurosecretory cells likewise more radioactive material is present in dehydrated animals than in normal ones. According to present results, the quantity of radioactive material present in pituicytes exceeds that in neurosecretory endings (table).

Table. *Relative $^{35}S$ concentration in normal and dehydrated rats*

| Rats | Thick sections | Pitui- cytes | Area $(\mu^2)$ | Nerve endings | Area $(\mu^2)$ | NS cells NSO | NPV | Area $(\mu^2)$ |
|---|---|---|---|---|---|---|---|---|
| Control | 5 | 2.10 | 100 | | | 1.08 | 0.96 | 1,000 |
| | 1 | 0.7 | 1,700 | 0.34 | 1,700 | | | |
| Dehydrated 7 days | 5 | 5.78 | 150 | | | 2.51 | 2.39 | 1,000 |
| | 1 | 1.88 | 1,700 | 1.26 | 1,700 | | | |

The values concern four animals of the ten hour interval group.

## Discussion

The results of the present study lead to the assumption that a transfer of NSM takes place from nerve endings to pituicytes. The quantity of material transferred and its ulterior degradation (ultraphagocytosis) probably determine the three different morpho-functional stages recognizable in the pituicytes (Krsulovic and Brückner, 1969). An active form of transport between nerve endings and pituicytes may be supposed. "Carrier molecules" (de Robertis, Nowinski and Saez, 1965), probably enzymes localized in the plasma membrane, may direct the entry of neurosecretory material into the endoplasmic reticulum of pituicytes. The process itself may occur by means of micropinocytosis (ultraphagocytosis).

In normal and hypertrophied pituicytes the "ingested material" and the concomitant need for hydrolytic enzymes may account for the presence of phagosomes, digestive vacuoles, or true lysosomes, i.e., the osmiophilic granules so numerous in the cytoplasm. Presumably, under normal conditions there is a balance between the material that the cell receives and its enzymatic capacity (within storage granules). In hypertrophied cells, the increase in free ribosomes and rough endoplasmic reticulum may be explained by the greater need for hydrolytic enzymes, since more NSM is taken up by this cell. Proteinases produced by these cells seem to exceed lipolytic enzymes, a fact which may account for the accumulation of lipids (Raviola and Raviola, 1963). Large vacuolated granules of moderate electron density, considerably increased in the damaged stage, probably represent "residual bodies" containing material that cannot be digested.

The incorporation of neurophysin macromolecules by pituicytes and the transport function of these cells was recently postulated by RODRÍGUEZ and LA POINTE (1969). Their views are thus in accord with those of the present authors. On the other hand, the high uptake of labelled tracers by pituicytes of dehydrated rats suggests that this material becomes a component of an enzyme rich in sulphur, and that the $^{35}S$ derives directly from the blood and not from hyperactive neurosecretory neurons. Perhaps a combination of these two possibilities exists.

## Summary

In the neurosecretory system of normal and dehydrated male albino rats the neural lobe was investigated, and special attention was payed to pituicytes and nerve endings. There was an inverse relation between the quantity of neurosecretory material (NSM) in the nerve endings and the number and size of osmiophilic granules within the cytoplasm of pituicytes. Hypertrophied pituicytes showed considerable polymorphism. There were peculiar changes in the vacuolar system of the cytoplasm which, in some areas, showed a morphologic relationship with the membranes of the osmiophilic granules. The assumption that macromolecules present in the nerve endings, such as parts of the NSM rich in cystine, may be transferred to pituicytes is in part supported also by results obtained in the autoradiographic experiments.

## References

BARGMANN, W., SCHARRER, E.: The site of origin of the hormones of the posterior pituitary. Amer. Scientist 39, 255–259 (1951).

DELLMANN, H. D., OWSLEY, P. A.: Investigations in the hypothalamo-neurosecretory system of the green frog (Rana pipiens) after transection of the proximal neurohypophysis. II. Light and electronmicroscopic findings in the disconnected neurohypophysis, with special emphasis on the pituicytes. Z. Zellforsch. 94, 325–336 (1969).

DE ROBERTIS, E., NOWINSKI, W., SAEZ, F.: The cytoplasmic vacuolar system and microsomes. In: Cell biology. Philadelphia: W. B. Saunders Company 1965.

FUJITA, H., HARTMANN, J. F.: Electron microscopy of the neurohypophysis in normal, adrenaline-treated and pilocarpine-treated rabbits. Z. Zellforsch. 54, 734–763 (1961).

HARTMANN, J.: Electron-microscopy of the neurohypophysis in normal and histamine-treated rats. Z. Zellforsch. 48, 291–308 (1958).

KRSULOVIC, J., BRÜCKNER, G.: Morphologic characteristics of pituicytes in different functional stages. Z. Zellforsch. 99, 210–220 (1969).

KUROSUMI, K., MATSUZAWA, T., KOBAYASHI, Y., SATO, S.: On the relation between the release of neurosecretory substance and lipid granules of pituicyte in the rat neurohypophysis. Gunma Symposia on Endocrinology, vol. 1, p. 87–118. Published from Institute of Endocrinology, Gunma University, Maebashi, Japan 1964.

ORTMANN, R.: Über experimentelle Veränderungen der Morphologie des Hypophysen-Zwischenhirnsystems und die Beziehung der sog. „Gomorisubstanz" zum Adiuretin. Z. Zellforsch. 36, 92–140 (1951).

POLENOV, A. L., BELENKII, M. A.: Electron-microscopic investigation of the ultrastructure of the neurosecretory elements of the posterior lobe of the hypophysis in albino mice. Dokl. Akad. Nauk SSSR 154, 940 (1964).

RAVIOLA, E., RAVIOLA, G.: Histochemistry of the rat neurohypophysial pituicyte lipid granules. Autooxidation of unsaturated fats during fixation. J. Histochem. Cytochem. 11, No 2 (1963).

REYNOLDS, E. S.: The use of lead citrate at high pH as an electron opaque stain in electron-microscopy. J. Cell Biol. 17, 208–215 (1963).

Rodríguez, E. M., la Pointe, J.: Histology and ultrastructure of the neural lobe of the lizard, *Klauberina riversiana*. Z. Zellforsch. **95**, 37–57 (1969).

Sterba, G., Brückner, G.: Zur Funktion der ependymalen Glia in der Neurohypophysis. Z. Zellforsch. **81**, 457–473 (1967).

— — Elektronenmikroskopische Untersuchungen über die Reaktion der Pituicyten nach Hypophysenstieldurchtrennung bei *Rana esculenta*. Z. Zellforsch. **93**, 74–83 (1969).

Wohlfarth-Bottermann, K. E.: Kontrastierung tierischer Zellen und Gewebe im Rahmen ihrer elektronenmikroskopischen Untersuchung an ultradünnen Schnitten. Naturwissenschaften **44**, 287–288 (1957).

# The Origin of "Synaptic" Vesicles in Neurosecretory Axons*

Lutz Vollrath

Department of Anatomy, University of Würzburg (Germany)

**Key words:** Neurosecretion — "Synaptic" vesicles.

It is generally accepted that the so-called synaptic vesicles found in terminals of neurosecretory axons are closely related to the release of neurosecretory material. It is, however, unclear whether these structures represent true synaptic vesicles containing acetylcholine which is needed for the liberation of neurohormones (DE ROBERTIS, 1964) or whether they are fragments of elementary granules (HOLMES and KNOWLES, 1960; BERN, 1963; KNOWLES, 1963, 1965; LEDERIS, 1965; HERLANT, 1967) or derivatives of multilamellar structures (LEDERIS, 1964; HOLMES and KIERNAN, 1964). Since the methods hitherto applied have not solved this problem (BARGMANN, 1967), the attempt was made (see also VOLLRATH, 1969) to study the origin of "synaptic" vesicles in fetal and newborn rats, for it was hoped that, by this ontogenetical approach, the formation of these structures might become more clearly visible than in adult rats whose neurohypophyseal axons contain large numbers of elementary granules and mitochondria.

## Material and Methods

In the present study 9 male and female Wistar rats from the 19th day of gestation to the 2nd postnatal day and 9 adult rats were used. The neurohypophyses were rapidly dissected out, cut into small pieces, fixed in 3% phosphate or cacodylate buffered glutaraldehyde for 3 h, postfixed in 1% phosphate or cacodylate buffered osmium tetroxide for 3 h, and embedded in Araldite. Sections, cut on a manual Porter-Blum microtome, were stained with 7% uranyl acetate and lead hydroxide according to MILLONIG. Electron microscope: Philips E.M. 300.

## Results and Discussion

The neurohypophyses of fetal and newborn rats differ from those of adult rats in that their axons contain only few elementary granules (1,000–2,000 Å in diameter) and few "synaptic" vesicles, i.e. electron-lucent vesicles of 300 to 600 Å in diameter. With regard to the formation of "synaptic" vesicles, tubules of up to 3,000 Å in length and 300 to 400 Å in width are of importance (Fig. 1). These structures are not identical with neurotubules, but occasionally were seen to be in continuity with them. These tubules, present mainly in terminals of neurosecretory axons, frequently show indentations at regular intervals and give rise to vesicles of the synaptic vesicle size range. As a results of this process "synaptic" vesicles may be found lying in rows.

* Supported by a grant of the Deutsche Forschungsgemeinschaft.

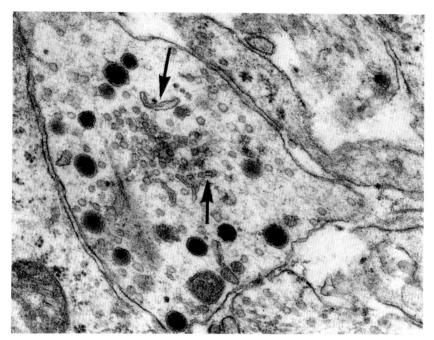

Fig. 1. Terminal of a neurosecretory axon containing tubulated structures (arrows) which are closely related to the formation of "synaptic" vesicles. Neurohypophysis of a 2 day old rat. ×47,900

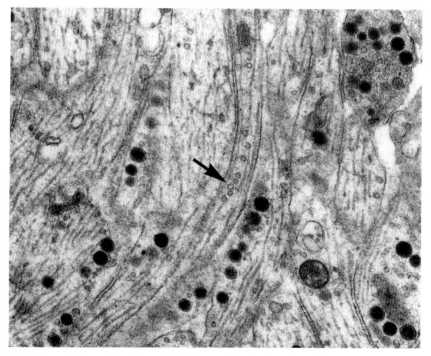

Fig. 2. "Synaptic" vesicles (arrow) in the preterminal region of a neurosecretory axon. Neurohypophysis of a 2 day old rat. ×32,000

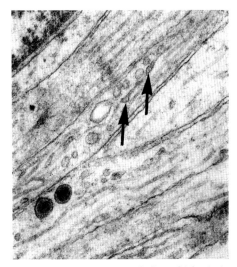

Fig. 3. Sac-like dilatations (arrows) of neurotubules which, it is suggested, give rise to "synaptic" vesicles. 20 day old rat fetus. ×44,500

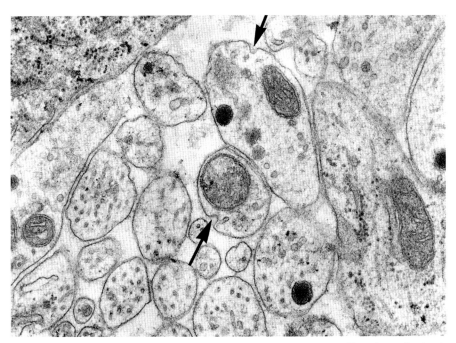

Fig. 4. Nerve fibres showing micropinocytotic invaginations (arrows). Neurohypophysis of a 1 h old rat. ×51,300

The nerve fibre terminals are not the only sites in which "synaptic" vesicles are present. They are also found in preterminal regions of neurosecretory axons (Fig. 2) and are thought to be derived from sack-like dilatations of neurotubules (Fig. 3).

Another possibility for the formation of "synaptic" vesicles is that micro-pinocytotic invaginations of the axolemma (Fig. 4) give rise to vesicles which are indistinguishable from "synaptic" vesicles if they are of the 300 to 600 Å size range.

A third possibility for the formation of "synaptic" vesicles in young rats corresponds to that described by Herlant (1967): small vesicles originate by budding from the membranes of elementary granules. This mechanism, however, does not seem to play an important role in young rats.

No indications were obtained in our material that "synaptic" vesicles occur within elementary granules.

From these results it is evident that "synaptic" vesicles, even within a single neurosecretory axon, are a heterogeneous group of vesicles and that this hetero-geneity has to be taken into account when a functional interpretation of these structures is attempted. It is not intended to give a new functional interpretation of the "synaptic" vesicles on the basis of the results described above. It has to be emphasized, however, that the functional interpretation of "synaptic" vesicles as given by de Robertis (1964) is more likely to be valid if these structure do not represent remnants of elementary granules. The observation that the majority of "synaptic" vesicles originate from neurotubules, in our opinion supports de Robertis' concept.

## References

Bargmann, W.: Schlußwort. In: Neurosecretion (ed. F. Stutinsky), p. 241–247. Berlin-Heidelberg-New York: Springer 1967.

Bern, H. A.: The secretory neuron as a doubly specialized cell. In: General physiology of cell specialization (D. Mazia and A. Tyler, eds.), p. 349–366. New York: McGraw-Hill 1963.

Herlant, M.: Mode de libération des produits de neurosécrétion. In: Neurosecretion (ed. F. Stutinsky), p. 20–35. Berlin-Heidelberg-New York: Springer 1967.

Holmes, R. L., Kiernan, J. A.: The fine structure of the infundibular process of the hedgehog. Z. Zellforsch. 61, 894–912 (1964).

— Knowles, F. G. W.: "Synaptic" vesicles in the neurohypophysis. Nature (Lond.) 185, 710 (1960).

Knowles, Sir F.: Techniques in the study of neurosecretion. In: Techniques in endocrine research (eds. P. Eckstein and F. Knowles), p. 57–65. London-New York: Academic Press 1963.

— Evidence for a dual control, by neurosecretion, of hormone synthesis and hormone release in the pituitary of the dogfish, Scylliorhinus stellaris. Phil. Trans. B 249, 435–455 (1965).

Lederis, K.: Fine structure and hormone content of the hypothalamo-neurohypophysial system of the rainbow trout (Salmo irideus) exposed to sea-water. Gen. comp. Endocr. 4, 638–661 (1964).

Robertis, E. D. P. de: Histophysiology of synapses and neurosecretion. Oxford-London-Edinburgh-New York-Paris-Frankfurt: Pergamon Press 1964.

Vollrath, L.: Über die Herkunft „synaptischer" Bläschen in neurosekretorischen Axonen. Z. Zellforsch. 99, 146–152 (1969).

# Hypothalamic Control of Anterior pituitary

## Dopaminergic Pathways and Gonadotropin Releasing Factors *

H. P. G. SCHNEIDER and S. M. McCANN

Department of Physiology, University of Texas Southwestern Medical School, Dallas (U.S.A.)

**Key words:** Anterior pituitary — Gonadotropin releasing factors — Dopaminergic pathways.

There is an imposing array of evidence which indicates that the anterior pituitary is a gland under neural control but lacking a secretomotor innervation. Instead, there is the hypophyseal portal system of veins which provides a specialized vascular link between hypothalamus and anterior pituitary. The first concept was that hypothalamic impulses for the discharge of trophic hormones might be some general synaptic mediators, released from nerve endings into capillary loops of the median eminence and then transported via the portal circulation into the sinusoids of the anterior lobe (HINSEY, 1937; GREEN and HARRIS, 1949). Stalk portal vessels and neural lobe portal vessels join the sinusoids in the pars distalis (for ref. see PORTER, HINES, SMITH, REPASS and SMITH, 1967). Although the interest has been focused on the stalk portal vessels (GREEN and HARRIS, 1949), the posterior lobe hormones were early considered as possible mediators for the release of the tropic hormones. This hypothesis was based partially on certain stimulating effects of the posterior lobe hormones on the adenohypophysis (MARTINI, 1954; McCANN and DHARIWAL, 1966).

Today it is evident, as a result of investigations over the past 15 years, that a whole new family of neurohormones called hypophysiotropic hormones or hypothalamic-releasing and -inhibiting factors control the secretion of each hormone from the adenohypophysis. Although the precise chemical nature of these hypophysiotropic hormones remains elusive, they have been prepared in highly purified form and separated chemically from each other (for ref. see McCANN and PORTER, 1969). With increased purification these releasing factors appeared to be smaller molecules than the neural lobe polypeptides, but most of them require the presence of peptide bonds for their activity. In 1968 however, WHITE, SCHALLY and their collaborators reported that following a variety of chromatographic procedures histamine, spermine and spermidine could be identified in the FSH-depleting fractions, as were lysine and putrescine. The polyamines were shown to be active in the pituitary hormone depletion assays employed by these workers at low doses and putrescine was even active at nanogram levels. The authors failed to apply these substances in other test systems than pituitary depletion assays. This has

* This study was supported by the Ford Foundation and Public Health Service Grant AM 10073–04.

been done by Kamberi (1969) in our laboratories who found that the amounts of spermine, spermidine and putrescine necessary to cause release of FSH *in vitro* from anterior pituitaries of normal male rats were far in excess of the amounts of these substances in hypothalamic extracts.

The idea however, that biogenic amines might nevertheless play a role in the regulation of the tropic hormones had just been strongly supported by the demonstration of serotonin and noradrenaline-containing neurons in the hypothalamus with the aid of fluorescence microscopy (Hillarp, Fuxe and Dahlström, 1966) and of dopamine-containing neurons, which have cell bodies located in the vicinity of the arcuate nucleus and axons which terminate near the primary plexus of the hypophyseal portal vessels in the median eminence (Fuxe and Hökfelt, 1967). The content of dopamine in these neurons is altered in situations associated with altered gonadotropin secretion (Fuxe, Hökfelt and Nilsson, 1967).

We therefore applied a variety of *in vitro* and *in vivo* test systems to elucidate the possible physiological role of monoaminergic pathways in the release of gonadotropins in particular.

## Materials and Methods

### In vitro Experiments

Adult male Sprague-Dawley or female Sherman rats were used as donors of hypothalami and pituitaries for incubation. Vaginal smear cytology of the Sherman rats was recorded six days a week, and animals were used for the experiments provided they displayed a clear-cut 4 day cyclicity in six consecutive cycles.

The incubation procedures were identical to those used in earlier studies (Schneider and McCann, 1969a). Wet weights of hypothalami ranged from 9.8–15.7 mg. The tissue was cut in one piece, limited by optic chiasm rostrally, hypothalamic fissures laterally and mamillary bodies posteriorly; the depth of the cut from the basal surface of the hypothalamus extended to about 1 mm. Either the anterior pituitaries alone or anterior pituitaries plus hypothalamic fragments were incubated in tissue culture medium 199. Each flask contained 12 pituitary halves, hypothalamic fragments were added in a 2:1 ratio to the glands. A 30 min preincubation followed by a 6 hr incubation period has been used throughout. LH released into the medium was measured by bioassay.

### In vivo Experiments

A stainless steel cannula, 22 gauge and 15 mm long, was implanted into the 3rd ventricle of female rats. A 28 gauge mandril was inserted into the cannula to prevent cerebrospinal fluid from leaking. Both the cannula and a small stabilizing screw driven into the skull near the implantation site were embedded in Nu Weld dental fixatives.

Two groups of animals have been subjected to this implantation procedure:

a) Adult normal or castrated female Sherman rats. Directly before and 15 min after intraventricular injection of a 2 µl solution of the drugs, blood samples were drawn by cardiac puncture in ether-anesthetized animals. In the interim between removal of the two blood samples the rats recovered from anesthesia. Plasma LH was measured by radioimmunoassay.

b) Hypophysectomized adult female Sprague-Dawley rats (Hormone Assay Lab, Chicago). These rats were maintained on a diet of beef heart and, at the time of the implantation and for the following 4 days were injected with 0.3 mg hydrocortisone sodium succinate (Solu-Cortef, Upjohn Co.) and 50,000 U potassium penicillin G (Squibb Co.) per animal as replacement and antiinflammatory therapy. The experiments were carried out in the week following this procedure.

Two ml of blood were drawn in the same fashion as before except by puncture of the jugular vein. The control and experimental plasma samples of the hypophysectomized rats were

injected into the jugular vein of estrogen-progesterone pretreated ovariectomized rats (RA-
MIREZ and McCANN, 1963) and plasma LH levels of these assay rats were measured by radioimmunoassay before and 10 min after the injections.

## LH- and FSH Assay

The incubation media were assayed for LH released from the AP's by the ovarian ascorbic
acid depletion method (PARLOW, 1961), using the one ovary four hour technique with a 3-point
design. Pooled incubation media were measured for their FSH concentration by the HCG-
augmentation method of STEELMAN and POHLEY (1953) as modified by PARLOW and REICHERT
(1963).

Plasma LH concentrations were measured by radioimmunoassay with antiovine LH serum
and ovine LH-$^{131}$I (NISWENDER, MIDGLEY, MONROE and REICHERT, 1968). The antiovine LH
serum was provided through the courtesy of Dr. A. R. MIDGLEY, University of Michigan
Medical School, Ann Arbor, Michigan, U.S.A.

The concentrations of LH have been expressed in terms of μg NIH-LH-S$_9$ (bioassay) and
NIH-LH-S$_1$ (radioimmunoassay), those of FSH in terms of NIH-FSH-S$_5$ (bioassay). The
bioassay data were calculated as μg LH-FSH equivalent released per 10 mg of pituitary tissue
per 6 hr or as percent of the control LH-FSH release, the control being set at 100%.

## Statistics

The relative potency, fiducial limits of error at $P = 0.95$ and the index of precision ($\lambda$) of
each assay were calculated as recommended by GADDUM (1953). Significance of differences
between control and experimental groups in the *in vivo* assays was calculated by Student's
test.

## Materials Tested

For the origin of crude or purified LRF, dopamine, epinephrine, norepinephrine, serotonin,
pronethalol, and phentolamine methanesulfonate we refer to SCHNEIDER and McCANN (1969a).

Phenoxybenzamine: -hydrochloride (source—Smith, Kline & French, Philadelphia, Pa.).

Haloperidol: supplied through the courtesy of Dr. L. I. GOLDBERG, Department of Internal Medicine, Division of Clinical Pharmacology, Emory University, Atlanta, Georgia,
U.S.A.

Estradiol: 17β-estradiol, Lot No. MI 22896 (source—Schering Corporation, Bloomfield,
N.J.), dissolved in a 0.1% alcohol solution.

# Results

## Effect of Mono- and Indolamines on Release of LRF by Stalk-Median Eminence (SME) Tissue in vitro

Doses of 0.5, 2.5 or 5.0 μg/ml of DA, NE or 5-HT failed to alter LH released
from pituitaries incubated alone, whereas 5 μg/ml E enhanced LH release to some
extent. DA at a 25.0 μg/ml dose significantly decreased assayable LH by inactivating it.

When anterior pituitaries (AP's) were incubated in the presence of stalk-
median eminence (SME) tissue (2 SME's per gland), LH release was stimulated
by an average of 20.7% ($P < 0.05$). If the combined SME + AP tissue was incubated with 0.5–5.0 μg/ml of either NE or 5-HT, this basal release of LH was
uneffected. E in a 5.0 μg/ml dose caused some inhibitory action in the presence of
SME fragments. LH release was significantly enhanced ($P < 0.01$) when DA was
added to the incubation medium in doses of 0.5–5.0 μg/ml, and a dose-response
could be obtained (Fig. 1). DA in similar doses failed to potentiate the LH-releasing

12*

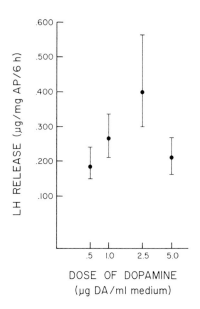

Fig. 1. Dose-response relationship between dose of dopamine and LH released into the medium of anterior pituitaries incubated with hypothalamic fragments. The dose of dopamine is on a logarithmic scale. Vertical bars give the 95% confidence limits

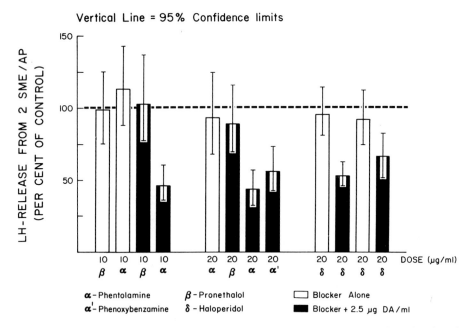

Fig. 2. Percentage changes of LH released into the medium of anterior pituitaries coincubated with hypothalamic fragments in the presence of dopamine and the blocking agents phentolamine, phenoxybenzamine, pronethalol, and haloperidol

action of crude rat hypothalamic extracts or of purified ovine LRF (SCHNEIDER and McCANN, 1969a).

DA had no effect on LH release when AP's were incubated with dorsal hypothalamic fragments which indicates that its action is localized to the basal tuberal region of the hypothalamus.

To determine if $\alpha$- or $\beta$-adrenergic receptors mediated the response of hypothalamic tissue to DA, phentolamine or phenoxybenzamine, $\alpha$-blocking agents, or pronethalol, a $\beta$-blocker, were added to the combined SME plus pituitary incubations at doses of 10.0 and 20.0 μg/ml. The basal release of LH was unaffected (Fig. 2, open bars). When the same dose of the blocking agents was tested in addition to 2.5 μg DA/ml (Fig. 2, solid bars), pronethalol did not alter the response to DA, whereas phentolamine and phenoxybenzamine, the $\alpha$-blocking agents, completely inhibited the DA-response. Haloperidol, a neuroleptic agent, had been shown to block specifically DA vascular receptors (YEH, McNAY and GOLDBERG, 1968). In a dose of 20 μg/ml haloperidol also blocked the DA response of SME tissue (Fig. 2). It should be mentioned that the adrenergic blocking agents failed to alter the LRF activity of crude SME extracts or purified ovine LRF.

### Effect of Mono- and Indolamines on Release of FRF by SME Tissue in vitro

This study was undertaken under identical *in vitro* conditions to determine if DA would act similarly to evoke release of FRF from hypothalamic fragments.

Again incubation of AP's in the presence of ME tissue resulted in a slight increase in FSH release ($P < 0.05$). When 1–5 μg/ml of NE, E and 5-HT were incubated in the presence of the combined SME and AP tissue, basal release of FSH was unaltered except for an increase with the highest dose of E. DA in the dose range of 2.5–5.0 μg/ml yielded a dose-related increase of FSH release into the medium ($P < 0.01$). The relative DA responses of LH and FSH release (% of control) into the medium of the coincubate were almost identical for the 2.0 μg/ml dose (KAMBERI, SCHNEIDER and McCANN, 1969).

DA in similar doses failed to alter FSH release from AP's incubated alone. Increased concentrations of DA (50–100 μg/ml) inactivate FSH (KAMBERI and McCANN, 1969). DA, NE, E or 5-HT at 5 μg/ml did not alter the FSH-releasing action of partially purified ovine FRF. The response to DA was completely inhibited by 20 μg/ml of the $\alpha$-adrenergic blocker, phentolamine, whereas pronethalol not only failed to suppress the DA response of the hypothalamic tissue but induced a further slight increase in FSH release (KAMBERI, SCHNEIDER and McCANN, 1969).

### Intraventricular Mono- or Indolamines and LH-Release in the Rat

Blood samples were drawn by cardiac puncture in ether-anesthetized animals bearing chronic cannulae in the 3rd ventricle (V) directly before and 15 min after intraventricular injection (4 μg of drug in 2 μl). In the interim between removal of the two blood samples the rats recovered from anesthesia. Plasma LH was measured by radioimmunoassay. Serotonin did not significantly alter plasma LH levels at any stage of 4-day estrous cycles (Table 1). Nor-epinephrine also did

Table 1. *Serotonin (5-HT) into 3rd ventricle of normal and castrated female rats*

| Injection (µg/2 µl) | Response (ng LH/ml plasma) | | | | Castrated | |
|---|---|---|---|---|---|---|
| | D$_1$ | D$_2$ | P | E | | |
| Control | 0.90 | 4.66 | 1.21 | 0.89 | 27.57 | 17.63 |
| 4.0 5-HT | 2.85 | 2.63 | 1.67 | 1.25 | 18.77 | 7.82 |
| Control | 3.38 | 1.30 | 4.01 | 3.45 | 22.12 | 21.00 |
| 4.0 5-HT | 2.49 | 0.80 | 4.55 | 1.58 | 4.20 | 8.17 |
| Control | 0.85 | 3.51 | 6.69 | 1.15 | 12.69 | 20.93 |
| 4.0 5-HT | 1.12 | 1.14 | 5.21 | 2.87 | 4.26 | 11.46 |
| Control | 1.11 | 2.02 | 2.52 | 3.51 | 35.84 | 26.88 |
| 4.0 5-HT | 1.05 | 1.82 | 2.03 | 3.35 | 24.53 | 13.78 |
| | n.s. | n.s. | n.s. | n.s. | $P < 0.001$ | |

Table 2. *Norepinephrine (NE) into 3rd ventricle of normal and steroid-blocked castrated female rats*

| Injection (µg/2 µl) | Response (ng LH/ml plasma) | | | | Castrated + block | |
|---|---|---|---|---|---|---|
| | D$_1$ | D$_2$ | P | E | | |
| Control | 1.27 | 1.48 | 2.17 | 3.53 | 7.02 | 6.62 |
| 4.0 NE | 1.50 | 2.30 | 1.93 | 5.52 | 12.00 | 13.31 |
| Control | 1.15 | 3.88 | 2.45 | 0.86 | | 5.78 |
| 4.0 NE | 1.32 | 4.89 | 3.45 | 4.62 | | 5.75 |
| Control | 0.87 | 3.39 | 2.39 | 1.21 | | 7.18 |
| 4.0 NE | 1.19 | 3.91 | 1.88 | 11.91 | | 8.37 |
| Control | 0.95 | 4.00 | 3.19 | 1.32 | | 12.61 |
| 4.0 NE | 1.76 | 6.02 | 2.97 | 4.27 | | 12.69 |
| Control | 0.84 | 4.24 | 3.25 | 1.42 | | 14.25 |
| 4.0 NE | 1.12 | 4.07 | 2.31 | 4.73 | | 18.22 |
| Control | | 4.32 | 3.98 | | | 10.11 |
| 4.0 NE | | 3.50 | 2.94 | | | 6.19 |
| Control | | 1.86 | | | | 6.07 |
| 4.0 NE | | 3.50 | | | | 15.00 |
| Control | | 2.95 | | | | 13.41 |
| 4.0 NE | | 4.43 | | | | 18.37 |
| | n.s. | n.s. | n.s. | $P < 0.05$ | n.s. | |

not produce overall significant changes in plasma LH although there were some positive responses (Table 2). Dopamine raised LH levels to 8 or 10 fold above controls ($P < 0.01$) in rats on the 2nd day of diestrus (D2) or in proestrus (P). DA proved to be less effective in estrus (E, Table 3) and least effective in D1. In normal males DA raised plasma LH in 5 out of 10 animals, whereas NE was ineffective. The DA effect in D2 and P rats could be blocked by simultaneous 3rd V. inj. of 30 µg phenoxybenzamine, but remained unaltered after the same dose of pronethalol (Table 4). In untreated spayed females NE or DA produced variable results independent of baseline LH levels; however, 5-HT significantly ($P<0.01$) decreased LH release in these animals (Table 1). Estrogen progesterone-blocked, castrated female rats responded with up to 10 fold increases ($P<0.01$) in plasma

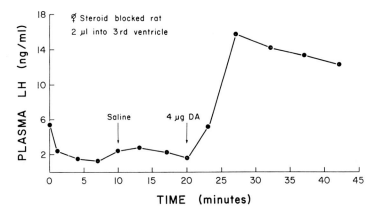

Fig. 3. Secretion pattern of plasma LH in the ovariectomized-steroid-blocked rat following saline control (2 µl) and dopamine injection (4 µg/2 µl) into the 3rd ventricle

Table 3. *Dopamine (DA) into 3rd ventricle of normal and steroid-blocked castrated female rats*

| Injection (µg/2 µl) | Response (ng LH/ml plasma) | | | | Castrated + block |
|---|---|---|---|---|---|
| | $D_1$ | $D_2$ | P | E | |
| Control | 0.85 | 5.21 | 2.53 | 0.35 | 7.07 |
| 4.0 DA | 0.70 | 12.71 | 8.40 | 3.76 | 56.73 |
| Control | 0.84 | 5.99 | 2.48 | 0.83 | 10.11 |
| 4.0 DA | 1.40 | 13.78 | 9.76 | 3.94 | 49.88 |
| Control | 0.94 | 3.38 | 2.70 | 1.55 | 5.85 |
| 4.0 DA | 1.85 | 7.02 | 8.00 | 4.07 | 65.50 |
| Control | 0.65 | 2.46 | 2.55 | 0.96 | 5.08 |
| 4.0 DA | 9.37 | 7.65 | 7.56 | 4.53 | 13.42 |
| Control | 1.21 | 1.88 | 2.26 | 1.22 | 10.78 |
| 4.0 DA | 14.86 | 8.34 | 4.95 | 3.98 | 51.14 |
| Control | 0.61 | 1.85 | 2.10 | | 14.75 |
| 4.0 DA | 1.22 | 5.31 | 6.99 | | 53.23 |
| Control | 0.62 | 2.12 | 2.24 | | 14.89 |
| 4.0 DA | 1.21 | 9.73 | 22.60 | | 55.50 |
| Control | | | 2.04 | | 9.76 |
| 4.0 DA | | | 16.18 | | 12.73 |
| Control | | | 2.06 | | 10.11 |
| 4.0 DA | | | 5.86 | | 8.87 |
| Control | | | 1.14 | | |
| 4.0 DA | | | 12.13 | | |
| | n.s. | $P<0.001$ | $P<0.001$ | $P<0.001$ | $P<0.001$ |

Table 4. *Dopamine (DA) and adrenergic blocking agents ($\alpha + \beta$) into 3rd ventricle of normal female rats*

| Injection ($\mu g/2\ \mu l$) | Response (ng LH/ml plasma) | |
|---|---|---|
| | $D_2$ | P |
| Control | 0.61 | 2.51 |
| 4.0 DA + 30.0 $\alpha$ | 1.08 | 2.78 |
| Control | 0.55 | 2.71 |
| 4.0 DA + 30.0 $\alpha$ | 0.44 | 3.10 |
| Control | 0.51 | 2.53 |
| 4.0 DA + 30.0 $\alpha$ | 0.48 | 2.22 |
| Control | 0.48 | 1.88 |
| 4.0 DA + 30.0 $\alpha$ | 0.45 | 2.21 |
| Control | 2.40 | |
| 4.0 DA + 30.0 $\alpha$ | 1.36 | |
| Control | 1.67 | |
| 4.0 DA + 30.0 $\alpha$ | 0.97 | |
| | n.s. | n.s. |
| Control | 1.67 | 1.12 |
| 4.0 DA + 30.0 $\beta$ | 6.90 | 11.72 |
| Control | 2.61 | 1.01 |
| 4.0 DA + 30.0 $\beta$ | 9.37 | 5.99 |
| Control | 1.89 | 1.03 |
| 4.0 DA + 30.0 $\beta$ | 4.25 | 7.19 |
| Control | 2.03 | 2.23 |
| 4.0 DA + 30.0 $\beta$ | 6.08 | 11.99 |
| | $P < 0.025$ | $P < 0.02$ |

LH following 3rd V. inj. of DA (Table 3), whereas NE produced only slight increases in 5 out of 9 rats (Table 2).

Monitoring an individual rat of this type by drawing blood from a carotid artery catheter at 3–7 min intervals revealed an 8 fold increase of plasma LH 7 min after intraventricular inj. of DA (Fig. 3). Saline (0.9%) did not produce an effect on LH release under any of the described conditions (Schneider and McCann, 1969 b).

## Intraventricular Mono- or Indolamines and LRF-Discharge in the Rat

LRF and other releasing factors appear in the blood of chronically hypophysectomized (hypox) rats (McCann and Porter, 1969).

Plasma samples were tested in the rat LH radioimmunoassay for possible LH contamination in all individual hypox rats being assayed for peripheral LRF. None of the rats revealed detectable plasma LH, which indicates completeness of the hypophysectomy.

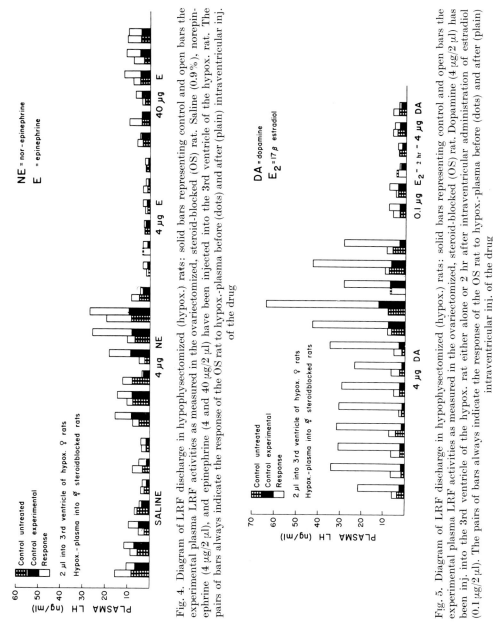

Fig. 4. Diagram of LRF discharge in hypophysectomized (hypox.) rats: solid bars representing control and open bars the experimental plasma LRF activities as measured in the ovariectomized, steroid-blocked (OS) rat. Saline (0.9%), norepinephrine (4 μg/2 μl), and epinephrine (4 and 40 μg/2 μl) have been injected into the 3rd ventricle of the hypox. rat. The pairs of bars always indicate the response of the OS rat to hypox.-plasma before (dots) and after (plain) intraventricular inj. of the drug

Fig. 5. Diagram of LRF discharge in hypophysectomized (hypox.) rats: solid bars representing control and open bars the experimental plasma LRF activities as measured in the ovariectomized, steroid-blocked (OS) rat. Dopamine (4 μg/2 μl) has been inj. into the 3rd ventricle of the hypox. rat either alone or 2 hr after intraventricular administration of estradiol (0.1 μg/2 μl). The pairs of bars always indicate the response of the OS rat to hypox.-plasma before (dots) and after (plain) intraventricular inj. of the drug

Plasma samples of female hypox rats (2–3 weeks post-hypophysectomy) have been assayed before (control) and 15 min after injection of the amines (experimental) into the 3rd V. The control samples of a total of 45 hypox rats from different assays significantly increased plasma LH of steroid-blocked spayed female test rats (*P* < 0.01–0.05). This is evidence for resting levels of peripheral LRF in hypox female rats and confirms the findings of NALLAR and McCANN (1965). A volume of 2 μl saline (0.9%) injected through an indwelling cannula into the 3rd V. of these hypox female rats did not alter peripheral LRF activity (Fig. 4).

NE injected intraventricularly at a dose of 4 μg elevated peripheral plasma LRF in a group of 7 animals when compared to the response in the control group ($P < 0.02$) (Fig. 4). DA (4 μg) boosted plasma LRF levels of the hypox rat up to 23 fold above controls. These responses were significant at the 0.1% level for a group of 13 animals (Fig. 5). When the DA and NE response of LRF discharge in the hypox rat are compared to each other, the activity of DA exceeds that of NE by a highly significant margin ($P < 0.001$). E at 4 and 40 μg doses did not produce any significant changes in peripheral LRF levels (Fig. 4).

### Feedback of Estradiol-17β ($E_2$) upon LRF Discharge

This was studied in both *in vitro* and *in vivo* experiments. LH release from AP's incubated alone was markedly enhanced by 0.5 or 1.0 μg/ml of $E_2$. This positive effect was blocked by puromycin (10.0 or 20.0 μg/ml) or by cycloheximide (10.0 μg/ml), although the antibiotics failed to influence basal release of LH from incubated glands. When AP's were incubated together with ME tissue, LH release was not altered by adding 0.5 or 1.0 μg $E_2$/ml to the medium; however, doses of 0.5 and 1.0 μg $E_2$/ml prevented the responsiveness of the ME to DA (2.5 μg DA/ml). This inhibitory effect of $E_2$ was again blocked by puromycin or cycloheximide. Small or high doses of $E_2$ (0.5, 1.0 or 25.0 μg/ml) did not alter the AP response to various concentrations of purified LRF and failed to affect assay of the LH released. AP and ME tissue of each sex appeared to give similar responses (Schneider and McCann, 1969c).

The *in vivo* experiments utilized hypox rats. When $E_2$ was injected into the 3rd V. 2 hr prior to the experiment at a dose of 0.1 μg in 2 μl, it completely blocked the DA-stimulated discharge of LRF in the hypox rat (Fig. 5). $E_2$ was dissolved in a 0.1% alcohol solution. This diluent was injected into the 3rd V. of control animals 2 hr prior to 4 μg of DA. The DA response was not impaired. Thus, both *in vivo* and *in vitro* experiments point to an inhibitory effect of $E_2$ on DA-induced LRF discharge.

### Discussion

Incubation *in vitro* of either anterior pituitaries alone or together with hypothalamic fragments proved to be an extremely useful methodological approach for the differential evaluation of the response of these tissues to various agents. The catechol- and indolamines tested (DA, NE, E and 5-HT) in doses known to be present in the hypothalamus, were without effect on pituitary LH- and FSH release.

E did not significantly stimulate release even at a high dose which was probably unphysiologic. In the presence of median eminence tissue, DA increased the release of LH and FSH, whereas the other monoamines again had little effect. Control studies revealed that DA failed to potentiate the action of LRF or FRF in releasing LH or FSH from pituitaries incubated alone. The conclusion drawn was that DA evoked a release of LRF and FRF from the hypothalamic fragments. DA appears to act on α-adrenergic receptors in discharging the gonadotropin-releasing factors since the response to the catecholamine was inhibited by α- and not $\beta$-receptor-blocking drugs. Haloperidol is considered to be a specific blocker of DA receptors; this neuroleptic drug also inhibited the DA-stimulated LRF discharge from hypothalamic tissue.

The similarity in the findings for LH- and FSH-release suggests that both gonadotropins may share, at least partially, a similar releasing or regulatory mechanism. Striking similarities in the changes in FSH and LH secretion during the rat estrous and human cycle have been pointed out just recently (McCLINTOCK and SCHWARTZ, 1968; SWERDLOFF and ODELL, 1968; PARLOW, DAANE and SCHALLY, 1969).

It has been known for years that antiadrenergic drugs will block ovulation in the rat (EVERETT, 1969). Reserpine, which depresses hypothalamic catecholamine content, also blocks ovulation, iproniazide prevents the blockade (LIPPMANN, LEONARDI, BALL and COPPOLA, 1967). We reported recently (SCHNEIDER and McCANN, 1969d) that reserpine blocks the response of the coincubated SME's plus AP's to DA, which was counteracted by addition of the monoamine-oxidase inhibitor, pargyline. MEYERSON and SAWYER (1968) demonstrated that the ovulation-blocking action of reserpine in the rat can be prevented by monoamine-oxidase inhibitors (pargyline, nialamide), which is in perfect agreement with our *in vitro* data.

Our effort to establish the role of DA as the transmitter to release both LRF and FRF led to a series of *in vivo* experiments in which infusion of the mono-amines into the 3rd V. was performed.

The results in the normal, castrated or steroid-blocked castrated rat provide evidence for the role of DA in LH release. Plasma LH concentrations monitored in the steroid-blocked spayed rat peaked as early as 7 min after intraventricular inj. of DA. The response of the female rat indicates cyclic variability in the sensitivity to DA. If DA is considered the transmitter for the release of LRF, then these findings can be interpreted as indicating an altered sensitivity to DA of the LRF neurosecretory neurons at various stages of the cycle. This could be caused by altered neuronal content of LRF or by an altered central excitatory state of the neurons imposed by activity in afferent neurons.

Another possibility would be an altered pituitary responsiveness to the LRF released by DA; however, ANTUNES-RODRIGUES, DHARIWAL and McCANN (1966) found little evidence for such cyclic fluctuations in pituitary response to LRF. This needs reinvestigation with present improved methodology.

Estradiol certainly is one of the factors, which are able to prevent DA from acting in its role as transmitter of the adrenergic tone responsible for LRF discharge. This was demonstrated first *in vitro*, and, furthermore, the inhibiting effect of $E_2$ appears to depend on protein synthesis. This is consistent with the hypothesis that $E_2$ is first taken up by a receptor and then transported to the nucleus where it induces specific m-RNA and in turn protein synthesis (Fig. 6).

An analogous negative $E_2$ feedback on the dopaminergic release of LRF into peripheral circulation resulted after injection of the steroid into the 3rd V. of hypox rats 2 hr prior to DA. DA failed to act in the presence of $E_2$. However, when the monoamine was injected into the 3rd V. of untreated hypox rats, peripheral LRF concentrations increased dramatically. Epinephrine failed to influence LRF discharge in the hypox rat and NE had only a feeble effect which points to the specificity of DA in releasing LRF. Since radioimmunological studies exclude any possible contamination of the hypox-blood with LH, it seems to us that the role of DA in discharging LRF is unquestionable.

In other experiments performed in this department DA elevated LRF in pooled portal vessel plasma from male pentobarbital-anesthetized rats when injected into the 3rd V. The LRF activity was measured *in vitro* as immuno-assayable LH released from one half AP and the activity in portal plasma was

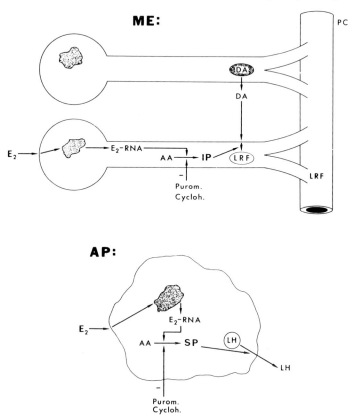

Fig. 6. Schematic representation of a hypothesis on the site and mode of action of estradiol at the anterior pituitary and median eminence

compared to that in peripheral plasma (Kamberi and Porter, 1969). This observation provides important confirmation of our peripheral plasma LRF data.

Although 5-HT failed to alter plasma LH levels in the normal rat, it significantly decreased plasma LH in the ovariectomized rat. This observation lends support to data from other laboratories on the possible inhibitory action of indolamines on LH release (Martini, Fraschini and Motta, 1969; Kordon, 1969).

The data presented seem to prove conclusively the existence of a dopaminergic transmission for LRF and indicate that this transmission might exist for FRF as well. This symposium, hopefully, will provide further information about the anatomical arrangement of a dopaminergic transmission to releasing factor neurons.

To our knowledge there exist three possibilities of information transfer: first, ordinary synaptic contact as known for most parts of the CNS; second, since the axons of the dopaminergic neurons appear to end in the ME itself at a point near the presumed terminals of the LRF-secreting neurons, there might exist axo-axonal contacts; and third, a final possibility is that the LRF-secreting neurons also contain DA granules and that intracellular release of DA may trigger release of LRF.

## Summary

Catechol- and indolamines (dopamine—DA, norepinephrine—NE, epinephrine—E, and serotonin— 5-HT) were tested *in vitro* on either anterior pituitaries alone or coincubated with hypothalamic fragments (SME). Only DA discharged LH- and FSH-releasing factors (LRF and FRF) from the SME tissue. DA failed to release gonadotropins when incubated with pituitaries alone. The other monoamines did not produce noticeable effects. Alpha-adrenergic receptors appeared to mediate the DA response. There was no interaction *in vitro* between DA and the gonadotropin-releasing factors. The DA effect on SME tissue was blocked specifically by haloperidol.

DA also was able to release LH *in vivo* as indicated by increased plasma LH levels in cycling and ovariectomized-steroid-blocked (OS) rats after injection of the catecholamine into the 3rd ventricle. Plasma LH concentrations in the OS rat peaked at levels 8 fold above controls as early as 7 min following intraventricular DA. In untreated, spayed females intraventricular NE or DA produced variable results; however, 5-HT significantly ($P < 0.001$) decreased LH release in these animals.

In chronically hypophysectomized rats E failed to stimulate discharge of LRF into the peripheral circulation, whereas NE slightly stimulated ($P < 0.02$) LRF discharge. On the other hand DA enhanced peripheral LRF concentrations to as much as 23 fold above controls ($P < 0.001$).

Estradiol-17$\beta$ (E$_2$) inhibited the dopaminergic release of LRF *in vivo* and *in vitro* indicating a possible site of the negative E$_2$-feedback at the median eminence.

The data are interpreted as indicating: (a) that monoamines do not act as releasing factors themselves, (b) DA seemingly is a transmitter for the gonadotropin-releasing factors, (c) indolamines such as 5-HT have inhibitory effects on LH release, and (d) the negative estradiol feedback is located at the site of the adrenergic transmission on the LRF secretory neurons.

## References

ANTUNES-RODRIGUES, J., DHARIWAL, A. P. S., McCANN, S. M.: Effect of purified luteinizing hormone-releasing factor (LH-RF) on plasma LH activity at various stages of the estrous cycle of the rat. Proc. Soc. exp. Biol. (N.Y.) **122**, 1001–1004 (1966).

EVERETT, J. W.: Neuroendocrine aspects of mammalian reproduction. Ann. Rev. Physiol. **31**, 383–416 (1969).

FUXE, K., HÖKFELT, T.: The influence of central catecholamine neurons on the hormone secretion from the anterior and posterior pituitary. In: Proc. 4th Intern. Symp. on Neurosecretion, edit. by F. STUTINSKY, p. 165–177. Berlin-Heidelberg-New York: Springer 1967.

— — NILSSON, O.: Activity changes in the tuberoinfundibular dopamine neurons of the rat during various states of the reproductive cycle. Life Sci. **6**, 2057–2061 (1967).

GADDUM, F. H.: Simplified mathematics for bioassays. J. Pharm. Pharmacol. 5, 345–358 (1953).

GREEN, J. D., HARRIS, G. W.: Observation of the hypophysioportal vessels of the living rat. J. Physiol. (Lond.) 108, 359–361 (1949).

HILLARP, N.-Å., FUXE, K., DAHLSTRÖM, A.: Demonstration and mapping of central neurons containing dopamine, noradrenaline and 5-hydroxytryptamine and their reactions to psychopharmaca. Pharmacol. Rev. 18, 727–741 (1966).

HINSEY, J. C.: The relation of the nervous system to ovulation and other phenomena of the female reproductive tract. Cold Spr. Harb. Symp. quant. Biol. 5, 269–279 (1937).

KAMBERI, I., MCCANN, S. M.: Effect of biogenic amines and other substances on the release of follicle stimulating hormone by pituitaries incubated in vitro. J. Reprod. Fertil. 18, 153 (1969).

— SCHNEIDER, H. P. G., MCCANN, S. M.: Action of dopamine to induce release of FSH-releasing factor (FRF) from hypothalamic tissue in vitro. Endocrinology 86, 278 (1970).

KORDON, C.: Effects of selective experimental changes in regional hypothalamic monoamine levels on superovulation in the immature rat. Neuroendocrinology 4, 129–138 (1969).

LIPPMANN, W., LEONARDI, R., BALL, J., COPPOLA, J. A.: Relationship between hypothalamic catecholamines and gonadotrophin synthesis in rats. J. Pharmacol. exp. Ther. 156, 258–266 (1967).

MARTINI, L., FRASCHINI, F., MOTTA, M.: Neural control of anterior pituitary functions. Recent Progr. Hormone Res. 24, 439–496 (1968).

MCCANN, S. M., PORTER, J. C.: Hypothalamic pituitary stimulating and inhibiting hormones. Physiol. Rev. 49, 240–284 (1969).

— DHARIWAL, A. P. S.: Hypothalamic releasing factors and the neurovascular link between brain and anterior pituitary, p. 261–296. In: Neuroendocrinology, edit. by L. MARTINI and W. F. GANONG. New York: Academic Press 1966.

MCCLINTOCK, J. A., SCHWARTZ, N. B.: Changes in pituitary and plasma follicle stimulating hormone concentrations during the rat estrous cycle. Endocrinology 83, 433–441 (1968).

MEYERSON, B. J., SAWYER, C. H.: Monoamines and ovulation in the rat. Endocrinology 83, 170–176 (1968).

NALLAR, R., MCCANN, S. M.: LH-releasing activity in plasma of hypophysectomized rats. Endocrinology 76, 272–294 (1965).

NISWENDER, G. D., MIDGLEY, A. R., JR., MONROE, S. E., REICHERT, L. E., JR.: Radioimmunoassay for rat luteinizing hormone with antiovine LH serum and ovine LH-[131]I. Proc. Soc. exp. Biol. (N.Y.) 128, 807–811 (1968).

PARLOW, A. F.: Bio-assay of pituitary luteinizing hormone by depletion of ovarian ascorbic acid. In: A. ALBERT, Human pituitary gonadotropins, p. 300–310. Springfield, Illinois: Ch. C. Thomas 1961.

— DAANE, T. A., SCHALLY, A. V.: Quantitative, differential measurement of rat serum FSH, LH and hypothalamic FSH-RH and LH-RH with specific radioimmunoassays. 51st Annual Meeting Amer. Endocr. Soc. 106, 83 (1969).

— REICHERT, L. E., JR.: Species differences in follicle stimulating hormone as revealed by the slope in the Steelman-Pohley assay. Endocrinology 73, 740–743 (1963).

PORTER, J. C., HINES, M. F. M., SMITH, K. R., REPASS, R. L., SMITH, A. J. K.: Quantitative evaluation of local blood flow of the adenohypophysis in rats. Endocrinology 80, 583–598 (1967).

RAMIREZ, V. D., MCCANN, S. M.: A new sensitive test for LH-releasing activity: the ovariectomized, estrogen progesterone-blocking rat. Endocrinology 73, 193–198 (1963).

SCHNEIDER, H. P. G., MCCANN, S. M.: Possible role of dopamine as transmitter to promote discharge of LH-releasing factor. Endocrinology 85, 121–132 (1969a).

— — Intraventricular mono- or indolamines and LH release in the rat. Physiologist (vol. 12, no. 3 1969b).

— — Feedback of estradiol upon median eminence and anterior pituitary in vitro. 51st Annual Meeting Amer. Endocr. Soc. 108, 84 (1969c).

— — Effect of dopamine on release of LH-releasing factor by stalk-median eminence tissue in vitro. Fed. Proc. 28, 381 (1969d).

STEELMAN, S. L., POHLEY, F. M.: Assay of the follicle stimulating hormone based on the augmentation with human chorionic gonadotropin. Endocrinology 53, 604–616 (1953).

SWERDLOFF, R. S., ODELL, W. D.: Some aspects of the control of secretion in LH and FSH in humans. In: Gonadotropins, edit. by E. ROSEMBERG, p. 155–162. Los Altos, Calif.: Geron-X, Inc. 1968.

WHITE, W. F., COHEN, A. I., RIPPEL, R. H., STOREY, J. C., SCHALLY, A. V.: Some hypothalamic polyamines that deplete pituitary follicle stimulating hormone. Endocrinology 82, 742–752 (1968).

YEH, B. K., McNAY, J. L., GOLDBERG, L. T.: Attenuation of dopamine renal and mesenteric vasodilation by haloperidol: evidence for a specific dopamine receptor. J. Pharmacol. exp. Ther. (in press).

# Participation of Central Monoamine Neurons in the Regulation of Anterior Pituitary Function with Special Regard to the Neuro-Endocrine Role of Tubero-Infundibular Dopamine Neurons*

KJELL FUXE and TOMAS HÖKFELT

Department of Histology, Karolinska Institutet, Stockholm (Sweden)

**Key words:** Anterior pituitary — Regulation — Aminergic neurons — Tubero-infundibular system.

Since the last neurosecretion meeting in 1966 (FUXE and HÖKFELT, 1967) our studies on the role of brain monoamines in neuroendocrine mechanisms have continued. It has been of special interest to further elucidate the neuroendocrine role of the tubero-infundibular dopamine (DA) neurons. This paper gives a summary of some of our recent work in this field, most of which has as yet not been published, and original findings will be described. The reader is also referred to two previous review articles (FUXE and HÖKFELT, 1969a, b) the contents of which will not be dealt with in the present paper.

## Tubero-Infundibular DA Neurons

### Anatomy

This system mainly originates from small DA cell bodies in the nuc. arcuatus and in the anterior periventricular hypothalamic nucleus, ventral part (FUXE, 1963, 1964). Thus, after amine loading experiments with nialamide-3,4-dihydroxy-phenylalanine (dopa) (FUXE and HÖKFELT, 1966) or α-methyl-noradrenaline (NA) (LICHTENSTEIGER and LANGEMANN, 1966) it has been possible to trace fibres from the arcuate cell bodies down to the DA nerve terminals in the median eminence. These findings have been confirmed by BARRY (1968). It cannot be excluded that a small percentage of the DA nerve terminals in the external layer of the median eminence arise from catecholamine cell bodies situated elsewhere in the hypothalamus, *e.g.* from CA cell bodies lying close to the nuc. mammillo-thalamicus or dorsal to the nuc. dorsomedialis hypothalami (A 13, FUXE and HÖKFELT, 1969a) and from some CA cell bodies within the area of the nuc. premammillaris ventralis (FUXE and UNGERSTEDT, 1968a). These latter cell bodies, which are about 20–25 μ in diameter, are hardly visible in the rat without amine-loading experiments, but easily found in the pigeon (FUXE and LJUNGGREN, 1965) or in the

---

* This study has been supported by a small Mental Health Grant (1-RO3-NH 16825–01) from the National Institute of Health, by the Swedish Medical Research Council (project No. 14X-715–05 B and 14X-2887–01) and by M. Bergwalls Stiftelse.

guinea-pig (BARRY, 1968; LEONARDELLI, 1968). The latter authors have suggested that these CA cell bodies in the premammillary area might participate in the dopaminergic innervation of the median eminence. However, this is not likely to be but a small percentage, since we have recently performed hypothalamic islands excluding the premammillary area and the CA cell group A 13 without being able to see any certain decrease in the number of fluorescent DA nerve terminals in the external layer. It may be, however, that some of these cell bodies give rise to the CA fibres innervating e.g. the intermediate lobe of the anterior pituitary and part of the posterior lobe. At least part of the CA nerve terminals in the pituitary gland contain NA, since the uptake of NA into at least part of them is diminished by pretreatment with desipramine (FUXE and HÖKFELT, 1969a). This drug does not block the uptake of CA into the DA neurons (CARLSSON et al., 1966).

So far available pharmacological evidence strongly indicates that all the CA nerve terminals in the external layer of the median eminence and the infundibular stem contain DA (see FUXE and HÖKFELT, 1969a).

However, the large droplet-like CA varicosities in the internal layer may very well contain NA since they decrease in number and intensity after treatment with repeated doses (25 mg/kg) of a potent dopamine-$\beta$-oxidase inhibitor (FLA 63) (CORRODI et al., to be published). Furthermore, after pretreatment with $\alpha$-methyl-dopa (400 mg/kg) the fluorescence remains after reserpine treatment, which strongly indicates that $\alpha$-methyl-NA has been formed in these varicosities (CARLSSON et al., 1965). These CA varicosities in the internal layer may arise from NA fibres running medially and ventrally from the lateral hypothalamic area innervating the retrochiasmatic area. Thus, after making small hypothalamic islands around the median eminence the CA varicosities in the internal layer decrease in number, and strong fluorescence accumulates in the NA fibres on the lateral side of the cut (FUXE et al., unpublished date). It cannot be excluded, however, that these varicosities may belong to fibres originating e.g. from the CA cell bodies in the ventral premammillary area.

## Function

At the previous meeting on neurosecretion we presented evidence that the tubero-infundibular DA neurons probably are involved in the regulation of gonadotrophin secretion but not adrenocorticotrophic hormone (ACTH) secretion from the anterior pituitary. Thus, during pregnancy and lactation it was found that the DA cell bodies in the arcuate nucleus showed marked increases in amine levels and that the turnover in the DA nerve terminals in the median eminence was markedly increased as revealed with the help of amine synthesis inhibitors (FUXE et al., 1967, 1969a). These changes are probably due to an increased neural activity in the tubero-infundibular DA neurons. The hypothesis was given that activation of this system participates in causing the blockade of follicle stimulating hormone (FSH) and/or luteinizing hormone (LH) secretion and ovulation found in these stages of the reproductive cycle. To obtain further evidence for this view and to link the system mainly to LH secretion, the turnover in this neuron system has been studied under various endocrinological conditions involving changes in gonadotrophin secretion.

## 1. Ovarian Cycle

It has been found that there is markedly increased turnover in diestrus compared to proestrus-estrus (Figs. 1, 2) (Fuxe *et al.*, 1969c). The CA cell bodies have also been found to undergo marked changes. Thus, in proestrus-estrus the DA cell bodies are increased in number and intensity as found both in guinea-pig (Leonardelli, 1968) and in rat (Lichtensteiger, 1968, 1969). A second peak of less magnitude in number and intensity or cell bodies seems to occur in diestrus (Fuxe *et al.*, 1967, 1969c; Leonardelli, 1968).

Thus, in contrast to what is the case in lactation and pregnancy, in proestrus-estrus the increased number and intensity of DA cell bodies are associated with decreased turnover and neural activity of the tubero-infundibular DA system.

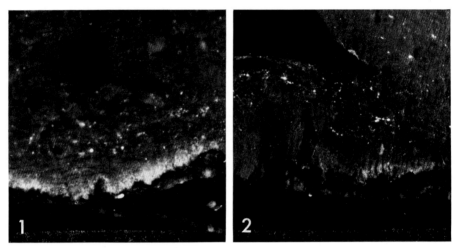

Fig. 1. Median eminence of rat in *proestrous* after treatment with H44/48 (250 mg/kg, $2^1/_2$ hours before killing). A fluorescence of moderate intensity remains in the external layer. $\times 200$

Fig. 2. Median eminence of rat in *diestrous* after treatment with H44/68 (250 mg/kg, $2^1/_2$ hours before killing). A fluorescence of very low intensity remains in the external layer. $\times 200$

The conclusion has to be drawn that from the appearance of the number and intensity of the DA cell bodies it is not possible to tell if the system is inactivated or activated.

Recently we have directly correlated the turnover changes occurring during the estrous cycle in the tubero-infundibular DA neurons with changes in pituitary LH contents during the estrous cycle (Ahrén *et al.*, unpublished data) using the lactic acid production test (Hamberger, 1967). A very good correlation was found between high pituitary LH levels and high DA turnover (diestrous) on one hand and low pituitary LH levels and low DA turnover (proestrous-early estrous) on the other hand. When the rat passed from diestrus to proestrus the decrease in pituitary LH levels appeared to be preceded by an inactivation of the tubero-infundibular DA neurons. In a similar manner, when the rat passed from estrus to diestrus, the increase in pituitary LH levels appeared to be preceded by an activation of the tubero-infundibular DA neurons. These results strongly underline

our previous view (FUXE *et al.*, 1967; FUXE and HÖKFELT, 1969a, b) that the
tubero-infundibular DA neurons participate in the control of gonadotrophin
secretion and suggest that they mainly participates in the control of LH secretion,
which has a marked and shortlasting peak in proestrus. The DA nerve terminals
in the median eminence probably exert an axo-axonic influence (HÖKFELT, 1967,
1968) on the terminals storing luteinizing hormone releasing factor (LRF) and act to
inhibit the nerve impulse induced release of LRF from these terminals by way
of presynaptic inhibition either by causing a hypo- or hyperpolarization (see
Fig. 3).

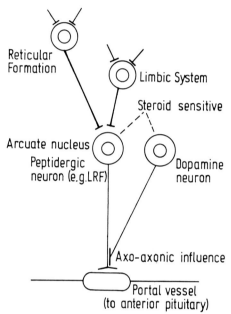

Fig. 3. *Principal diagram on nervous and hormonal inputs to the peptidergic neurons, releasing
hormones into the portal vessels.* Only the large nervous inputs from the limbic system and the
reticular formation onto the peptidergic cell body are illustrated. These areas are heavily
innervated by NA and 5-HT nerve terminals. The tubero-infundibular DA neurons are shown
to interfere with the transmission in the peptidergic neuron at another level *i.e.* at the level
of the nerve terminal by way of axo-axonic contacts. Both the peptidergic and the tubero-
infundibular DA neurons may be sensitive to steroids

## 2. Castration and Effect of Sex Hormones

After castration the cyclic changes in DA turnover are lost and the turnover
remains low as in proestrus-estrus (FUXE *et al.*, 1967, 1969c). Also the cyclic
changes in the number and intensity of DA cell bodies are lost and they appear as
found in diestrus (LICHTENSTEIGER *et al.*, 1969).

When castrated male or female rats are treated with low doses (at least down
to 0.15 µg) of estradiol benzoate or testosterone (at least down to 0.3 mg) there is
a marked increase in the DA turnover in the tubero-infundibular DA neurons
(FUXE *et al.*, 1967, 1969b). Progesterone (15 mg/rat) caused only a slight increase
and hydrocortisone caused no certain changes in the DA turnover. LICHTEN-

Steiger et al. (1969) have described a disappearance of fluorescence from the DA cell bodies during treatment with estradiol, which further illustrates the necessity of performing turnover studies before interpreting changes in amine levels in cell bodies. The marked activation obtained after treatment with estrogen or testosterone suggests that the negative feedback on LH secretion exerted by these hormones may at least partly be mediated via an activation of the tubero-infundibular DA neurons (see Fig. 3).

Higher doses of sexhormones are needed in normal rats to cause an activation similar to that found in castrated rats. This may be due to an increased reactivity of the tubero-infundibular DA neurons or to a decreased breakdown of the sex hormones in the castrated animal (Lehmann and Breuer, 1969).

### 3. Some Endocrine States with Blocked Ovulation

If it is true that the tubero-infundibular DA neurons participate in inhibiting the release of LRF from the median eminence this neuron system should be activated also in pseudopregnant rats, androgen-sterilized rats and constant estrous rats, in which ovulation is blocked but not the secretion of estrogen or prolactin (pseudopregnancy). This was also found to be the case.

*a) Pseudopregnancy.* The pseudopregnant state was produced either by mechanical stimulation at estrous or by way of salpingectomy after normal mating (Fuxe et al., 1969a). The pseudopregnant state was found to be associated with a marked activation of the tubero-infundibular DA neurons which subsided when normal cycling started after 12–13 days of pseudopregnancy (Fuxe et al., 1969a). This study illustrates the importance of mechanical stimuli for the subsequent activation of the tubero-infundibular DA neurons and that the hypothalamic neurons may be sensitized to the effects of the mechanical stimuli by estrogen which has been shown to activate the tubero-infundibular DA system (see above).

*b) Androgen-Sterilized and Constant Estrous Rats.* In androgen-sterilized rats ovulation is blocked, but estrogen secretion remains unimpaired (see review by Barraclough, 1967). A similar situation exists in constant light (3 months) rats (see review by Wurtman, 1967). No cyclic changes in DA turnover were found, but the activity remained constantly high as in diestrous (Fuxe et al., 1969c). Furthermore, in several rats exposed to constant light the turnover in the tubero-infundibular DA neurons was increased even above that found in diestrous, and the number and intensity of DA cell bodies were markedly increased. This activation may be due to the constant high secretion of estrogen which will activate the DA system directly or indirectly. In support of this view castration of e.g. androgen-sterilized rats leads to a considerable decrease in turnover of DA in the median eminence. Higher doses of sex hormones have to be given to castrated androgen-sterilized rats than to normal, castrated rats in order to obtain activation of the tubero-infundibular DA system again. This finding may be due to a decreased sensitivity of the hypothalamic nerve cells of the androgen-sterilized rats to sex hormones as compared to normal, castrated rats.

It is important to point out that FSH secretion must be relatively high in these rats, since high amounts of estrogen were being formed, whereas the peak secretion of LH was blocked. Thus, the activation of the tubero-infundibular DA neurons may be associated with blockade of LRF release necessary for ovulation but not with follicle stimulating hormone releasing factor (FSHRF) release from

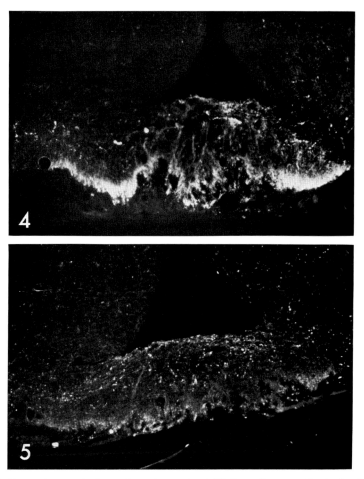

Fig. 4. Median eminence of a hypophysectomized rat (10 days after operation) after treatment with H44/68 (250 mg/kg, 3 hours before killing). A fluorescence of strong intensity remains in the external layer. ×120

Fig. 5. Median eminence of a hypophysectomized rat (10 days after operation). The rat has been treated with prolactin (0.5 mg/day, i.v.) for 3 days, the last injection made 2 hours before the H44/68 treatment, which was performed as described in text to Fig. 3. A fluorescence of very low to low intensity remains in the external layer. ×120

the median eminence. These findings may be interpreted to support the view that the tubero-infundibular DA neurons mainly act to inhibit the release of LRF without necessarily affecting FSHRF release. However, it has to be considered that in these two states the blockade of ovulation may simply be due to the inability of storing LRF in sufficient concentrations in the peptidergic nerve terminals.

### 4. Hypophysectomy and Effect of Pituitary Hormones

Following hypophysectomy there is a marked decrease in DA turnover in the median eminence (Fuxe and Hökfelt, 1969a, b) to a degree of activity below that found in castration and proestrous-estrous. This marked decrease in activity is probably due to the removal of prolactin secretion, since injections of prolactin (in doses at least down to 0.3 mg/rat) in hypophysectomized and/or castrated rats cause a dose-dependent activation of the tubero-infundibular DA neurons (Figs. 4, 5) which is of the same order of magnitude as found after treatment with estrogen or testosterone (Fuxe and Hökfelt, unpublished data). A similar activation is also found when anterior pituitary transplants are made into the anterior chamber of the eye (Olson et al., unpublished data). In view of these results it is probable that the marked activation of the tubero-infundibular DA neurons found in pregnancy, pseudopregnancy and lactation is due to the increased secretion of prolactin found in these endocrine states. Injections of FSH, LH, ACTH and vasopressin have not been found to influence the activity in the tubero-infundibular DA neurons of hypophysectomized and/or castrated rats.

In agreement with the view that prolactin maintains the high activation of the tubero-infundibular DA neurons in the endocrine states mentioned above, it has been found that hypophysectomy in lactation or pregnancy cause a marked decrease in activity of the tubero-infundibular DA neurons (Fuxe and Hökfelt, unpublished data). Furthermore, antiprogestational compounds such as ergocornine and 2-Br-α-ergo-kryptine (3 mg/kg, i.p.) given in early pregnancy or in lactation cause a similar marked decrease in activity of the tubero-infundibular DA neurons (Fuxe and Hökfelt, unpublished data). This effect of the drugs could be caused by an interference with prolactin secretion. In consequence to this prolactin blood levels decline. The high activity of the tubero-infundibular DA neurons can no longer be maintained and LRF release occurs in significant amounts to cause ovulation.

The important role played by prolactin in the regulation of the activity in the tubero-infundibular DA neurons also explains why the activity of this neuron system is highest in diestrous, at which stage prolactin secretion is high (Sar and Meites, 1967). The switch in activity from low to high activity in the tubero-infundibular DA neurons in late estrous-early diestrous is therefore probably partly due to the increase in prolactin secretion and partly to the maximum secretion of estrogen occurring at this time. The switch from high to low activity in late diestrous-early proestrous is accordingly at least partly due to a decrease in prolactin secretion.

### 5. General Discussion

It is obvious from the present results that the claim by Schneider and McCann (1969) from their in vitro studies that DA in the median eminence acts to stimulate LRF secretion is in marked opposition to our results. This may indicate that results obtained from in vitro studies have to be interpreted with great caution. It is also remarkable that the effects of DA on LRF can be blocked by treatment with α-adrenergic blocking agents (McCann, 1969), since α-adrenergic blocking agents block NA receptors in the CNS and do not seem to have any certain actions on DA receptors (ANDÉN et al., 1969). SAWYER (1969), on the other hand, reported at the Stresa meeting that in his laboratory using injections into the third ventricle adrenaline induced ovulation, whereas DA proved to be relatively ineffective. McCANN (1969) reported the opposite results after intraventricular injections with DA, which by him was claimed to cause release of LRF (see SCHNEIDER, this symposium). The only results obtained with local monoamine implantation into the median eminence which are in agreement with the evidence presented here and in an earlier review (FUXE and HÖKFELT, 1969a) are those reported by KOBAYASHI and MATSUI (1969). They found prolonged diestrous phases with intermittent estrous after DA and NA implantation. Thus, since several workers report different results no strong conclusions can at the present time be drawn from studies based on implantation and intraventricular injections as to the actions of the monoamines in the median eminence region.

The evidence obtained from our own studies, summarized in the present paper, are based on turnover studies using two different techniques. Thus, both rate of decline of amine following synthesis inhibition (α-methyl-p-tyrosine-methylester, α-propyldopacetamide) and rate of decline of labelled DA have been studied and been found to give essentially the same results.

Our view that the tubero-infundibular DA neurons inhibit the release of LRF from the median eminence is further strengthened by the fact that in estrogen-treated castrated rats reserpine or a potent DA receptor blocking agent clothiapine (0.1 mg/kg, i.p.) causes increased LH secretion from the anterior pituitary as revealed in vitro with the help of the lactic acid production test (HAMBERGER et al., unpublished data). Incubations of anterior pituitaries with DA (12 µg/ml) have never been found to change the secretion of LH into the medium. Thus, DA in all probability acts at the median eminence level and not at the pituitary level to influence LH secretion (HAMBERGER et al., to be published). Results indicating that DA acts at the hypothalamic level have also been obtained by other workers (McCANN, 1969; KORDON, 1969).

In view of the above discussion it is of great interest to know which neuron systems are involved in the control of prolactin inhibitory factor (PIF) secretion from the median eminence. There exist findings from the use of drugs interfering with central monoamine neurotransmission (see SAWYER, 1963; EVERETT, 1964; COPPOLA et al., 1965) that central catecholaminergic mechanisms are involved in this control. There now exist data that mainly a noradrenergic mechanism is involved (FUXE and HÖKFELT, 1969c and see below).

## Central NA Neurons

### Morphology

See previous reviews by FUXE and HÖKFELT (1969a, b). It should only be pointed out that the hypothalamus with the preoptic area and large parts of the limbic system is innervated by a ventral NA pathway arising mainly from group A 1, A 2, A 5 and A 7 in the medulla oblongata and pons (DAHLSTRÖM and FUXE, 1964; UNGERSTEDT, unpublished data; FUXE and HÖKFELT, unpublished data). The neocortex is mainly innervated by a dorsal NA pathway originating from the NA cell bodies in the locus coeruleus (Olson and Fuxe, 1969; Ungerstedt, unpublished data; Hökfelt and Fuxe, to be published). It should be remembered that in view of the very large number of collaterals formed by one single NA neuron there is probably no selective activation of e.g. the hypothalamic NA nerve terminals, but the NA nerve terminals in many parts of the brain are usually activated.

## Function

The reader is mainly referred to recent reviews (Fuxe and Hökfelt, 1969a, b, c) and especially to the review by Fuxe et al. (1969d) in which mainly our present view on the neuroendocrine role of the central NA neurons is summarized. In the present review mainly the role of the central NA neurons in the regulation of prolactin secretion, but not their possible direct influence on LHRF and/or FSHRF secretion, will be discussed, since by influencing prolactin secretion central noradrenergic mechanisms could influence indirectly the activity in the tubero-infundibular DA neurons.

After treatment with drugs which selectively block NA neurotransmission such as phenoxybenzamine, which causes blockade of NA but not of DA receptors (Andén et al., 1969) and a potent dopamine-$\beta$-oxidase inhibitor FLA 63 (Corrodi et al., unpublished data) there is a marked activation of the tubero-infundibular DA neurons with increased DA turnover and marked increases in number of DA cell bodies in the arcuate nucleus (Fuxe and Hökfelt, 1969a, and unpublished data). It is well known that phenoxybenzamine causes blockade of ovulation and induces pseudopregnancy (Markee et al., 1948). After hypophysectomy phenoxybenzamine and FLA 63 could no longer elicit their marked activation of the tubero-infundibular DA neurons. This might suggest that the effects of the noradrenergic drugs were primarily to cause release of prolactin from the anterior pituitary by way of directly or indirectly blocking release of PIF into the portal vessels, in this way causing pseudopregnancy. In agreement with this, monoamine depleting agents have been found to cause pseudopregnancy with increased prolactin-secretion (Coppola et al., 1965).

In view of these results the following hypothesis can be made: Central NA neurons participate in the neural mechanism controlling PIF secretion exerting a stimulatory influence on PIF secretion, e.g. by way of disinhibition. When central NA neurotransmission is blocked prolactin secretion and thus prolactin blood levels will increase. This leads to a marked activation of the tubero-infundibular DA neurons and subsequent blockade of LRF release from the LRF storing neurons, probably by way of axo-axonic inhibition induced by the released DA. In this way prolactin secretion can influence LH secretion and control it. In agreement with this the activation of the tubero-infundibular DA neurons in late estrous-early diestrous seems to be associated with and rather preceded by a decreased neural activity in and release from the hypothalamic NA nerve terminals (Fuxe and Hökfelt, unpublished). The inactivation of the DA neurons in late diestrous-proestrons, on the other hand, seems to associated with or rather preceded by an increased neural activity in and increased release from the hypothalamic NA nerve terminals.

# Central 5-HT Neurons

## Anatomy

See previous reviews (FUXE et al., 1968; FUXE and HÖKFELT, 1969c). It should only here be pointed out that also each central 5-HT neuron in the same way as each central NA neuron gives rise to a large number of collaterals. Therefore activation of only a few 5-HT cell bodies will cause release of 5-HT from nerve terminals in many areas of the brain. Furthermore, the ascending 5-HT pathways to the tel- and diencephalon mainly arise from the raphe cell bodies of the mesencephalon [nuc. raphe dorsalis (B7), nuc. raphe medianus (B8), see DAHLSTRÖM and FUXE, 1964]. Thus, e.g. the hypothalamus and the preoptic area mainly receive mesencephalic 5-HT afferents.

## Function

As to their possible role in gonadotrophin regulation, see previous reviews by FUXE and HÖKFELT (1969b, c). In a previous article evidence was presented that both central NA and 5-HT neurons could participate in the regulation of ACTH secretion and that pituitary-adrenal activity in turn could influence the activity in the NA and 5-HT neurons (FUXE et al., 1969e). Thus, in agreement with the findings of JAVOY et al. (1968), adrenalectomy caused an increase in the NA turnover. This increased turnover was found in many areas of the brain and could be changed to normal again by treatment with cortisol. The interpretation was given in view of results e.g. on the effect of adrenergic drugs on ACTH secretion that the dexamethasone-sensitive nerve cells (at least partly identical with CRF containing neurons) in the hypothalamus (STEINER et al., 1969) change their activity after adrenalectomy. Hereby a neural feedback is induced to the NA cell bodies in the rhombencephalon increasing the activity in the NA neurons, possibly to avoid excessive stimulation of ACTH secretion. After treatment with cortisol the activity in the dexamethasone sensitive neurons is restored to a normal level and as a consequence of this also the activity in the central NA neurons.

The turnover in some 5-HT neurons, may possibly be decreased after adrenalectomy and restored to normal or above normal after repeated treatment with cortisol or dexamethasone (FUXE et al., unpublished data). This has been indicated both in studies with amine-synthesis inhibitors (α-propyl-dopacetamide) and in studies on the accumulation of 5-HT in the neurons following nialamide treatment. In agreement with this McEWEN (pers. comm.) has recently found an increased tryptophan hydroxylase activity following treatment with cortisol. Since 5-HT nerve terminals are present in high numbers in hypothalamus where dexamethasone-sensitive neurons exist and injections of 5-HT into hypothalamus cause marked effects on ACTH secretion (NAUMENKO, 1968) the present results could suggest that the 5-HT neurons may also participate in the regulation of ACTH secretion. The inactivation of the 5-HT neurons may be indirect by way of a neural feedback elicited from glycocorticoid-sensitive neurons in the hypothalamus as suggested in the case of the NA neurons. It cannot be excluded, however, that the 5-HT cell bodies in the mesencephalon themselves are sensitive to glycocorticoids such as cortisol and dexamethasone. If this is the case, these steroids could then directly decrease the membrane resting potential of the 5-HT neurons either by way of increasing membrane conductance or *e.g.* decreasing the efficiency of the sodium-pump by an intraneuronal action. It is possible that steroids *e.g.* via an effect on RNA or DNA turnover and/or by the activation of the adenylcyclase could increase protein-synthesis and in this way increase the activity of the tryptophan hydroxylase.—These results may explain why there are only shortlasting decreases in 5-HT in response to stress (CORRODI *et al.*, 1968). Thus, this decrease which probably is due to an activation of the tryptophan pyrrolase by the cortisol released from the adrenal medulla (GREEN and CURZON, 1970), is soon counteracted by the direct actions of cortisol on the brain, causing the activation of the 5-HT neurons as described above. This activation of the 5-HT neurons could at least partly indicate that the negative feedback exerted by glycocorticoids on ACTH secretion is mediated via an activation of the central 5-HT neurons.—Since the activation of 5-HT neurons by glycocorticoids occurs in many parts of the brain, this action could have important effects on mood. It is known from several studies that a decrease in central 5-HT neurotransmission is at least one of the biochemical factors causing depression (COPPEN, 1967; CARLSSON *et al.*, 1968; FUXE and UNGERSTEDT, 1968b; CARLSSON *et al.*, 1969). Treatment with dexamethasone has recently also been found to cause good therapeutical effects in depressed patients (McQUIRE, pers. comm.).

## Summary

Evidence has been presented that the tubero-infundibular DA neurons act by inhibiting the release of at least LRF from the median eminence, probably by way of axo-axonic influence on the terminals storing LRF. Evidence has also been given that the central NA neurons participate in the regulation of PIF secretion. In the absence of NA neuro-transmission PIF secretion is diminished and prolactin secretion markedly increased. Since prolactin markedly activates the tubero-infundibular DA neurons, the results may explain why high prolactin secretion is often associated with a decrease in LH secretion.—Evidence has also been presented that central NA and 5-HT neurons may participate in the control of ACTH secretion and that the negative feedback exerted by glycocorticoids on ACTH secretion may partly be mediated via an increased 5-HT neurotransmission. This latter finding also explains why glycocorticoids have effects on mood in man, since many findings support the view that there is a decreased 5-HT neurotransmission in depression. Accordingly glycocorticoids should alleviate depression by activating the central 5-HT neurons.

## References

ANDÉN, N.-E., CORRODI, H., FUXE, K.: Turnover studies using synthesis inhibition. In: Metabolism of amines in the brain (ed. G. HOOPER), p. 38–47. London: MacMillan 1969.
BARRACLOUGH, C. A.: Modifications in reproductive function after exposure to hormones during the prenatal and early postnatal period. In: Neuroendocrinology (eds. L. MARTINI and W. F. GANONG), vol. II, p. 61–99. New York-London: Academic Press 1967.
BARRY, M. J.: Recherches sur l'origine et les sites de terminaison des fibres monoaminergiques du tractus hypothalamo-hypophysaire. C. R. Soc. Biol. (Paris) 162, 1946–1948 (1968).
CARLSSON, A., DAHLSTRÖM, A., FUXE, K., HILLARP, N.-Å.: Failure of reserpine to deplete noradrenaline neurons of α-methyl noradrenaline formed from α-methyl-DOPA. Acta pharmacol. (Kbh.) 22, 270–276 (1965).

CARLSSON, A., CORRODI, H., FUXE, K., HÖKFELT, T.: Effect of antidepressant drugs on the depletion of intraneuronal brain 5-hydroxytryptamine stores caused by 4-methyl-α-ethyl-meta-tyramine. Europ. J. Pharmacol. 5, 357–366 (1969).

— FUXE, K., HAMBERGER, B., LINDQVIST, M.: Biochemical and histochemical studies on the effects of imipramine-like drugs and (+)-amphetamine on central and peripheral catecholamine neurons. Acta physiol. scand. 67, 481–497 (1966).

— — UNGERSTEDT, U.: The effect of imipramine on central 5-hydroxy-tryptamine neurons. J. Pharm. Pharmacol. 20, 150–151 (1968).

COPPEN, A.: The biochemistry of affective disorders. Brit. J. Psychiat. 113, 1237–1241 (1967).

COPPOLA, J. A., LEONARDI, R. G., LIPPMAN, W., PERRINE, J. W., RINGLER, I.: Induction of pseudopregnancy in rats by depletors of endogenous catecholamines. Endocrinology 77, 485–490 (1965).

CORRODI, H., FUXE, K., HÖKFELT, T.: The effect of immobilization stress on the activity of central monoamine neurons. Life Sci. 7, 107–112 (1968).

DAHLSTRÖM, A., FUXE, K.: Evidence for the existence of monoamine neurons in the central nervous system. I. Demonstration of monoamines in the cell bodies of brain stem neurons. Acta physiol. scand. 62, Suppl. 232, 1–55 (1964).

EVERETT, J. W.: Central neural control of reproductive functions of the adenohypophysis. Physiol. Rev. 44, 373–431 (1964).

FUXE, K.: Cellular localization of monoamines in the median eminence and infundibular stem of some mammals. Acta physiol. scand. 58, 383–384 (1963).

— Cellular localization of monoamines in the median eminence and infundibular stem of some mammals. Z. Zellforsch. 61, 710–724 (1964).

— CORRODI, H., HÖKFELT, T., JONSSON, G.: Central monoamine neurons and pituitary-adrenal activity. Paper read at conference on "The pituitary-adrenal axis and the nervous system", Vierhouten, The Netherlands, July 1969 (1969e).

— HÖKFELT, T.: Further evidence for the existence of tubero-infundibular dopamine neurons. Acta physiol. scand. 66, 243–244 (1966).

— — The influence of central catecholamine neurons on the hormone secretion from the anterior and posterior pituitary. In: Neurosecretion (ed. F. STUTINSKY), p. 165–177. Berlin-Heidelberg-New York: Springer 1967.

— — Catecholamines in the hypothalamus and the pituitary gland. In: Frontiers in neuroendocrinology (eds. W. F. GANONG and L. MARTINI), p. 47–96. New York-London-Toronto: Oxford University Press 1969a.

— — Monoaminergic afferent input to the hypothalamus and the dopamine afferent input to the median eminence. In: Progress in endocrinology (ed. C. GUAL), p. 495–502. Amsterdam: Excerpt. Med. Int. Congr. Ser. 184. 1969b.

— — Central monoaminergic neurons and hypothalamic function. Paper read at conference on "Integration of endocrine and non-endocrine mechanisms in the hypothalamus", Stresa, May 1969 (1969c).

— — JONSSON, G.: Participation of central monoamine neurons in the regulation of the anterior pituitary secretion. Paper read at "2nd. Int. Meet. Int. Soc. Neurochem.", Milan, Italy, September 1969 (1969d).

— — NILSSON, O.: Activity changes in the tubero-infundibular dopamine neurons of the rat during various states of the reproductive cycle. Life Sci. 6, 2057–2061 (1967).

— — — Factors involved in the control of the activity of the tubero-infundibular dopamine neurons during pregnancy and lactation. Neuroendocrinology 5, 257–270 (1969a).

— — — Castration, sex hormones and tubero-infundibular dopamine neurons. Neuroendocrinology 5, 107–120 (1969b).

— — — Tubero-infundibular dopamine neurons and the estrous cycle. To be published (1969c).

— — UNGERSTEDT, U.: Localization of indolealkylamines in CNS. Adv. Pharmacology 6A, 235–251 (1968).

— LJUNGGREN, L.: Cellular localization of monoamines in the upper brain stem of the pigeon. J. comp. Neurol. 125, 355–382 (1965).

Fuxe, K., Ungerstedt, U.: Histochemical studies on the distribution of catecholamines and 5-hydroxytryptamine after intraventricular injections. Histochemie 13, 16–28 (1968a).
— — Histochemical studies on the effect of (+)-amphetamine, drugs of the imipramine group and tryptamine on central catecholamine and 5-hydroxytryptamine neurons after intraventricular injections of catecholamines and 5-hydroxytryptamine. Europ. J. Pharmacol. 4, 135–144 (1968b).
Green, A. R., Curzon, G.: Decrease of 5-hydroxytryptamine in the brain provoked by hydrocortisone and its prevention by allopurinol. Nature (Lond.), in press (1970).
Hamberger, L.: Effects of gonadotrophins on the metabolism of the rat ovary. M. D. Thesis, Gothenburg, Sweden (1968).
Hökfelt, T.: The possible ultrastructural identification of tubero-infundibular dopamine containing nerve endings in the median eminence of the rat. Brain Res. 5, 121–123 (1967).
— Electron microscopic studies on peripheral and central monoamine neurons. M. D. Thesis, Stockholm, Sweden (1968).
Javoy, F., Glowinski, J., Kordon, C.: Effects of adrenalectomy on the turnover of norepinephrine in the rat brain. Europ. J. Pharmacol. 4, 103–104 (1968).
Kobayashi, H., Matsui, T.: Fine structure of the median eminence and its functional significance. In: Frontiers in neuroendocrinology (eds. W. F. Ganong and L. Martini), p. 3–46. New York-London-Toronto: Oxford University Press 1969.
Kordon, C.: Discussion remark at conference on "Integration of endocrine and non-endocrine mechanisms in the hypothalamus", Stresa, May 1969.
Lehmann, W. D., Breuer, H.: Stoffwechsel von Östrogenen in der Rattenleber vor und nach Kastration sowie nach Verabreichung verschiedener Steroidhormone. Hoppe-Seylers Z. physiol. Chem. 350, 191–200 (1969).
Leonardelli, J.: Modifications des fibres et cellules monoaminergiques de la région infundibulo-tubérienne du Cobaye au cours du cycle oestral. C. R. Soc. Biol. (Paris) 162, 1937–1940 (1968).
Lichtensteiger, W.: Mikrofluorimetrische Studien an katecholaminhaltigen hypothalamischen Nervenzellen der Ratte in den verschiedenen Phasen des viertägigen Östruszyklus. Helv. physiol. pharmacol. Acta 25, 423–425 (1968).
— Cyclic variations of catecholamine content in hypothalamic nerve cells during the estrous cycle of the rat, with a concomitant study of the substantia nigra. J. Pharm. exp. Ther. 165, 204–215 (1969).
— Korpela, K., Langemann, H.: Mikrofluorimetrische Studien an katecholaminhaltigen hypothalamischen Nervenzellen der Ratte. Der Einfluß von Ovariektomie und gonadalen Steroiden. Helv. physiol. pharmacol. Acta 26, 360–361 (1969).
— Langemann, H.: Uptake of exogenous catecholamines by monoamine-containing neurons of the central nervous system: Uptake of catecholamines by arcuato-infundibular neurons. J. Pharm. exp. Ther. 151, 400–408 (1966).
Markee, J. E., Sawyer, C. H., Hollinshead, W. H.: Adrenergic control of the release of luteinizing hormone from the hypophysis of the rabbit. Recent Progr. Hormone Res. 2, 117–131 (1948).
McCann, S. M.: Chemistry and physiological aspects of the releasing factors. Paper read at conference on "Integration of endocrine and non-endocrine mechanisms in the hypothalamus", Stresa, May 1969.
Naumenko, E. V.: Hypothalamic chemoreactive structures and the regulation of pituitary adrenal function. Effects of local injections of norepinephrine, carbachol and serotonin into the brain of guinea-pigs with intact brains and after mesencephalic transection. Brain Res. 11, 1–10 (1968).
Olson, L., Fuxe, K.: Development of central monoamine neurons. To be published (1969).
Sar, M., Meites, J.: Changes in pituitary prolactin release and hypothalamic PIF content during the estrous cycle of rats. Proc. Soc. exp. Biol. (N.Y.) 125, 1018–1021 (1967).

SAWYER, C. H.: Discussion of paper by P. L. MUNSON: Pharmacology of neuroendocrine blocking agents. In: Advances in neuroendocrinology (ed. A. V. NALBANDOV), p. 444–459. Urbana: University of Illinois Press 1963.
— Some endocrinological applications of electrophysiology. Paper read at conference on "Integration of endocrine and non-endocrine mechanisms in the hypothalamus", Stresa, May 1969.
SCHNEIDER, H. P. G., McCANN, S. M.: Possible role of dopamine as transmitter to promote discharge of LH-releasing factor. Endocrinology 85, 121–132 (1969).
STEINER, F. A., RUF, K., AKERT, K.: Steroid-sensitive neurons in rat brain: anatomical localization and responses to neurohumors and ACTH. Brain Res. 12, 74–85 (1969).
WURTMAN, R. J.: Effects of light and visual stimuli on endocrine function. In: Neuroendocrinology (eds. L. MARTINI and W. F. GANONG), vol. II, p. 19–59. New York-London: Academic Press 1967.

# Brain Catecholamines and Growth Hormone Release*

Eugenio E. Müller**

Department of Pharmacology, School of Pharmacy, University of Pavia, Pavia (Italy)

**Key words:** Brain catecholamines — Growth hormone releasing factor — Growth hormone release. — Noradrenaline and growth hormone release.

There is much evidence, based on physiological, chemical and biochemical studies, that the central nervous system (CNS) participates in the control of growth hormone (GH) secretion (Pecile and Müller, 1966; Glick, 1969). The hypothalamus of many animal species contains a specific neurohormone (growth hormone-releasing factor, GRF) controlling GH secretion (see Schally and Kastin, 1969). However, much work has yet to be done to clarify all aspects of CNS control over GH release.

The introduction, in the last years, of a highly specific and sensitive histo-chemical fluorescence method for the demonstration of noradrenaline and dopamine (Falck, Hillarp, Thieme and Torp, 1962; Hillarp, Fuxe and Dahlström, 1966), has demonstrated in the hypothalamus of many species neural fibers containing primary catecholamines (CA) terminating close to hypothalamic nuclei or portal capillaries in the median eminence (Fuxe, 1965; Fuxe and Hök-felt, 1967). Since these are the places where neurohormones controlling anterior pituitary function are in operation (McCann and Dhariwal, 1966), our main interest was to investigate whether brain CA might mediate the influence of peripheral stimuli on the hypothalamic-hypophysial unit controlling GH secretion.

## Material and Methods

### Animals

Intact male or female Sprague-Dawley rats weighing 130–140 g were used as experimental animals. Hypophysectomized assay animals 26–28 days old (Falconi and Rossi, 1964) were used for "tibia test" assay 14–16 days after surgery. Some rats were hypophysectomized one week before the experiment and treated by intraventricular injection with various drugs (see below). Six to eight rats were used for each experimental group.

### Procedures

The influence of reserpine on pituitary GH content and on the release of growth hormone induced by insulin administration was studied. All animals were deprived of food overnight

* Supported by USPHS Grant HD 01109–04. The participation of Dr. A. Pecile in this research project is gratefully acknowledged. The author wishes also to express his gratitude to the Endocrinology Study Section of the National Institutes of Health for the supply of growth hormone and to Miss Vannisa Albrici for the skilful technical assistance.

** Present address: Department of Pharmacology, School of Medicine, University of Milan, Milan, Italy.

before the treatment. The following day they were injected with the drug suspended in special reserpine diluent. In addition to reserpine (1 mg/kg i.p.), the following central or peripheral norepinephrine and serotonin depletors were studied for their capacity to suppress insulin-induced GH release: α-methyl-dopa (300 mg/kg), α-methyl-m-tyrosine (300 mg/kg), tetra-benazine (15 mg/kg), guanethidine (30 mg/kg), tyramine (15 mg/kg) and brethylium (50 mg/kg). Three hours after these treatments, the rats were injected intraperitoneally with 2 U/kg of regular insulin (Iletin, Lilly) and were sacrificed 1 hr later. Control animals were injected with saline or with special reserpine diluent. In the experiments in which an attempt was made to counteract the suppressive action of reserpine on GH secretion, iproniazid (150 mg/kg) was given subcutaneously 18–21 hr prior to the injection of reserpine.

When the GH-releasing activity of hypothalamic tissue was tested, the following substances were administered by intraventricular injection, dissolved in 20 μl volume of pyrogen-free saline: epinephrine (E) (0.5 and 0.1 μg), norepinephrine (NE) (0.5 and 0.1 μg), dopamine (DA) (0.5 and 0.1 μg), serotonin (0.5 μg), histamine (0.5 μg), acetylcholine (0.5 μg), vasopressin (8 mU), oxytocin (8 mU). When salts of drugs were used, doses were expressed in terms of the drug base. In experiments in which the GRF activity was determined in the hypothalamus and plasma of intact or hypophysectomized rats the following substances were administered by intraventricular injection dissolved in 20 μl of pyrogen-free saline: NE(0.5 μg); DA (0.5 μg); serotonin (0.5 μg). When the minimal dose of CA which still induces GH release was investigated both NE and DA were injected intraventricularly into intact rats at the doses of 0.05, 0.01, 0.005 μg.

### Intraventricular Injection

The method recently described by Noble, Wurtman and Axelrod (1967) was used.

### GH Assay

The experimental animals subjected to the various treatments described above were killed by decapitation. Their anterior pituitaries were removed and weighed to the nearest 0.02 mg on a microtorsion balance; adenohypophysial tissue was then pooled by groups (6–8 animals/group) and homogenized in 0.9% saline. The diluted material was kept frozen until immediately before injection. GH activity of the samples was measured by the "tibia test" method of Greenspan et al. (1949). Significance of differences in epiphysial cartilage width was determined by Student's t test.

### Test of Hypothalamic GRF Activity

The stalk median eminence region (SME) of intact or hypophysectomized rats was removed 30 min after the intraventricular injection. Acid extracts of the SME were prepared by the method previously described (Pecile, Müller, Falconi and Martini, 1965). Thirty-day-old female Sprague-Dawley rats were used as recipient animals. They were given the equivalent of 2.5 or 2.0 SME (see Tables) in 0.5 ml of saline by intracarotid injection under ether anesthesia. The control recipient rats were injected with 0.5 ml saline only. Fifteen or 30 min after injection the recipient rats were decapited. GH activity of their anterior pituitary glands was measured as described above. The depletion of pituitary GH in recipient animals was used as an index of GRF activity present in the SME extract injected.

### Test of Plasma GRF Activity

Blood was collected from the trunk of intact or hypophysectomized rats 30 min after the treatment. Blood from each group of 6–8 rats was pooled in a chilled heparinized plastic tube and the plasma separated by centrifugation. The pooled plasma samples were kept frozen until immediately before injection. One ml of the plasma was injected into the carotid artery of recipient rats. GRF activity of the plasma was determined in a way similar to that for hypothalamic GRF.

### Blood Glucose

A sample of venous blood was withdrawn from experimental rats at the time of sacrifice for blood glucose determinations (Glucostat, Worthington Biochemicals).

*Temperature*

Body temperature was recorded using a rectally-inserted probe, and displayed on an electrical thermometer calibrated at 0.1 intervals. Temperature was recorded before the intraventricular injection of test substances (see Table 2) and just before decapitation. All temperature measurements were carried out in a room at a temperature of 21–23° C.

Table 1. *Growth hormone-releasing activity of stalk median eminence (SME) extracts of rats submitted to insulin hypoglycemia, with and without pretreatment with reserpine*

| Groups | Treatment[a] of SME donor animals (dose and no. in parentheses) | Material administered to pituitary donor animals | Growth hormone evaluation | | $p$ value vs group 1 |
|--------|--------|--------|--------|--------|--------|
| | | | Epiphyseal width $\mu$ (mean $\pm$ S.E.)[b] | Pituitary GH content ($\mu$g GH/mg wet pituitary) | |
| 1 | — | Saline | $273 \pm 5.3$ | 82.5 | — |
| 2 | (15) Saline | 2.5 SME | $247 \pm 6.9$ | 52.1 | 0.01 |
| 3 | (15) Insulin (2 U/kg i.p.) | 2.5 SME | $261 \pm 6.3$ | 71.6 | NS |
| 4 | (15) Reserpine (1 mg/kg i.p.) | 2.5 SME | $243 \pm 1.7$ | 47.7 | 0.001 |
| 5 | (15) Reserpine + Insulin | 2.5 SME | $230 \pm 4.2$ | 29.4 | 0.001 |

[a] Saline given 1 hour before sacrifice. Insulin given 1 hour before sacrifice. Reserpine given 4 hours before sacrifice.

[b] 6–8 hypophysectomized animals per group.

# Results

## Central or Peripheral Depletors of Catecholamines and GH Release from the Pituitary

From the results obtained, it appears that only brain norepinephrine depletors were able to suppress insulin-induced GH release. Single intraperitoneal injections of reserpine, α-methyl-dopa, α-methyl-m-tyrosine or tetrabenazine blocked the release of growth hormone induced by the administration of insulin. Tetrabenazine alone induced a significant depletion of pituitary GH, whereas slight but significant reductions of pituitary GH content were noted after the administration of all brain norepinephrine depletors. The values of blood glucose found in control or treated animals appear to be similar: only α-methyl-m-tyrosine and tetrabenazine induced a significant increase in blood sugar.

At variance with the action of brain norepinephrine-depletors, peripheral depletors of catecholamines, guanethidine, tyramine and brethylium were unable to suppress the GH releasing effect of insulin hypoglycemia.

In another series of experiments an attempt was made to reverse the blockade of GH induced by reserpine. Iproniazid, which given alone was unable to block the GH release induced by insulin, completely antagonized the suppressive action of reserpine.

It has been previously shown that the suppressive action of reserpine on insulin-induced GH release occurs at the level of the CNS and not on the pituitary

Table 2. *Effect on pituitary growth hormone (GH) activity, blood glucose and body temperature of epinephrine, norepinephrine and dopamine given by intraventricular injection*

| Treatment (dose and no. of animals in parentheses) | Epiphyseal width μ (mean ± S.E.)[e] | Blood glucose (mg/100 ml) | Temperature (°C ± S.E.) initial | Temperature (°C ± S.E.) final | Difference (°C ± S.E.)[f] |
|---|---|---|---|---|---|
| 6) Saline (0.02 ml) | 230 ± 4.7 | 103 ± 1.5 | 37.00 ± 0.037 | 37.55 ± 0.148 | +0.26 ± 0.068 |
| 6) Norepinephrine (0.5 μg/0.02 ml) | 212 ± 4.3[b] | 106 ± 2.8 | 37.62 ± 0.452 | 37.00 ± 0.540 | −0.62 ± 0.147 |
| 6) Dopamine (0.5 μg/0.02 ml) | 202 ± 10.7[a] | 67 ± 5.1[d] | 37.78 ± 0.069 | 37.41 ± 0.171 | −0.42 ± 0.125 |
| 6) Saline (0.02 ml) | 246 ± 3.5 | 104 ± 1.1 | 38.12 ± 0.106 | 37.58 ± 0.146 | −0.54 ± 0.144 |
| 6) Norepinephrine (0.5 μg/0.02 ml) | 209 ± 4.2[d] | 98 ± 1.7 | 38.16 ± 0.206 | 37.38 ± 0.076 | −0.86 ± 0.143 |
| 6) Saline (0.02 ml) | 237 ± 8.8 | 103 ± 0.6 | 38.07 ± 0.069 | 37.52 ± 0.188 | −0.55 ± 0.720 |
| 6) Dopamine (0.5 μg/0.02 ml) | 199 ± 9.6[c] | 77 ± 1.1[c] | 37.88 ± 0.064 | 37.22 ± 0.174 | −0.64 ± 0.598 |
| 5) Saline (0.02 ml) | 254 ± 2.1 | 100 ± 2.1 | — | — | — |
| 5) Norepinephrine (0.1 μg/0.02 ml) | 235 ± 2.2[d] | 108 ± 4.2 | — | — | — |
| 5) Dopamine (0.1 μg/0.02 ml) | 229 ± 2.9[d] | 104 ± 6.5 | — | — | — |
| 5) Saline (0.02 ml) | 252 ± 4.6 | 88 ± 4.4 | 37.55 ± 0.226 | 36.88 ± 0.374 | −0.65 ± 0.520 |
| 5) Epinephrine (0.5 μg/0.02 ml) | 233 ± 5.2[b] | 121 ± 8.7[a] | 38.02 ± 0.181 | 37.32 ± 0.126 | −0.69 ± 0.221 |
| 5) Epinephrine (0.1 μg/0.02 ml) | 242 ± 4.8 | 109 ± 4.0 | 37.84 ± 0.065 | 37.21 ± 0.222 | −0.55 ± 0.723 |

[a] $p < 0.05$ vs saline.
[b] $p < 0.02$ vs saline.
[c] $p < 0.01$ vs saline.
[d] $p < 0.001$ vs saline.
[e] 6–8 hypophysectomized assay animals were used per group.
[f] Difference was calculated as the mean of the differences of temperature values of each animal.

(MÜLLER, SAITO, ARIMURA and SCHALLY, 1967). Thus, in the last series of these experiments we have investigated the possibility that the blockage of GH release induced by reserpine involves the impairment of synthesis and/or release of hypothalamic GRF. From the results reported in Table 1, it appears that a single injection of reserpine (1 mg/kg i.p.) does not affect the GRF content of rat SME, since the depletion of pituitary growth hormone content induced by SME extracts of animals injected with reserpine is of the same order of magnitude as that induced by SME extracts of saline injected animals (group 4 vs 2). However, this drug, when given three hours before insulin is able to prevent completely the release of GRF from the hypothalamus evoked by insulin treatment, as evidenced by the absence of GRF activity in the SME extracts of animals treated with insulin (group 3 vs 1) and by the presence of GRF activity in the SME extracts of animals pretreated with reserpine and subsequently given insulin (group 5 vs 3).

### Intraventricular Administration of Hypothalamic Substances

All data dealing with the effects of catecholamines were grouped in Table 2. It appears that epinephrine, norepinephrine and dopamine, given by intraventricular injection at the dose of 0.5 µg, induce depletion of the pituitary growth hormone content. This is apparent from the narrower epiphysial cartilage in hypophysectomized rats receiving pituitary homogenates from animals injected with E, NE and DA. While NE and DA were active also at doses of 0.1 µg, E did not show any GH releasing effect at this lower dose. On the contrary, the GH activity of the pituitaries taken from animals injected intraventricularly with serotonin, histamine, acetylcholine, vasopressin or oxytocin appeared to be similar to that of pituitaries from control animals. Blood glucose levels in animals injected with NE were not significantly different from controls; they were significantly lower in animals injected with DA (0.5 µg), serotonin, vasopressin or oxytocin, while they were significantly higher than control levels in rats injected with E (0.5 µg only), histamine or acetylcholine. A decrease of body temperature was observed after the intraventricular injection of all substances used; however, only that consequent to serotonin injection appeared to be significant.

### Hypothalamic GRF Activity in Intact and Hypophysectomized Rats after Administration of Brain Amines

The results summarized in Tables 3 and 4 show that administration of pituitary homogenates from saline-treated control rats (Table 3, expl. 1 and 2, group A), when given to the assay rats, widened the epiphyseal cartilage. By contrast, when the pituitaries of animals given SME extracts from intact rats treated intraventricularly with saline were used (exp. 1, group B; exp. 2, group B), the widening of the epiphyseal cartilage was much smaller, indicating the presence of GRF activity. This GRF activity was no longer present in the SME extracts of intact rats given intraventricularly NE (0.5 µg) or DA (0.5 µg), since in this instance the epiphyseal widening induced by the administration to the assay rats of pituitaries from the recipient animals was comparable in degree to that induced by pituitaries from saline-treated control rats (exp. 1 and 2, groups C and D vs A). In the SME extracts of intact animals receiving serotonin intraventricularly, GRF activity appeared not to be modified (exp. 2, group E vs B). Results similar to those obtained in normal rats were obtained in hypophysectomized animals. Table 4 shows, in fact, that no GRF activity was present in the SME extracts of hypophysectomized rats 30 min after intraventricular administration of norepinephrine (0.5 µg) or dopamine (0.5 µg) (groups C and D vs B and A), while GRF activity was still present in the SME extracts of animals treated intraventricularly with saline or serotonin (groups B and E vs A).

Table 3. *Effect on hypothalamic growth hormone releasing activity of norepinephrine (NE), dopamine (DA) or serotonin (5-HT) given by intraventricular injection (i.v.) into normal rats*

| Exp. | Groups | Treatment of SME donor animals | Material administered to pituitary donor animals | Epiphyseal width μ[a] (mean ± S.E.) | Blood glucose (mg/100 ml) |
|---|---|---|---|---|---|
| 1 | A | — | Saline (0.5 ml/rat i.c.) | $255 \pm 3.1$ | — |
| | B | Saline (0.02 ml i.v.) | SME (2 SME/rat i.c.) | $229 \pm 3.3$ [c] | $103 \pm 1.5$ |
| | C | NE (0.5 μg/0.02 ml i.v.) | SME (2 SME/rat i.c.) | $257 \pm 2.1$ | $106 \pm 2.8$ |
| | D | DA (0.5 μg/0.02 ml i.v.) | SME (2 SME/rat i.c.) | $253 \pm 1.6$ | $67 \pm 5.1$ [c] |
| 2 | A | — | Saline (0.5 ml/rat i.c.) | $253 \pm 3.65$ | — |
| | B | Saline (0.02 ml i.v.) | SME (2 SME/rat i.c.) | $224 \pm 1.46$ [c] | $82 \pm 2.2$ |
| | C | NE (0.5 μg/0.02 ml i.v.) | SME (2 SME/rat i.c.) | $247 \pm 5.0$ | $90 \pm 3.0$ |
| | D | DA (0.5 μg/0.02 ml i.v.) | SME (2 SME/rat i.c.) | $250 \pm 3.61$ | $64 \pm 3.8$ [b] |
| | E | 5-HT (0.5 μg/0.02 ml i.v.) | SME (2 SME/rat i.c.) | $223 \pm 10.1$ [c] | $94 \pm 5.1$ |

[a] 6–8 hypophysectomized assay animals were used per group.
[b] $p < 0.01$ vs group A (epiphyseal width) or group B (blood glucose).
[c] $p < 0.001$ vs group A (epiphyseal width) or group B (blood glucose).

Table 4. *Effect on hypothalamic growth hormone releasing activity of norepinephrine (NE), dopamine (DA) or serotonin (5-HT) given by intraventricular injection (i.v.) into hypophysectomized rats*

| Groups | Treatment of SME donor animals[c] | Material administered to pituitary donor animals | Epiphyseal width μ[a] (mean ± S.E.) | Blood glucose (mg/100 ml) |
|---|---|---|---|---|
| A | — | Saline (0.5 ml/rat i.c.) | $252 \pm 1.6$ | — |
| B | Saline (0.02 ml i.v.) | SME (2 SME/rat i.c.) | $216 \pm 4.4$ [b] | $76 \pm 6.0$ |
| C | NE (0.5 μg/0.02 ml i.v.) | SME (2 SME/rat i.c.) | $252 \pm 3.7$ | $103 \pm 9.8$ |
| D | DA (0.5 μg/0.02 ml i.v.) | SME (2 SME/rat i.c.) | $246 \pm 2.8$ | $36 \pm 3.7$ [b] |
| E | 5-HT (0.5 μg/0.02 ml i.v.) | SME (2 SME/rat i.c.) | $204 \pm 3.9$ [b] | $24 \pm 9.6$ [b] |

[a] 6–8 hypophysectomized assay animals were used per group.
[b] $p < 0.001$ vs group A (epiphyseal width) or group B (blood glucose).
[c] Rats hypophysectomized one week before were used as donor animals (6–8 per group).

Table 5. *Lack of growth hormone releasing activity in plasma of normal rats injected intraventricularly (i.v.) with norepinephrine (NE), dopamine (DA) or serotonin (5-HT)*

| Groups | Treatment of plasma donor animals | Material administered to pituitary donor animals | Epiphyseal width μ[a] (mean ± S.E.) | Blood glucose (mg/100 ml) |
|---|---|---|---|---|
| A | — | Saline (1 ml/rat i.c.) | 252 ± 3.5 | — |
| B | Saline (0.02 ml i.v.) | Plasma (1 ml/rat i.c.) | 256 ± 2.0 | 82 ± 2.2 |
| C | NE (0.5 μg/0.02 ml i.v.) | Plasma (1 ml/rat i.c.) | 256 ± 4.2 | 90 ± 3.0 |
| D | DA (0.5 μg/0.02 ml i.v.) | Plasma (1 ml/rat i.c.) | 244 ± 10.1 | 64 ± 3.8[b] |
| E | 5-HT (0.5 μg/0.02 ml i.v.) | Plasma (1 ml/rat i.c.) | 254 ± 2.3 | 94 ± 5.1 |

[a] 6–8 hypophysectomized assay animals were used per group.
[b] $p < 0.01$ vs saline.

Table 6. *Growth hormone releasing activity in plasma of hypophysectomized rats injected intraventricularly (i.v.) with norepinephrine (NE), dopamine (DA) or serotonin (5-HT)*

| Exp. | Groups | Treatment of plasma donor animals[c] | Material administered to pituitary donor animals | Epiphyseal width μ[d] (mean ± S.E.) | Blood glucose (mg/100 ml) |
|---|---|---|---|---|---|
| 1 | A | — | Saline (1.0 ml/rat i.c.) | 258 ± 1.6 | — |
| | B | Saline (0.02 ml i.v.) | Plasma (1.0 ml/rat i.c.) | 252 ± 4.6 | 76 ± 6.0 |
| | C | NE (0.5 μg/0.02 ml i.v.) | Plasma (1.0 ml/rat i.c.) | 219 ± 5.6[b] | 103 ± 9.8 |
| | D | DA (0.5 μg/0.02 ml i.v.) | Plasma (1.0 ml/rat i.c.) | 203 ± 7.1[b] | 36 ± 3.7[b] |
| | E | 5-HT (0.5 μg/0.02 ml i.v.) | Plasma (1.0 ml/rat i.c.) | 248 ± 4.3 | 24 ± 9.6[b] |
| 2 | A | — | Saline (1.0 ml/rat i.c.) | 257 ± 4.2 | — |
| | B | Saline (0.02 ml i.v.) | Plasma (1.0 ml/rat i.c.) | 251 ± 3.2 | — |
| | C | NE (0.5 μg/0.02 ml i.v.) | Plasma (1.0 ml/rat i.c.) | 236 ± 3.0[a] | — |
| | D | 5-HT (0.5 μg/0.02 ml i.v.) | Plasma (1.0 ml/rat i.c.) | 245 ± 5.0 | — |

[a] $p < 0.01$ vs group A.
[b] $p < 0.001$ vs group A (epiphyseal width) or group B (blood glucose).
[c] Animals hypophysectomized one week before were used (6–8 per group).
[d] 6–8 hypophysectomized assay animals were used per group.

Blood glucose levels in the intact animals injected with NE were not significantly different from controls (Table 3, exp. 1 and 2, group C vs B), while they
were significantly higher in hypophysectomized rats (Table 4, group C vs B). Blood
glucose levels were significantly lower than controls in intact animals treated with
DA (Table 3, exp. 1 and 2, group D vs B) and in hypophysectomized rats treated
with DA or serotonin (Table 4, groups D and E vs B).

## Plasma GRF Activity in Intact and Hypophysectomized Rats after Administration of Brain Amines

In the second series of experiments plasma samples obtained from intact or
hypophysectomized animals in which the intraventricular administration of CA
had caused disappearance of GRF from the hypothalamus (Table 5, same animals

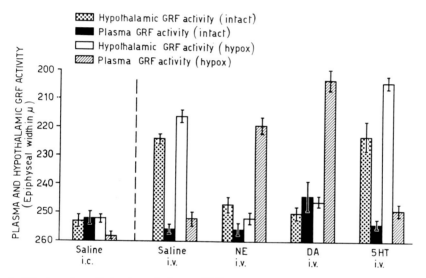

Fig. 1. Effect on hypothalamic and plasma GRF activity of norepinephrine ($NE$), dopamine
($DA$) or serotonin ($5$-$HT$) given by intraventricular injection (i.v.) to intact or hypophysectomized (hypox) rats. Left side of the figure shows the effect of saline given by intracarotid
injection

as exp. 2, Table 3, Table 6, exp. 1, same animals of the experiment reported in
Table 4) were tested for their GRF activity.

As shown in Table 5 neither injection of plasma from intact saline treated rats
nor from intact rats treated with NE (0.5 μg) or DA (0.5 μg) induced depletion of
pituitary GH of recipient rats (groups B, C and D vs A). By contrast the injection
of plasma obtained from hypophysectomized rats treated intraventricularly with
NE (0.5 μg) or DA (0.5 μg), induced a significant depletion of pituitary GH
activity of recipient rats (Table 6, exp. 1, groups C and D vs A, B and E; exp. 2,
group C vs A, B and D), indicating the presence of GRF in the plasma.

Results described in Tables 3–6 are summarized in Fig. 1.

## Comparison at Lower Dose Levels between Norepinephrine and Dopamine as to their Ability of Releasing GH

It has been previously shown by us that, while NE and DA were active in releasing GH also at doses of 0.1 μg, epinephrine did not show any effect at this lower dose (see Table 2). In the last series of experiments a comparison between the ability of NE and DA of releasing GH at lower dose levels was made.

Table 7. *Effect on pituitary GH activity of small amounts of norepinephrine (NE) or dopamine (DA) given by intraventricular injection*

| Exp. | Groups | Treatment (i. v.) | Epiphyseal width (mean ± S.E.) | Blood glucose (mg/100 ml) |
|------|--------|-------------------|-------------------------------|---------------------------|
| 1 | A | Saline (0.02 ml) | $254 \pm 1.22$ | $79 \pm 7.3$ |
|   | B | NE (0.05 μg/0.02 ml) | $211 \pm 2.6^a$ | $69 \pm 4.0^b$ |
|   | C | DA (0.05 μg/0.02 ml) | $214 \pm 4.6^a$ | $92 \pm 5.1^b$ |
| 2 | A | Saline (0.02 ml) | $257 \pm 3.0$ | — |
|   | B | NE (0.01 μg/0.02 ml) | $211 \pm 5.5^a$ | — |
|   | C | NE (0.005 μg/0.02 ml) | $207 \pm 3.2^a$ | — |
|   | D | DA (0.01 μg/0.02 ml) | $217 \pm 1.2^a$ | — |
|   | E | DA (0.005 μg/0.02 ml) | $246 \pm 3.1^b$ | — |

[a] $p < 0.001$ vs saline.
[b] $p$ NS.

From Table 7 it appears that NE at doses of 0.05, 0.01 and 0.005 μg induced a clearcut depletion of pituitary GH activity (exp. 1, group B vs A; exp. 2, groups B and C vs A), while dopamine at a dose of 0.005 μg was ineffective (exp. 2, group E vs A).

## Discussion

The present study indicates that, in addition to reserpine, α-methyl-dopa, α-methyl-m-tyrosine and tetrabenazine are able to suppress the release of growth hormone which follows insulin-induced hypoglycemia. Tetrabenazine, when given alone, is able to induce GH release. In contrast to these substances, guanethidine, tyramine and brethylium are unable to block the effect of the hypoglycemic stimulus on the release of GH. It can be excluded that the blockage induced by reserpine, α-methyl-dopa, α-methyl-m-tyrosine and tetrabenazine takes place through a reduction or suppression of the hypoglycemic effect of insulin. In fact, in animals treated with these drugs, blood glucose levels after insulin administration did not significantly differ from the values found in animals treated with insulin alone. Reserpine and α-methyl-dopa share the ability to deplete brain and peripheral tissue of norepinephrine, dopamine and serotonin in rats (SHORE, SILVER and BRODIE, 1955; HESS, CONNAMACHER, OZAKI and UDENFRIEND, 1961). α-methyl-m-tyrosine markedly reduces brain and peripheral levels of norepinephrine, without reducing to any appreciable extent those of serotonin (CARLSSON, FALCK and HILLARP, 1962). Tetrabenazine causes depletion mainly of brain norepinephrine (QUINN, SHORE and BRODIE, 1959). Guanethidine, tyramine and brethylium mainly deplete peripheral stores of norepinephrine in rats (Cass and Spriggs, 1961; Trendelenburg, 1961). That insulin acts at the level of the CNS in releasing GH is supported by many observations (Abrams, Parker, Blanco, Reichlin and Daughaday, 1966; Katz, Krulick and McCann, 1966; Müller, Sawano, Arimura, Schally, 1967a). Our results suggest that the presence of intact stores of catecholamines in the brain is necessary for GH release after the stimulus of insulin hypoglycemia. This finding is supported by the observation that pretreatment with a monoamine oxidase inhibitor like iproniazid reverses the block of GH release by protecting brain stores of norepinephrine from the depletion caused by reserpine. By contrast, the absence of peripheral stores of catecholamines does not abolish the ability of the hypoglycemic stimulus to trigger GH release.

Lack of the central sympathetic tone might result in impairment of the release of neural mediators controlling the adenohypophysis. The finding that after reserpine administration, the release of GRF from the hypothalamus evoked by insulin is completely abolished is in keeping with this view. The suppressive effect of acute reserpine administration on GH release appears, therefore, to be mediated by an impairment of the release of the hypothalamic neurohormone governing GH secretion.

While a role of brain CA in the process leading to release of growth hormone was suggested by these data, it appeared from previous studies that epinephrine, was unable to elicit release of growth hormone when administered by intracarotid injection (Müller, Pecile and Smirne, 1965; Krulich, Dhariwal and McCann, 1965). If peripherally administered norepinephrine does not gain ready access to the brain, due to the presence of a blood-brain barrier (Axelrod, 1965), this handicap can be circumvented by intraventricular administration (Noble, Wurtman and Axelrod, 1967).

The present experiments confirmed our previous data on the ineffectiveness as GH releasers of serotonin, histamine, acetylcholine, vasopressin, or oxytocin administered by intracarotid injection (Müller, Smirne and Pecile, 1965), but demonstrated that minute amounts of epinephrine, norepinephrine or dopamine, when injected into the ventricle, have a GH releasing effect. No explanation can be given for the lack of activity of E at the lower dose used, although it may be recalled that at the hypothalamic level catecholamine stores consist mainly of NE and dopamine (Paton, 1958). Our previous failure to evoke release of GH by injecting epinephrine into the carotid (Müller, Smirne and Pecile, 1965) and the negative results obtained with epinephrine by Roth, Glick, Yalow and Berson (1963) in humans, may be explained on the basis of the relative impermeability of the blood brain barrier to this amine (Axelrod, 1965).

The observed release of GH induced by E, NE and DA might be related to changes of blood glucose levels. This possibility, however, appears to be remote. In fact, while E (0.5 µg) by intraventricular injection enhanced blood glucose levels, NE did not modify them and dopamine induced only a small decrease of blood glucose, which is not within the range necessary for GH release in the rat (Müller, Saito, Arimura and Schally, 1967b). On the other hand serotonin, vasopressin and oxytocin, which induced a significant decrease of blood glucose, did not affect the pituitary growth hormone content. Recalling that exposure to cold (Müller, Saito, Arimura and Schally, 1967b; Machlin, Takahashi, Horino, Hertelendy, Gordon and Kipnis, 1967) or cooling of the hypothalamus (Gale and Jobin, 1967) causes a release of GH from the pituitary, the GH releasing effect of E, NE and DA might be interpreted as a result of such an effect.

This hypothesis seems, however, to be excluded since, of the many substances tested in our experiments, only serotonin, which was ineffective in releasing GH, induced a significant decrease of body temperature.

Since it is known that the majority of stimuli able to induce release of growth hormone do so by triggering hypothalamic GRF mobilization (Katz, Dhariwal and McCann, 1967; Müller, Sawano, Arimura and Schally, 1967a; Müller, Arimura, Sawano, Saito and Schally, 1967c) it was felt urgently needed to ascertain if CA acted directly at the pituitary level or through GRF mobilization. The latter possibility seemed more probable since reserpine impairment of the adrenergic tone blocked GRF release.

Intraventricular administration of norepinephrine or dopamine at doses which induced release of pituitary GH, caused disappearance of GRF activity from the hypothalamus of intact rats. Serotonin which does not induce release of pituitary GH, left unaffected hypothalamic GRF activity. This finding implies that the two CA released pituitary GH by triggering the discharge of hypothalamic GRF, and not simply by acting on the pituitary following diffusion into the portal vessels. Release of hypothalamic GRF after intraventricular administration of NE or DA occurred not only in intact, but also in hypophysectomized animals. Simultaneous determinations of GRF activity in the hypothalamus and plasma of intact or hypophysectomized rats, showed that only in the latter was depletion of GRF from the hypothalamus accompanied by its appearance in the plasma. Our observation may be interpreted to mean either that in the hypophysectomized rats the degree of GRF release after CA administration is higher than in intact rats, so that GRF becomes detectable in the peripheral blood, or that in the intact animals GRF released from the hypothalamus is taken up by the pituitary (Krulich and McCann, 1966). The possibility that in the case of dopamine-treated hypophysectomized rats, the release of GH induced by plasma may be merely related to the changes of glucose levels appears to be remote. In fact plasma from hypophysectomized, noradrenaline treated rats with high glucose levels released pituitary GH and samples from hypophysectomized serotonin treated rats did not affect pituitary GH, although their glucose levels were very low.

From the last series of experiments at lower dose levels, it appears that NE is active at the very small dose of 5 ng, while at this dose dopamine is inactive. This suggests that of the two amines, NE is primarily concerned with the control of GH secretion and dopamine, given intraventricularly, might be active in releasing GH, since it is partially converted to noradrenaline (50%) in the hypothalamus (Glowinski and Iversen, 1966). Recalling, however, that DA is the chief amine present in the nerve fibers surrounding the primary capillary plexus (Fuxe and Hökfelt, 1967), such an interpretation of the present results must be made cautiously.

It might be clarifying in this context to study the effect on growth and development of 6 OH-DA, a drug which, when given intraventricularly, selectively destroys hypothalamic NE neurons, with little effect on structures containing dopamine

(URETSKY and IVERSEN, 1969). As to the site of action of CA in triggering the release of GRF, since the amines were injected into the lateral ventricle, they could have acted almost anywhere in the brain. It is premature to attribute their primary action to be on the hypothalamus. However, a hypothalamic site is suggested by the reported presence of NE-containing nerve fibers around the supraoptic nucleus (FUXE and HÖKFELT, 1967), an area whose destruction has been associated with stunted growth and impairment of GH secretion (BERNARDIS, BOX and STEVENSON, 1963). The peculiar relationship that an area recognized important for GH secretion, i.e., the ventromedial nucleus of the hypothalamus (FROHMAN and BERNARDIS, 1968a; FROHMAN, BERNARDIS and KANT, 1968b), is one of the few catecholamine-poor areas of the hypothalamus (FUXE and HÖKFELT, 1969; LEWIS, 1966), renders it unlikely that this nucleus is directly stimulated by adrenergic neurons, but it does not exclude the possibility that the adrenergic tone of other areas of the hypothalamus might exert an influence on it.

On the other hand, the presence of high concentrations of CA in nerve terminals surrounding the primary capillary plexus of the portal system (FUXE, 1965) offers another fascinating alternative, i.e., that amines might trigger the release of GRF by acting on the terminals of neurosecretory cells located elsewhere in the hypothalamus. Synaptic contacts between adrenergic or cholinergic neurons and typical neurosecretory neurons have been recently described by BAUMGARTEN and WARTENBERG (1970) in the neurohypophysis of lower vertebrates. A final possibility is that the GRF secreting neurons also contain NE and that the intracellular release of this neurochemical mediator may trigger the release of GRF. A similar mechanism has been suggested (GERSCHENFELD, TRAMEZZANI and DE ROBERTIS, 1960; KOELLE and GEESEY, 1961) for the acetylcholine induced release of vasopressin from the posterior lobe.

## Summary

These studies substantiate the view that the central adrenergic system plays a significant role in the neurochemical control of growth hormone (GH) secretion. In addition to reserpine, other norepinephrine depletors suppress the release of growth hormone that follows insulin induced hypoglycemia. Peripheral depletors of catecholamines were unable to block the effect of the hypoglycemic stimulus in releasing GH.

The blockage of GH release induced by reserpine was reversed by a monoamine oxidase drug, iproniazid. After reserpine treatment the release of growth hormone releasing factor (GRF) from the hypothalamus induced by insulin was abolished.

Epinephrine (0.5 µg), norepinephrine (0.5 and 0.1 µg) and dopamine (0.5 and 0.1 µg), when injected into the lateral ventricle of the rat brain, caused a depletion of pituitary GH activity.

Unlike adrenergic compounds, other hypothalamic constituents, i.e. serotonin (0.5 µg), acetylcholine (0.5 µg), vasopressin (8 mU) and oxytocin (8 mU) did not show any GH releasing activity when given by the intraventricular route.

Norepinephrine and dopamine, at doses known to be effective in depleting GH from the pituitary (0.5 µg), induced in intact and hypophysectomized rats disappearance of GRF activity from the hypothalamus and its appearance in plasma from hypophysectomized rats but not from intact rats. In intact rats NE given intraventricularly induced a depletion of pituitary GH activity at 0.005 µg, while DA at this dose was inactive.

It is suggested that NE is the synaptic transmitter for the release of GRF. Three possibilities regarding the interaction between noradrenergic neurons and neurosecretory neurons secreting GRF are considered.

## References

ABRAMS, R. L., PARKER, M. L., BLANCO, S., REICHLIN, S., DAUGHADAY, W. H.: Hypothalamic regulation of growth hormone secretion. Endocrinology 78, 605–613 (1966).

AXELROD, J.: The metabolism, storage and release of catecholamines. Recent Progr. Hormone Res. 21, 597–622 (1965).

BAUMGARTEN, H. G., WARTENBERG, H.: Adrenergic neurons in the lower spinal cord of the pike (Esox lucius) and their relation to the neurosecretory system of the neurophysis spinalis caudalis. Proc. of this Symposium, 1970, p. 104.

BERNARDIS, L. L., BOX, B. M., STEVENSON, J. A. F.: Growth following hypothalamic lesions in the weanling rat. Endocrinology 72, 684–692 (1963).

CARLSSON, A., FALCK, B., HILLARP, N.-Å.: Cellular localization of brain monoamines. Acta physiol. scand., Suppl. 196, 1–28 (1962).

CASS, R., SPRIGGS, T. L. B.: Tissue amine levels and sympathetic blockade after guanethidine and brethylium. Brit. J. Pharmacol. 17, 442–450 (1961).

FALCK, B., HILLARP, N.-Å., THIEME, G., TORP, A.: Fluorescence of catecholamines and related compounds condensed with formaldehyde. J. Histochem. Cytochem. 10, 348–354 (1962).

FALCONI, G., ROSSI, G.: Transauricular hypophysectomy in rats and mice. Endocrinology 75, 301–303 (1964).

FROHMAN, L. A., BERNARDIS, L. L.: Growth hormone and insulin levels in weanling rats with ventromedial hypothalamic lesions. Endocrinology 82, 1125–1132 (1968a).

— — KANT, K. J.: Hypothalamic stimulation of growth hormone secretion. Science 162, 580–582 (1968b).

FUXE, K.: Evidence for the existence of monoamine neurons in the central nervous system. IV. The distribution of monoamine nerve terminals in the central nervous system. Acta physiol. scand. 64, Suppl. 247, 39–85 (1965).

— HÖKFELT, T.: The influence of central catecholamine neurons on the hormone secretion from the anterior and posterior pituitary. In: Neurosecretion, IV. Internat. Symposium on Neurosecretion. Berlin-Heidelberg-New York: Springer 1967.

— — Catecholamines in the hypothalamus and the pituitary gland. In: Frontiers in neuro-endocrinology (W. F. GANONG and L. MARTINI, eds.). Oxford: Oxford University Press, Inc. 1969.

GALE, C. C., JOBIN, M.: CNS-endocrine responses to hypothalamic cooling in unanesthetized baboons. Fed. Proc. 26, 211 (1967) (Abstract).

GERSCHENFELD, H. M., TRAMEZZANI, J., DE ROBERTIS, E.: Ultrastructure and function in neurohypophysis of the toad. Endocrinology 66, 741–762 (1960).

GLICK, S. M.: The regulation of growth hormone secretion. In: Frontiers in neuroendocrinology (W. F. GANONG and L. MARTINI, eds.). Oxford: Oxford University Press, Inc. 1969.

GLOWINSKI, J., IVERSEN, L. L.: Regional studies of catecholamines in the rat brain. I. The disposition of [³H] norepinephrine, [³H] dopamine and [³H] dopa in various regions of the brain. J. Neurochem. 13, 655–669 (1966).

GREENSPAN, F. S., LI, C., SIMPSON, H., EVANS, H. M.: Bioassay of hypophyseal growth hormone: the tibia test. Endocrinology 54, 455–459 (1949).

HESS, S. M., CONNAMACHER, H., OZAKI, M., UDENFRIEND, S.: The effects of α-methyl-dopa and α-methyl-meta-tyrosine on the metabolism of norepinephrine and serotonin "in vivo". J. Pharmacol. exp. Ther. 134, 129–138 (1961).

HILLARP, N.-Å., FUXE, K., DAHLSTRÖM, A.: Central monoamine neurons. In: Mechanisms of release of biogenic amines (U. S. VON EULER, S. ROSELL, and B. UVNÄS, eds.). Stockholm: Pergamon Press 1966.

KATZ, S., DHARIWAL, A. P. S., McCANN, S. M.: Effect of hypoglycemia on the content of pituitary growth hormone (GH) and hypothalamic growth hormone releasing factor (GHRF) in the rat. Endocrinology 81, 337–339 (1967).
— KRULICH, L., McCANN, S. M.: Effect of insulin-induced hypoglycemia on the concentration of growth hormone releasing factor (GHRF) in plasma and hypothalamus. Fed. Proc. 25, 191 (1966).
KOELLE, G. B., GEESEY, C. N.: Localization of acetylcholinoesterase in the neurohypophysis and its functional implications. Proc. Soc. exp. Biol. (N.Y.) 106, 625–628 (1961).
KRULICH, L., DHARIWAL, A. P. S., McCANN, S. M.: Growth hormone releasing activity of crude ovine hypothalamic extracts. Proc. Soc. exp. Biol. (N.Y.) 120, 180–184 (1965).
— McCANN, S. M.: Evidence for the presence of growth hormone-releasing factor in blood of hypophysectomized rats. Proc. Soc. exp. Biol. (N.Y.) 122, 668–671 (1966).
MACHLIN, L. J., TAKAHASHI, Y., HORINO, M., HERTELENDEY, F., GORDON, R. S., KIPNIS, D.: Regulation of growth hormone secretion in non-primate species. In: Growth hormone, Internat. Symposium on Growth Hormone (A. PECILE and E. E. MÜLLER, eds.). Amsterdam: Excerpta Medica 1968.
McCANN, S. M., DHARIWAL, A. P. S.: Hypothalamic releasing factors and the neurovascular link between the brain and the anterior pituitary. In: Neuroendocrinology (L. MARTINI and W. F. GANONG, eds.). New York and London: Academic Press 1966.
MÜLLER, E. E., ARIMURA, A., SAWANO, S., SAITO, T., SCHALLY, A. V.: Growth hormone releasing activity in the hypothalamus and plasma of rats subjected to stress. Proc. Soc. exp. Biol. (N.Y.) 125, 874–879 (1967 c).
— SAITO, T., ARIMURA, A., SCHALLY, A. V.: Hypoglycemia, stress and growth hormone release: blockade of growth hormone release by drugs acting on the central nervous system. Endocrinology 80, 109–117 (1967 b).
— SAWANO, S., ARIMURA, A., SCHALLY, A. V.: Blockade of release of growth hormone by brain norepinephrine depletors. Endocrinology 80, 471–476 (1967 a).
— SMIRNE, S., PECILE, A.: Substances present at hypothalamic level and growth hormone releasing activity. Endocrinology 77, 390–392 (1965).
NOBLE, E. P., WURTMAN, R. J., AXELROD, J.: A simple and rapid method for injecting $^3$H-norepinephrine into the lateral ventricle of the rat brain. Life Sci. 6, 281–291 (1967).
PATON, W. D. M.: Central and synaptic transmission in the nervous system (pharmacological aspects). Ann. Rev. Physiol. 20, 431–470 (1958).
PECILE, A., MÜLLER, E. E.: Control of growth hormone secretion. In: Neuroendocrinology (L. MARTINI and W. F. GANONG, eds.). New York and London: Academic Press 1966.
— — FALCONI, G., MARTINI, L.: Growth hormone releasing activity of hypothalamic extracts at different ages. Endocrinology 77, 241–246 (1965).
QUINN, G. P., SHORE, P. A., BRODIE, B. B.: Biochemical and pharmacological studies of RO 1-9569 (Tetrabenazine), a non-indole tranquilizing agent with reserpine-like effects. J. Pharm. exp. Ther. 127, 103–109 (1959).
ROTH, J., GLICK, S. M., YALOW, R. S., BERSON, S. A.: Hypoglycemia: a potent stimulus to secretion of growth hormone. Science 140, 987–988 (1963).
SCHALLY, A. V., KASTIN, A. J.: The present concept of the nature of hypothalamic hormones stimulating and inhibiting the release of pituitary hormones. Triangle 9, 19–25 (1969).
SHORE, P. A., SILVER, S. L., BRODIE, B. B.: Interaction of reserpine, serotonin and lysergic acid diethylamide in brain. Science 122, 284–285 (1955).
TRENDELENBURG, U.: Modifications of the effect of tyramine by various agents and procedures. J. Pharmacol. exp. Ther. 134, 8–17 (1961).
URETSKY, N. J., IVERSEN, L. L.: Effects of 6-hydroxydopamine on noradrenaline-containing neurones in the rat brain. Nature (Lond.) 221, 557–559 (1969).

# Experimental Electron Microscopic Studies on the Neurovascular Link between the Hypothalamus and Anterior Pituitary*

U. K. Rinne

Department of Neurology, University of Turku, Turku 3 (Finland)

**Key words:** Hypothalamus — Anterior pituitary — Neurovascular connexions — Ultrastructure.

Histological, histochemical and, recently, electron microscopic studies have demonstrated that a great number of hypothalamic nerve fibres terminate on the capillaries of the hypophysial portal vessels in the median eminence (for lit. cf. Bargmann, 1953; Szentágothai, 1964; Rinne, 1960, 1966; Fuxe, 1964). From the morphological point of view, electron microscopic examinations have shown that these perivascular nerve endings contain a large number of granular and/or agranular vesicles (Rinne, 1966; Monroe, 1967; Rodríguez, 1969). The nature and functional significance of these inclusions is not exactly known, but increasing numbers of current experimental studies aim at clarifying the matter (Rinne and Arstila, 1966; Akmayev et al., 1967; Rinne et al., 1967; Pellegrino de Iraldi and Jaim Etcheverry, 1967; Kobayashi et al., 1967, 1968; Sano et al., 1967; Streefkerk, 1967; Zambrano and de Robertis, 1968; Zambrano, 1969).

Histochemical (Fuxe, 1964; Lichtensteiger and Langemann, 1966; Fuxe and Hökfelt, 1966) and biochemical (Laverty and Sharman, 1965; Rinne and Sonninen, 1968) demonstrations of monoamines in the median eminence have led investigators to ask whether these inclusions are the storage sites of monoamines. Indeed, in some experimental studies a clear correspondence has been found to exist between the monoamine content and the number of granular vesicles in the nerve endings of the median eminence (Rinne and Arstila, 1966; Rinne et al., 1967; Pellegrino de Iraldi and Jaim Etcheverry, 1967; Sano et al., 1967; Streefkerk, 1967; Kobayashi et al., 1968), but not all workers have found this correspondence (Mazzuca, 1965; Monroe, 1967). Experiments designed to throw further light on this point form the first part of this paper.

Concerning the hypothalamic control of corticotrophin secretion, I and my co-workers (Arko, Kivalo and Rinne, 1962, 1963) showed several years ago that bilateral adrenalectomy caused the appearance of very many aldehyde-fuchsin-staining nerve fibres in the outer layer of the median eminence of the rat. Recently, this finding has been confirmed by several other workers (Bock and aus der Mühlen, 1968; Goebel, 1968; Stöhr, 1969; Bock and v. Forstner, 1969; Bock et al., 1969). The aim of the second part of this paper is to link this phenomenon

* Aided by a grant from the Sigrid Jusélius Foundation.

to the ultrastructural alterations in the granular vesicles of the nerve endings and in the histochemical fluorescence reaction for monoamines.

## Material and Methods

The material consisted of male rats. Experimental conditions are summarised in Table 1.

Depletion of dopamine was induced by treatment with α-methyl dopa and reserpine (CARLSSON et al., 1965) (2 doses of 400 mg/kg i.p. with a 3-hour interval and 10 mg/kg i.p., respectively) and that of noradrenaline by diethyldithiocarbamate (COLLINS, 1965; CARLSSON et al., 1966) (2 doses of 500 mg/kg i.p. with a 2-hour interval) and by α-methyl-m-tyrosine (HESS et al., 1961; CARLSSON et al., 1962) (2 doses of 400 mg/kg i.p. with a 2-hour interval).

Bilateral adrenalectomy was performed 21 days before sacrifice of the animals.

For the histological studies the region of the median eminence was fixed in BOUIN's fluid and treated in the usual way, and the sections were stained with GOMORI's (1950) aldehyde-fuchsin after acid permanganate oxidation (LANDING et al., 1956). The histochemical demonstration of monoamines was performed by the fluorescence method from the freeze-dried tissue according to FALCK (FALCK, 1962; FALCK and OWMAN, 1965). For the electron microscopic studies the region of the median eminence was fixed in cold 5 per cent glutaraldehyde, post-fixed in osmium tetroxide and embedded in Epon. The ultrathin sections were examined in a Siemens Elmiskop I. The quantitative evaluation of the number and diameter of the granular vesicles was carried out from micrographs enlarged 30,000 times. For the measurement, the basal region of the outer layer of the median eminence was charted planimetrically into areas of 20–40 sq.μ and, in all, 400 sq.μ, except 800 sq.μ in the adrenalectomy group, were measured in micrographs taken at random from control and experimental animals. This area extended for an average of 3–4 μ dorsally from the perivascular space. All the granular inclusions present in the nerve endings were measured. The correction for the distribution of particle sizes from a distribution of section diameters was calculated according to SALTYKOV (UNDERWOOD, 1968).

Table 1. *Summary of experimental conditions*

| Experiment | Dose | Interval between experiment and killing |
|---|---|---|
| 1. Depletion of DA | | |
| α-methyl dopa | 400 mg/kg i.p. twice with a 3-hour interval | 24 hours |
| and reserpine | 10 mg/kg i.p. 24 h later | |
| 2. Depletion of NA | | |
| Diethyldithio-carbamate | 500 mg/kg i.p. twice with a 3-hour interval | 4 hours |
| α-methyl-m-tyrosine | 400 mg/kg i.p. twice with a 2-hour interval | 24 hours |
| 3. Bilateral adrenalectomy | — | 21 days |

## Results

### I. Relation between Monoamines and Granular Vesicles in the Nerve Endings of the Median Eminence

The results showed that experimental depletion of dopamine with α-methyl dopa and reserpine caused almost total loss of the fluorescent material in the median eminence (Fig. 1). But electron microscopic examination did not reveal any significant changes in the numbers of granular vesicles (Table 2).

Table 2. *Number of granular vesicles per surface unit in the perivascular nerve endings and changes in the fluorescent material in the median eminence under conditions of experimental interference with monoamine metabolism*

| Group | Number of granular vesicles per 10 sq.μ (mean ± S.E.M.) | | | | Fluorescent material in the median eminence |
|---|---|---|---|---|---|
| | Total | 500 to 600 Å | 1,000 Å | 1,300 to 1,600 Å | |
| 1. Control | 53.2 ± 4.1 | 6.9 ± 0.7 | 23.2 ± 2.9 | 7.7 ± 0.7 | |
| 2. Depletion of DA | | | | | |
| α-methyl dopa and reserpine | 57.4 ± 4.3 | 9.3 ± 1.6 | 24.2 ± 2.2 | 14.3 ± 2.0 | Almost total depletion |
| 3. Depletion of NA | | | | | |
| Diethyldithio-carbamate | 37.8 ± 4.5 ($P < 0.05$) | 2.6 ± 0.6 ($P < 0.01$) | 16.1 ± 2.1 | 9.4 ± 1.8 | Slight depletion |
| α-methyl-m-tyrosine | 46.1 ± 3.2 | 3.6 ± 0.7 ($P < 0.05$) | 19.7 ± 1.6 | 10.3 ± 1.8 | Slight depletion |

On the other hand, depletion of noradrenaline caused only a slight decrease of the fluorescence in the median eminence. However, this was associated with a significant decrease in the number of small granular vesicles about 500–600 Å in diameter in the nerve endings of the median eminence. According to the size distribution values corrected by the method of SALTYKOV, there was no population of small granular vesicles at all. The total number of granular vesicles decreased significantly after diethyldithiocarbamate treatment, too (Table 2).

## II. Relation between Corticotrophin Secretion and Aldehyde-Fuchsin-Staining Substance, Monoamines and Granular Vesicles in the Nerve Endings of the Median Eminence

Bilateral adrenalectomy resulted in the appearance of a great number of aldehyde-fuchsin-staining nerve fibres in the outer layer of the median eminence

Table 3. *Number of granular vesicles per surface unit in the perivascular nerve endings and changes in the fluorescent material in the median eminence in control and bilaterally adrenalectomised rats*

| Group | Number of granular vesicles per 10 sq.μ (mean ± S.E.M.) | | | | Fluorescent material in the median eminence |
|---|---|---|---|---|---|
| | Total | 500 to 600 Å | 1,000 Å | 1,300 to 1,600 Å | |
| 1. Control | 53.2 ± 4.1 | 6.9 ± 0.7 | 23.2 ± 2.9 | 7.7 ± 0.7 | |
| 2. Bilateral adrenalectomy | 40.0 ± 2.1 | 3.2 ± 0.3 | 13.2 ± 0.8 | 14.0 ± 1.4 | No certain changes |
| | $P < 0.01$ | $P < 0.001$ | $P < 0.001$ | $P < 0.01$ | |

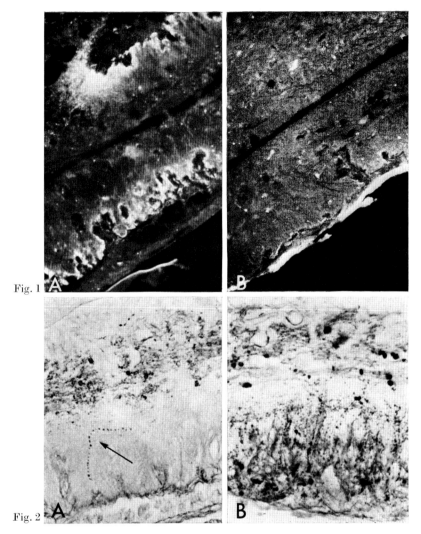

Fig. 1 A and B. Sagittal sections of the median eminence. The fluorescent material is depleted after treatment with α-methyl dopa and reserpine (B) as compared to the section of a control rat (A). ×200

Fig. 2 A and B. Sagittal sections of the median eminence. Note only one aldehyde-fuchsin-staining nerve fibre (arrow) running towards the hypophysial portal vessels in the section of a control rat (A) but a great number of these nerve fibres after bilateral adrenalectomy (B). Aldehyde-fuchsin. ×300

terminating on the hypophysial portal vessels (Fig. 2). However, there were no clear changes in the fluorescence of monoamines in the median eminence (Table 3).

Electron microscopic examination showed that after bilateral adrenalectomy the total number of granular vesicles decreased significantly ($P < 0.01$). This decrease took place in the numbers of small granular vesicles. In contrast, the

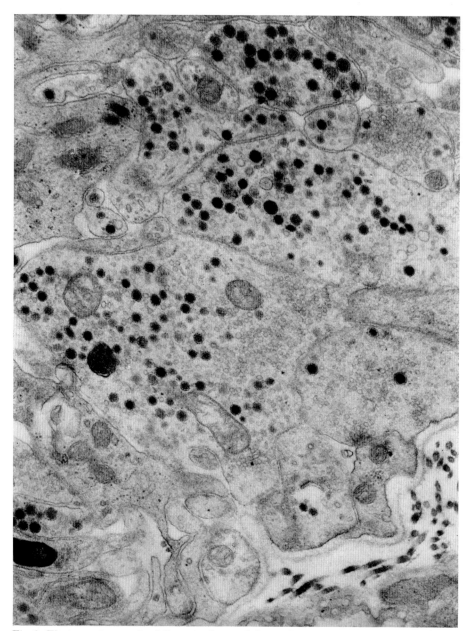

Fig. 3. Electron micrograph of the outer layer of the median eminence of a control rat. The perivascular nerve endings contain a great number of granular and agranular vesicles. ×30,000

number of large granular vesicles about 1,300–1,600 Å in size increased significantly ($P < 0.01$). In the corrected histogram we can see a new population of large granular vesicles which did not exist in the control material. Correspondingly, the proportion of large agranular vesicles had risen somewhat (Table 3, Figs. 3 and 4).

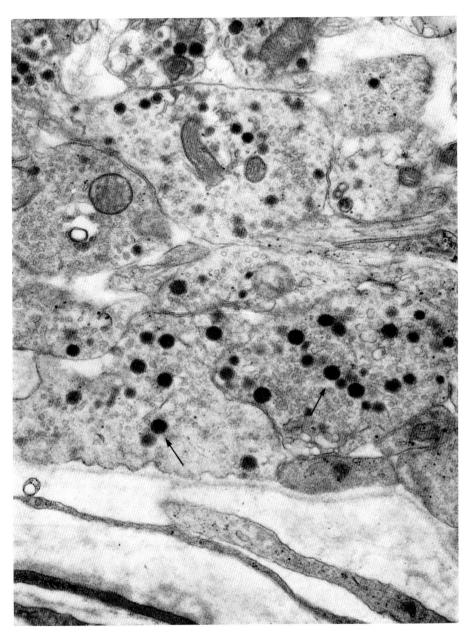

Fig. 4. Electron micrograph of the outer layer of the median eminence of a bilaterally adrenal-ectomised rat. Note the appearance of large granular vesicles (arrows) and the decrease of the total number of the granular vesicles as compared to the control section. ×30,000

## Conclusions

The results of the experimental studies described in the first part of this paper indicate that in the median eminence dopamine is not contained in the granular vesicles rendered visible by glutaraldehyde and osmium. However, small granular vesicles may be involved in the storage or metabolism of noradrenaline in the median eminence. Correspondingly, using potassium permanganate as fixative, it has been shown recently by Hökfelt (1967, 1968) that both in the peripheral and central nervous system monoamines are stored mainly in the small granular vesicles about 500 Å in diameter.

The results obtained after bilateral adrenalectomy support the view that the aldehyde-fuchsin-staining substance and the large granular vesicles may be concerned with the neurohumoral control of corticotrophin secretion. But there is still no evidence that dopamine plays a role in this process. The large granular vesicles may act as the storage site of corticotrophin-releasing factor and may be the subcellular structures corresponding to the aldehyde-fuchsin-staining substance in the median eminence. Obviously the increased number of large granular vesicles found in the present study corresponds to the abundance of large empty vesicles described by Akmayev et al. (1967) 10 to 17 days after bilateral adrenalectomy.

## References

Akmayev, I. G., Réthelyi, M., Majorossy, K.: Changes induced by adrenalectomy in nerve endings of the hypothalamic median eminence (Zona palisadica) in the albino rat. Acta biol. Acad. Sci. hung. 18, 187–200 (1967).

Arko, H., Kivalo, E., Rinne, U. K.: The hypothalamo-hypophysial neurosecretion after various endocrine gland extirpations. Acta pathol. microbiol. scand., Suppl. 154, 91–92 (1962).

— — — Hypothalamo-neurohypophysial neurosecretion after the extirpation of various endocrine glands. Acta endocr. (Kbh.) 42, 293–299 (1963).

Bargmann, W.: Neurosekretion und hypothalamisch-hypophysäres System. Anat. Anz., Erg.-Bd. 100, 30–45 (1953).

Bock, R., aus der Mühlen, K.: Beiträge zur funktionellen Morphologie der Neurohypophyse. I. Über eine „gomoripositive" Substanz in der Zona externa infundibuli beidseitig adrenalektomierter weißer Mäuse. Z. Zellforsch. 92, 130–148 (1968).

— Forstner, R. v.: Beiträge zur funktionellen Morphologie der Neurohypophyse. II. Vergleichsuntersuchung histologischer Veränderungen im Infundibulum der Ratte nach beidseitiger Adrenalektomie und nach Hypophysektomie. Z. Zellforsch. 94, 434–440 (1969).

— — aus der Mühlen, K., Stöhr, Ph. A.: Beiträge zur funktionellen Morphologie der Neurohypophyse. III. Über die Wirkung einer Corticoid- oder ACTH-Behandlung auf das Auftreten „gomoripositiver" Granula in der Zona externa infundibuli von Ratten und Mäusen nach beidseitiger Adrenalektomie oder Hypophysektomie. Z. Zellforsch. 96, 142–150 (1969).

Carlsson, A., Dahlström, A., Fuxe, K., Hillarp, N.-Å.: Failure of reserpine to deplete noradrenaline neurons of α-methylnoradrenaline formed from α-methyl dopa. Acta pharmacol. (Kbh.) 22, 270–276 (1965).

— Falck, B., Fuxe, K., Hillarp, N.-Å.: Cellular localization of brain monoamines. Acta physiol. scand., Suppl. 196, 1–28 (1962).

— Lindqvist, M., Fuxe, K., Hökfelt, T.: Histochemical and biochemical effects of diethyl-dithiocarbamate on tissue catecholamines. J. Pharm. Pharmacol. 18, 60–62 (1966).

Collins, G. G. S.: Inhibition of dopamine-β-oxidase by diethyl-dithiocarbamate. J. Pharm. Pharmacol. 17, 526–527 (1965).

Falck, B.: Observations on the possibilities of the cellular localization of monoamines by a fluorescence method. Acta physiol. scand., Suppl. 197, 1–26 (1962).

— Owman, C.: A detailed methodological description of the fluorescence method for the cellular demonstration of biogenic monoamines. Acta Univ. Lund. 2, No 7, 1–23 (1965).

FUXE, K.: Cellular localization of monoamines in the median eminence and the infundibular stem of some mammals. Z. Zellforsch. **61**, 710–724 (1964).

— HÖKFELT, T.: Further evidence for the existence of tubero-infundibular dopamine neurons. Acta physiol. scand. **66**, 245–246 (1966).

GOEBEL, F. D.: Neue Ergebnisse zur Morphologie neurosekretorischer Systeme in Hypothalamus und in der Neurohypophyse der normalen und adrenalektomierten Maus. Inaug.-Diss. Med. Fak. Bonn 1968.

GOMORI, G.: Aldehyde-fuchsin: a new stain for elastic tissue. Amer. J. clin. Path. **20**, 665–666 (1950).

HESS, S. M., CONNAMACHER, R. H., OZAKI, M., UDENFRIEND, S.: The effects of α-methyldopa and α-methyl-meta-tyrosine on the metabolism of norepinephrine and serotonin *in vivo*. J. Pharmacol. exp. Ther. **134**, 129–138 (1961).

HÖKFELT, T.: On the ultrastructural localization of noradrenaline in the central nervous system of the rat. Z. Zellforsch. **79**, 110–117 (1967).

— *In vitro* studies on central and peripheral monoamine neurons at the ultrastructural level. Z. Zellforsch. **91**, 1–74 (1968).

KOBAYASHI, T., KOBAYASHI, T., YAMAMOTO, K., KAIBARA, M., AJIKA, K.: Electron microscopic observation on the hypothalamo-hypophyseal system in the rat. III. Effect of reserpine treatment on the axonal inclusions in the median eminence. Endocr. jap. **15**, 321–335 (1968).

— — — KAMEYA, Y., KAIBARA, M.: Electron microscopic observation on the hypothalamo-hypophyseal system in the rat. II. Ultrafine structure of the median eminence and of the nerve cells of the arcuate nucleus. Endocr. jap. **14**, 158–177 (1967).

LANDING, B. H., HALL, H. E., WEST, C. D.: Aldehyde-fuchsin-positive material of the posterior pituitary. Its nature and significance. Lab. Invest. **5**, 256–266 (1956).

LAVERTY, R., SHARMAN, D. F.: The estimation of small quantities of 3,4-dihydroxyphenylethylamine in tissues. Brit. J. Pharmacol. **24**, 538–548 (1965).

LICHTENSTEIGER, W., LANGEMANN, H.: Uptake of exogenous catecholamines by monoamine-containing neurons of the central nervous system: Uptake of catecholamines by arcuato-infundibular neurons. J. Pharmacol. (Baltimore) **151**, 400–408 (1966).

MAZZUCA, M.: Structure fine de l'éminence médiane du cobaye. J. Microsc. **4**, 225–238 (1965).

MONROE, B. G.: A comparative study of the ultrastructure of the median eminence infundibular stem and neural lobe of the hypophysis of the rat. Z. Zellforsch. **76**, 405–432 (1967).

PELLEGRINO DE IRALDI, A., JAIM ETCHEVERRY, G.: Ultrastructural changes in the nerve endings of the median eminence after nialamide-DOPA administration. Brain Res. **6**, 614–618 (1967).

RINNE, U. K.: Neurosecretory material around the hypophysial portal vessels in the median eminence of the rat. Studies on its histological and histochemical properties and functional significance. Acta endocr. (Kbh.) **35**, Suppl. 57, 1–108 (1960).

— Ultrastructure of the median eminence of the rat. Z. Zellforsch. **74**, 98–122 (1966).

— ARSTILA, A. U.: Electron microscopic evidence on the significance of the granular and vesicular inclusions of the neurosecretory nerve endings in the median eminence of the rat. Med. Pharmacol. exp. **15**, 357–369 (1966).

— SONNINEN, V.: The occurrence of dopamine and noradrenaline in the tubero-hypophysial system. Experientia (Basel) **24**, 177–178 (1968).

— — HELMINEN, H.: Ultrastructural alterations and changes in the catecholamine content of the neurosecretory nerve endings in the median eminence of the rat after oxypertine injection. Med. Pharmacol. exp. **17**, 108–118 (1967).

RODRÍGUEZ, E. M.: Ultrastructure of the neurohaemal region of the toad median eminence. Z. Zellforsch. **93**, 182–212 (1969).

SANO, Y., ODAKE, G., TAKETOMO, S.: Fluorescence microscopic and electron microscopic observations on the tuberohypophyseal tract. Neuroendocrinology **2**, 30–42 (1967).

STÖHR, PH. A.: Über quantitative Veränderungen „gomoripositiver" Substanzen in Infundibulum und Hypophysenhinterlappen der Ratte nach beidseitiger Adrenalektomie. Z. Zellforsch. **94**, 425–433 (1969).

Streefkerk, J. G.: Functional changes in the morphological appearance of the hypothalamo-
    hypophyseal neurosecretory and catecholaminergic neural system, and in the adenohypo-
    physis of the rat. Acad. Diss., Amsterdam, 1967.
Szentágothai, J.: The parvicellular neurosecretory system. In: Progress in brain research,
    vol. 5, Lectures on the diencephalon, p. 135–146, ed. by W. Bargmann and J. P. Schadé.
    Amsterdam-London-New York: Elsevier 1964.
Underwood, E. E.: Particle-size distribution. In: Quantitative microscopy, p. 149–199, ed.
    by R. T. de Hoff and F. N. Rhines. New York: McGraw-Hill Book Co. 1968.
Zambrano, D.: The arcuate complex of the female rat during the sexual cycle. An electron
    microscopic study. Z. Zellforsch. **93**, 560–570 (1969).
— de Robertis, E.: The effect of castration upon the ultrastructure of the rat hypothalamus.
    II. Arcuate nucleus and outer zone of the median eminence. Z. Zellforsch. **87**, 409–421
    (1968).

# Lichtmikroskopische Untersuchungen zur Frage eines morphologischen Äquivalentes des Corticotropin-releasing factor

Rudolf Bock

Abteilung für Experimentelle Biologie im Anatomischen Institut der Universität
(Direktor: Prof. Dr. K. Fleischhauer) Bonn (Germany)

**Key words:** Releasing factors — Corticotropin = RF — Structural equivalent — Light microscopy.

Im Infundibulum der Säugerhypophyse kommen — ähnlich wie bei Vögeln und Amphibien (z. B. Dierickx und van den Abeele, 1959; Oksche, Laws, Kamemoto und Farner, 1959) — sowohl in der Zona interna als auch in der Zona externa „Gomori-positive" Substanzen (GpS) vor. Die Menge der in der Zona externa zu beobachtenden „Gomori-positiven" Substanzen (GpSZe) unterliegt erheblichen Speziesdifferenzen (Lit. bei Bock und aus der Mühlen, 1968).

Es kann heute als gesichert betrachtet werden, daß es sich bei den GpS der Zona interna um ein Neurosekret handelt, das als Trägerprotein der Hinterlappenhormone fungiert. Die Rolle der GpSZe war dagegen bisher weitgehend unklar. Neuere Untersuchungen haben gezeigt, daß ihre Menge in Beziehung zum Funktionszustand der Nebennierenrinde bzw. zur Höhe des Corticoid-Spiegels steht.

Bilaterale Adrenalektomie führt bei Ratten (Abb. 1) und Mäusen zu einer erheblichen Vermehrung der GpSZe (Arko, Kivalo und Rinne, 1963; Bock und aus der Mühlen, 1968; Bock und v. Forstner, 1969; Stöhr, 1969). Die gleiche Reaktion wurde nach Hypophysektomie bei der Ratte beobachtet (Bock und v. Forstner, 1969). Demgegenüber erfolgt keine oder nur eine geringere Zunahme der GpSZe, wenn hypophysektomierte Tiere mit ACTH oder adrenalektomierte Tiere mit Corticoiden behandelt werden (Bock, v. Forstner, aus der Mühlen und Stöhr, 1969). Nach Absetzen der Substitutionsbehandlung steigt die Menge der GpSZe jedoch auch in diesem Fall an (Bach, 1970). Die Substitution mit Corticoiden verhindert die Vermehrung der GpSZe nach bilateraler Adrenalektomie allerdings nur dann, wenn sie unmittelbar nach der Operation begonnen wird. Eine Corticoid-Applikation, die erst einige Zeit nach Entfernung der Nebennieren erfolgt, scheint eher eine weitere Zunahme der GpSZe zu bewirken (Hennes, 1970).

Neben ihrer eindeutigen Beziehung zum Corticoid-Haushalt sprechen eine Reihe weiterer Gründe dafür, die GpSZe als morphologisches Äquivalent eines Corticotropin-releasing factor (CRF) oder seines Trägerproteins anzusehen:

1. Die GpSZe sind in einem Gebiet lokalisiert, das als Ort des Übertrittes von releasing factors in das Pfortader-System des Hypophysenvorderlappens angesehen wird.

2. Die Vermehrung der GpSZe setzt ein in der 2. Woche nach bilateraler Adrenalektomie (Bock und aus der Mühlen, 1968; Stöhr, 1969), d. h. zu einem Zeitpunkt, zu dem im biologischen Test erstmals ein Anstieg der CRF-Aktivität in der Eminentia mediana nachzuweisen ist (Vernikos-Danellis, 1965).

3. Die GpSZe verhalten sich aufgrund ihres relativen Reichtums an Disulfidgruppen färberisch ähnlich wie das Neurosekret des supraoptico-hypophysären Systems (Bock und aus der Mühlen, 1968), was nahelegt, in ihnen ebenfalls

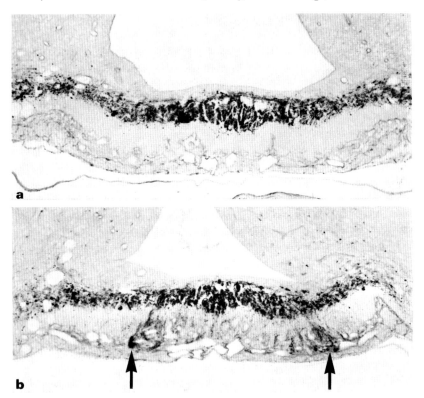

Abb. 1a u. b. Frontalschnitte durch die ventrale Infundibulumwand einer normalen (a) und einer bilateral adrenalektomierten Ratte, 14 Tage p.o. (b). Pikrinsäure-Formol-Fixierung. Crotonaldehydfuchsin-Färbung. Vergr. 100×. Pfeile: „Gomori-positive" Substanzen in der Zona externa infundibuli

ein Trägerprotein zu sehen. Ebenso wäre denkbar, daß die GpSZe den (oder einen) CRF selbst repräsentieren, da eine der aus Neurohypophysen-Extrakten gewonnenen Fraktionen mit CRF-Wirkung ein Disulfidgruppen-reiches Peptid darstellt (Schally, Arimura, Bowers, Kastin, Sawano und Redding, 1968).

Die bisher vorliegenden lichtmikroskopischen Untersuchungen haben noch nicht klären können, ob die GpSZe Nerven- oder Ependymfasern angehören. Verteilung und Anordnung der Substanzen sprechen jedoch eher dafür, daß sie in Nervenfasern lokalisiert sind. Auf Frontalschnitten durch das Infundibulum erkennt man, daß die GpSZe vorwiegend die paramedianen Bereiche einnehmen und die Infundibulum-Mitte weitgehend freilassen. Ihre Anordnung erweckt dabei den Eindruck zweier sich in der Medianebene überkreuzender Fasersysteme (Abb. 1 b). Da diese jedoch bisher noch keinem hypothalamischen Kerngebiet zugeordnet werden konnten, muß eine endgültige Klärung der Frage, ob auch die GpSZe neurosekretorischen Ursprungs sind, elektronenmikroskopischen Untersuchungen vorbehalten bleiben.

## Literatur

ARKO, H., KIVALO, E., RINNE, U. K.: Hypothalamo-neurohypophysial neurosecretion after the extirpation of various endocrine glands. Acta endocr. (Kbh.) **42**, 293–299 (1963).

BACH, H. H.: In Vorbereitung, 1970.

BOCK, R., FORSTNER, R. v.: Beiträge zur funktionellen Morphologie der Neurohypophyse. II. Vergleichsuntersuchung histologischer Veränderungen im Infundibulum der Ratte nach beidseitiger Adrenalektomie und nach Hypophysektomie. Z. Zellforsch. **94**, 434–440 (1969).

— — AUS DER MÜHLEN, K., STÖHR, PH. A.: Beiträge zur funktionellen Morphologie der Neurohypophyse. III. Über die Wirkung einer Corticoid- oder ACTH-Behandlung auf das Auftreten „gomoripositiver" Granula in der Zona externa infundibuli von Ratten und Mäusen nach beidseitiger Adrenalektomie oder Hypophysektomie. Z. Zellforsch. **96**, 142–150 (1969).

— AUS DER MÜHLEN, K.: Beiträge zur funktionellen Morphologie der Neurohypophyse. I. Über eine „gomoripositive" Substanz in der Zona externa infundibuli beidseitig adrenalektomierter weißer Mäuse. Z. Zellforsch. **92**, 130–148 (1968).

DIERICKX, K., ABEELE, A. VAN DEN: On the relations between the hypothalamus and the anterior pituitary in *Rana temporaria*. Z. Zellforsch. **51**, 78–87 (1959).

HENNES, H.: In Vorbereitung, 1970.

OKSCHE, A., LAWS, D. F., KAMEMOTO, F. I., FARNER, D. S.: The hypothalamo-hypophysial neurosecretory system of the white-crowned sparrow, *Zonotrichia leucophrys gambelii*. Z. Zellforsch. **51**, 1–42 (1959).

SCHALLY, A. V., ARIMURA, A., BOWERS, C. Y., KASTIN, A. J., SAWANO, S., REDDING, T. W.: Hypothalamic neurohormones regulating anterior pituitary function. In: Recent progress in hormone research (ed. E. B. ASTWOOD), p. 497–581. New York and London: Academic Press 1968.

STÖHR, PH. A.: Über quantitative Veränderungen „gomoripositiver" Substanzen in Infundibulum und Hypophysenhinterlappen der Ratte nach beidseitiger Adrenalektomie. Z. Zellforsch. **94**, 425–433 (1969).

VERNIKOS-DANELLIS, J.: Effect of stress, adrenalectomy, hypophysectomy and hydrocortison on the corticotropin-releasing activity of rat median eminence. Endocrinology **76**, 122–126 (1965).

# La localisation fine des terminaisons nerveuses fixant la noradrénaline H³ dans les différents lobes de l'Adénohypophyse de l'Epinoche. (*Gasterosteus aculeatus* L.)

Ernest Follenius

Laboratoire de Zoologie et d'Embryologie Expérimentale, 12, Rue de l'Université à
Strasbourg et
Laboratoire des Applications Biologiques du C.N.R.S. (France)

**Key words:** Adenohypophysis — Teleost — aminergic innervation.

Chez les Poissons téléostéens, les relations hypothalamo-hypophysaires présentent quelques particularités dues aux rapports spéciaux qui existent entre la neurohypophyse et l'adénohypophyse. Leur juxtaposition très étroite va de pair, comme l'ont montré de nombreux travaux d'histologie (BARGMANN, 1953; DIEPEN, 1953–1954; STUTINSKY, 1953; STAHL, 1953; DA LAGE, 1958; BILLENSTIEN, 1962), et de microscopie électronique (FOLLENIUS, 1962; VOLLRATH, 1966, 1967), avec une innervation directe de certaines catégories de cellules hypophysaires par des fibres se détachant des prolongements de la neurohypophyse et pénétrant profondément dans le parenchyme glandulaire. Comme nous l'avions précédemment montré (FOLLENIUS, 1962) des terminaisons péricapillaires situées sur la partie rostrale du réseau vasculaire complètent, chez certaines espèces, l'innervation directe. Ces relations neurovasculaires rostrales évoquent un système porte rudimentaire.

Plusieurs travaux (BARGMANN, 1953; STUTINSKY, 1953; BUGNON et LENYS, 1960; LENYS, 1962) avaient abordé le problème de la nature de l'innervation et de sa répartition dans les différents lobes. Avec les méthodes alors disponibles ils avaient montré que la méta- et la mésoadénohypophyse recevaient l'essentiel de l'innervation Gomori-positive alors que la proadénohypophyse était innervée par des fibres Gomori-négatives.

Au microscope électronique, l'hétérogénéité de l'innervation hypophysaire a été confirmée par plusieurs auteurs (FOLLENIUS, 1963–1967; VOLLRATH, 1966, 1967; KNOWLES et VOLLRATH, 1966a, b), posant ainsi le problème de la distinction des fibres nerveuses allant dans les trois secteurs de l'adénohypophyse.

Les critères ultrastructuraux, notamment la taille des grains de neurosécrétions permettent, chez certaines espèces, de distinguer les fibres d'origine préoptique de celles qui proviennent du noyau latéral du tuber (FOLLENIUS, 1962), mais pour les fibres adrénergiques, on considère également l'aspect des grains (V. KNOWLES, 1965). Les fibres à catécholamines contiendraient, comme les fibres sympathiques, de fins granules marginés. Ces critères ultrastructuraux, utiles pour les études morphologiques ne sont cependant pas suffisants. L'identification des différents types de fibres sur ces bases resterait assez aléatoire, car la taille et l'aspect des grains de neurosécrétions ne sont pas assez spécifiques des neurotransmetteurs qu'ils renferment.

Pour les catécholamines et les indolamines, on dispose depuis peu de méthodes histochimiques applicables en microscopie électronique (WOOD et coll., 1964), mais par leur principe même celles-ci attachent plus de valeur à la spécificité histochimique qu'à la visualisation des structures. D'autres comme la fluorescence secondaire d'après FALCK et coll. (1962) ne s'appliquent qu'en microscopie optique et connaissent de ce fait les limitations propres à ce mode d'observation.

L'autoradiographie au microscope électronique, par contre, autorise à la fois l'identification des fibres adrénergiques et l'étude de leur localisation exacte. Certaines fibres nerveuses absorbent sélectivement la noradrénaline H³ exogène selon un processus étudié aussi bien sur des fractions granulaires (V. EULER, 1965) que par autoradiographie au microscope électronique sur des terminaisons sympathiques des capillaires du tube digestif (DEVINE et SIMPSON, 1968) ou sur celles de l'épiphyse (TAXI et DROZ, 1967).

En partant de ces données, nous avons envisagé de différencier les terminaisons nerveuses hypophysaires susceptibles de fixer la noradrénaline tritiée et d'en étudier la localisation dans l'hypophyse de l'Epinoche.

## Matériel et méthodes

18 Epinoches out reçu une injection intrapéritonéale de 25 µCi/g de DL noradrénaline 7 H³ (Act. spécifique 1,2 Ci/mM) ce qui représente une dose de 30 µg par poisson.

Les poissons ont été sacrifiés par groupes de trois: 2 min, 5 min, 10 min, 1 h, 3 h, 5 h, après l'injection. L'hypophyse et l'hypothalamus ventral ont été prélevés en une seule pièce, fixés dans le glutaraldéhyde à 5% tamponné à pH 7,2 au cacodylate de sodium et postfixés dans le liquide de Palade.

Après inclusion dans le Maraglas, 2 séries de 5 autoradiographies ont été réalisées dans chaque pièce préalablement orientée; l'une parasagittale contenant le noyau latéral du tuber et les parties latérales de l'hypophyse, l'autre pratiquement dans le plan sagittal contient l'ensemble des lobes hypophysaires et une partie de l'hypothalamus située au voisinage. Dans ces conditions, des comparaisons valables peuvent être faites concernant l'activité des différentes structures présentes sur la même coupe. Des autoradiographies sur des coupes semifines adjacentes complètent l'ensemble et permettent de localiser les secteurs étudiées au M.E.

Pour la microscopie électronique les autoradiographies ont été réalisées d'après la technique de GRANDBOULAN (1965) et contrastées par double coloration à l'acétate d'uranyle et au citrate de plomb.

## Resultats

Les données concernant la fixation de noradrénaline exogène dans le complexe neuro-adénohypophysaire des poissons et dans la partie basse de l'hypothalamus sont des plus réduites. Sur nos autoradiographies nous avons été amenés à explorer l'ensemble de ce complexe en vue de déceler l'intégration de la noradrénaline tritiée.

Dès deux minutes après l'injection, les capillaires hypophysaires et cérébraux sont fortement marqués et dans l'hypophyse s'amorce la diffusion du produit marqué qui se traduit par l'apparition de halos de marquage autour des capillaires.

Dans le cerveau, par contre, la noradrénaline marquée ne franchit pas la basale péricapillaire qui semble représenter la structure responsable de l'effet

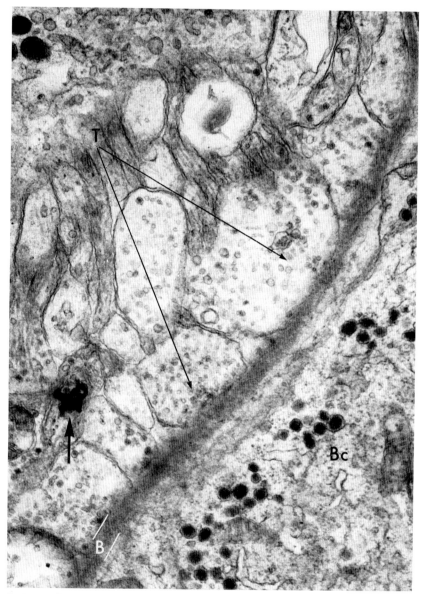

Fig. 1. Autoradiographie au microscope électronique de la zone de contact rostrale. Les terminaisons nerveuses (*T*.) situées à gauche de la basale (*B*.) sont pratiquement dépourvues de marquages autoradiographiques. Les cellules de la «bandelette chromophobe» (*B.C.*) sont situées à droite de la basale. ↑ = grain autoradiographique isolé. Gr. 30000

barrière. Cette barrière hémato-encéphalique très efficace quelle que soit la durée de l'expérience empêche toute diffusion de noradrénaline vers les tissus nerveux du système nerveux central ou vers les cavités des ventricules. Dans ces conditions, il est normal de constater l'absence de marquage au-dessus du noyau latéral du tuber que nous avons étudié en particulier.

Dans le complexe hypophysaire même, la diffusion s'opère rapidement et après 10 minutes, les premiers marquages apparaissent au-dessus de certaines fibres nerveuses. Après 5 heures il subsiste encore une quantité appréciable du produit radioactif ou de ses dérivés dans les sites d'intégration. TAXI et DROZ (1967) avaient décrit une évolution analogue au niveau des fibres sympathiques épiphysaires. En culture, ce comportement n'est pas propre aux terminaisons nerveuses, mais à l'ensemble des cellules ganglionnaires sympathiques (BURDMAN, 1968).

Chez l'Epinoche (FOLLENIUS, 1965, 1967) comme chez les autres espèces de poissons téléostéens, la neurohypophyse dans son ensemble est au contact des différents lobes de l'adénohypophyse. Les articulations entre fibres nerveuses et cellules glandulaires ne sont pas identiques dans les trois principaux secteurs que nous envisagerons successivement :

Dans la zone rostrale, au-dessus de la bandelette chromophobe, se terminent un grand nombre de fibres nerveuses renfermant des vésicules synaptiques et des grains très fins (environ 685 Å). Aucune de ces fibres ne pénètre dans le parenchyme glandulaire sous-jacent. Elles s'arrêtent côte à côte sur la basale séparant la neurohypophyse antérieure de la «bandelette chromophobe» proprement dite.

Précédemment, nous avons (FOLLENIUS, 1967) évoqué les problèmes posés par cette innervation particulière, bien localisée, mettant au contact la partie rostrale de la neurohypophyse et un secteur particulier de la proadénohypophyse. L'examen de cette zone au microscope électronique, nous avait conduit à mettre en doute l'origine tubérienne (NLT) classiquement admise (V. FOLLENIUS, 1962; KNOWLES et VOLLRATH, 1966b) de ces fibres. Ces terminaisons contiennent, en effet, des granules denses beaucoup plus fins que ceux élaborés par les neurones géants de la pars lateralis du noyau latéral du tuber. Comme KNOWLES et VOLLRATH (1966b) nous avions signalé l'analogie d'aspect de ces granulations et des grains à catécholamines décrits par GRILLO et PALAY (1962) et par TAXI (1965) dans les fibres sympathiques. Or, l'étude des autoradiographies au microscope électronique après injection de noradrénaline tritiée montre que ces terminaisons nerveuses sont dépourvues de tout marquage. Dans tous les cas étudiés et quel que soit la durée de l'expérience, les résultats sont négatifs (Fig. 1). On peut toutefois noter que si les terminaisons proprement dites sont négatives, il y a quelques marquages sur de rares fibres passant à une certaine distance de la basale. La bordure de la bandelette chromophobe a été explorée sur toute sa longueur, sans qu'une variation régionale ait été mise en évidence. Il semble que toutes les terminaisons touchant la basale aient les mêmes propriétés physiologiques comme elles présentent d'ailleurs la même structure au microscope électronique. Ces deux critères militent en faveur d'une innervation homogène de ce secteur de l'adénohypophyse. L'absence d'affinité pour la noradrénaline exogène, si elle ne permet pas d'exclure formellement leur nature aminergique, semble plutôt indiquer qu'elles appartiennent à une autre catégorie de fibres nerveuses, ayant des caractéristiques ultrastructurales voisines.

Dans la mésoadénohypophyse de l'Epinoche (FOLLENIUS, 1967) l'innervation pénètre le parenchyme glandulaire à partir des prolongements neurohypophysaires. Elles cheminent entre les cellules en formant de place en place des renflements ayant des caractéristiques d'une terminaison. On y décèle des vésicules synap-

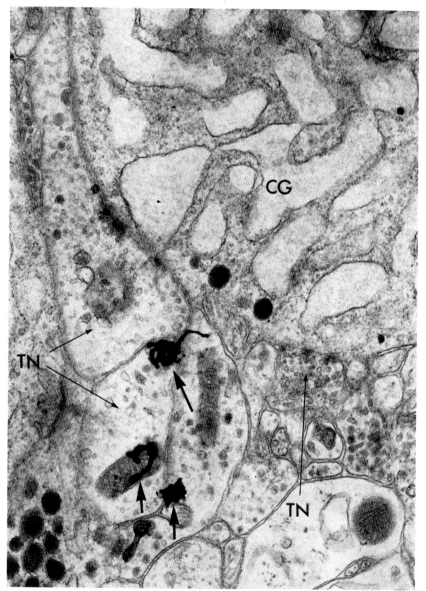

Fig. 2. Terminaisons nerveuses (*T.N.*) marquées et non marquées au voisinage d'une cellule
gonadotrope (*C.G.*) de la mésoadénohypophyse. Gr. 30000

tiques, des grains de neurosécrétion et des mitochondries. Les sites actifs sont
relativement rares sur nos clichés, bien que chez d'autres espèces Bargmann et
coll. (1967) ont montré que des encroûtements existent entre les fibres nerveuses et
les cellules glandulaires hypophysaires.

Ces terminaisons sont assez abondantes dans les zones périphériques de la
mésoadénohypophyse où elles abordent surtout des cellules ayant toutes les caractéristiques des cellules gonadotropes.

Après injection de DL-noradrénaline H³, certaines fibres de ce type se marquent, mais il semble que le contingent de fibres marquées ne soit pas très important (Fig. 2). Plusieurs facteurs pourraient expliquer ce fait: l'innervation complexe de ce lobe faisant intervenir des fibres nerveuses de types différents ou la variation des propriétés physiologiques en ce qui concerne l'aptitude de stockage des catécholamines exogènes. La première hypothèse est surtout basée sur le fait que dans cette région de l'hypophyse il existe une riche vascularisation cheminant d'abord dans les prolongements neurohypophysaires et dans le parenchyme glandulaire ensuite. L'innervation propre de la vascularisation est mélangée à celle des cellules glandulaires. Dans ces conditions il est difficile de savoir dans quelle mesure l'innervation aminergique aboutit sur les capillaires ou sur les cellules glandulaires.

Le marquage signalant l'intégration de la noradrénaline H³ a été décelé au-dessus de segments renflés des fibres nerveuses. Dans ces expansions pré-terminales ou terminales, plus ou moins enroulées autour des cellules gonadotropes, se trouvent, à la fois des vésicules synaptiques et des grains denses de faible diamètre (environ 600–900 Å). Souvent les marquages sont associés aux mitochondries.

Le marquage n'est pas exclusivement limité à la partie terminale présentant ces caractéristiques. Dans les prolongements neurohypophysaires mêmes, des faisceaux de fibres se marquent sélectivement bien qu'elles soient dépourvues, à ce niveau, de grains à coeur dense ou de vésicules synaptiques. Leur comportement vis à vis de la noradrénaline exogène tend à montrer qu'il s'agit de trajets nerveux allant se terminer plus loin dans le parenchyme glandulaire comme nous l'avons décrit.

Ce fait, déjà signalé par d'autres chercheurs, semble montrer que l'intégration de la noradrénaline exogène n'est pas nécessairement associée à la présence de vésicules synaptiques ou de grains de catécholamines à coeur dense. Mais il convient de se rappeler que l'autoradiographie au M.E. ne décèle pas forcément la noradrénaline, mais également tous les métabolites ayant conservé le H³. En gardant cette restriction à l'esprit, on peut considérer que les marquages décelés pourraient au moins, en partie, provenir du pool des catécholamines libres non associés aux grains à coeur dense. Du point de vue pratique, cette propriété particulière permet de suivre les trajets des fibres adrénergiques sur une certaine distance.

Les cellules glandulaires de la métaadénohypophyse (lobe intermédiaire des autres Vertébrés) reçoivent une innervation complexe (BARGMANN et KNOOP, 1960; FOLLENIUS, 1967). Au microscope électronique on observe chez l'Epinoche, des fibres nerveuses pénétrant entre les cellules glandulaires. Elles ne se terminent pas sur la basale comme chez la Truite et chez la Perche (BARGMANN, 1953; FOLLENIUS, 1962). Du point de vue morphologique, trois types de fibres avaient été différenciés. Chez cette espèce les fibres à granules neurosécretoires de forte taille ( ∅ environ 1580 Å) qui correspondent aux fibres Gomori-positives visibles sur les préparations histologiques, des fibres à granulations fines ( ∅ 600–800 Å) et des fibres sans inclusions remarquables au niveau de la coupe.

L'autoradiographie révèle un fort contingent de fibres fixant la noradrénaline tritiée. Dès 10 minutes après l'injection l'autoradiographie est positive au-dessus des fibres et des terminaisons (Fig. 3), cheminant entre les cellules de ce lobe. Le

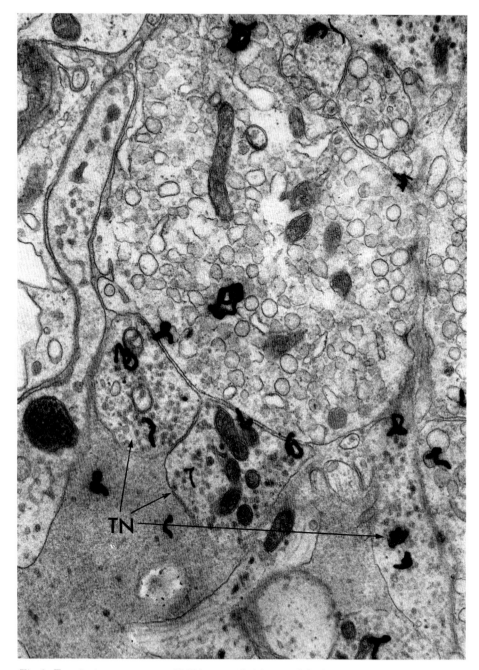

Fig. 3. Terminaisons nerveuses (*T.N.*) ayant fixé la noradrénaline tritiée situées contre une cellule claire de la métaadénohypophyse. Quelques grains autoradiographiques sont situés sur la cellule. Gr. 21000

marquage intéresse les fibres à granulations fines. Il est plus intense au niveau des renflements contenant les vésicules synaptiques, les granules et les mitochondries. Elles cheminent d'abord parallèlement en des faisceaux fins groupant quelques

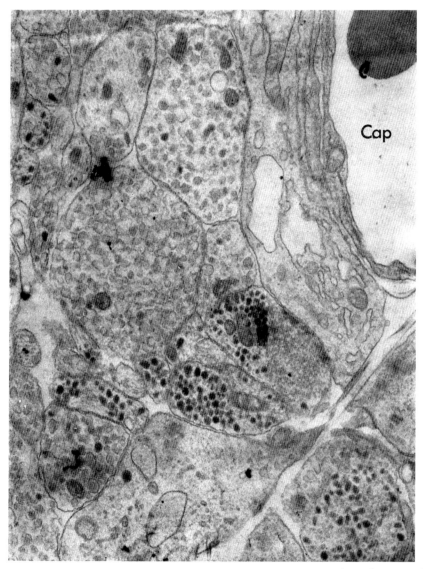

Fig. 4. Autoradiographie d'une plage de la partie postérieure de la neurohypophyse avec les deux types de fibres neurosécrétrices. Absence de marquages spécifiques. *Cap* capillaire.
Gr. 15000

axones qui s'écartent ensuite pour cheminer entre les cellules en les contournant plus ou moins. Certains clichés suggèrent qu'elles peuvent s'enrouler autour de l'un des pôles des cellules. Elles s'appliquent étroitement contre la membrane des cellules glandulaires mais il est rare d'observer des sites actifs bien définis. Dans les

cellules glandulaires aucune différenciation particulière ne peut être décelée en face
des terminaisons. D'après ces images, les relations entre terminaisons nerveuses et
cellules glandulaires ressemblent plus à celles qui existent au niveau des muscles
lisses qu'aux terminaisons classiques. A ce point de vue elles sont moins caractéristiques que celles décrites par Bargmann et coll. (1967) dans le lobe intermédiaire du Chat.

Dans le lobe nerveux proprement dit, on distingue, comme chez d'autres
espèces des fibres du type A 1 et A 2, mais aucune des catégories de fibres nerveuses
qui s'y terminent ne semble présenter une affinité particulière pour la noradrénaline
exogène (Fig. 4). Dans les zones médianes et paramédianes que nous avons speciale-
ment explorées, aucun marquage net de fibres ou de terminaisons n'a été observé.
Quelques grains autoradiographiques isolés représentent tout au plus un voile de
diffusion. Dans nos conditions d'expériences, les résultats sont négatifs, mais une
exploration de tous les secteurs est indispensable avant de donner des conclusions
définitives.

## Discussion

L'ensemble des résultats obtenus par autoradiographie au microscope électronique après injection de noradrénaline $H^3$ est basé sur l'existence d'un mécanisme
d'absorption et de stockage spécifique au niveau de certaines catégories de fibres
nerveuses. Plusieurs travaux (Taxi et Droz, 1967) tendent à montrer que les fibres
adrénergiques possèdent la propriété d'absorber la noradrénaline exogène. Mais
Björklund et coll. (1968) ont notamment montré que des fibres aminergiques se
terminant dans l'éminence médiane sont capables d'absorber et de stocker des
catécholamines et leurs précurseurs. Il semble donc que le fait d'absorber de la
noradrénaline exogène ne permette pas de définir d'une façon stricte les seules
fibres contenant normalement de la noradrénaline endogène. Cette propriété pourrait être commune à l'ensemble des fibres aminergiques.

Inversement les fibres adrénergiques absorbent non seulement la noradrénaline,
mais également des faux neurotransmetteurs (Tranzer et coll., 1967), ou des
indolamines (Snipes et coll., 1968). Il s'avère, par contre, que plusieurs catégories
de fibres dont celles de la neurohypophyse postérieure venant du noyau préoptique
et transportant des peptides et celles de la neurohypophyse rostrale aboutissant
sur la bandelette chromophobe n'absorbent pas la noradrénaline exogène; elles
appartiennent à la catégorie de fibres non aminergiques Gomori-positives comme
celles venant du noyau préoptique ou Gomori-négatives comme celles se terminant
sur la bandelette chromophobe. Pour l'instant, seules les fibres Gomori-positives
sont bien étudiées aussi bien quant à leur origine, leur trajet, qu'en ce qui concerne
leur contenu. Il n'est est pas ainsi pour les fibres à granules très fins de la zone de
contact proximale dont ni l'origine, ni le contenu ne sont encore définis. Comme
nous l'avons souligné précédemment elles ne proviennent pas des neurones géants
de la pars lateralis du noyau latéral du tuber.

Il semble, dans ces conditions difficiles d'homologuer d'une façon précise cette
zone de contact rostrale de la neurohypophyse des poissons à l'un des secteurs de
l'éminence médiane des tétrapodes où Kobayashi et coll. (1966) ont décelé en plus
des catécholamines de l'acétylcholine.

Malgré de nombreux travaux la répartition exacte des différents types de fibres nerveuses dans l'eminence médiane est encore peu connue. Même chez les Oiseaux, où l'on distingue une zone rostrale et une zone caudale dans l'éminence médiane de plusieurs espèces, on ne signale guère que chez le Pigeon, une distribution particulière des axones à l'échelle de la structure fine (MATSUI, 1966). Cette subdivision, non signalée chez les Mammifères, serait en rapport avec la subdivision de la pars distalis en un lobe rostral et un lobe caudal. On peut penser que chez les Poissons la différenciation d'une zone rostrale particulière de la neurohypophyse soit également en rapport avec la zonation hypophysaire. Toutes les cellules corticotropes (BALL et OLIVEREAU, 1966) sont réunies dans la bandelette chromophobe qui fait face à la zone des terminaisons nerveuses rostrales. Il s'agit dans ce cas d'une innervation spécifique d'une seule catégorie de cellules hypophysaires. On dispose ainsi d'un système neuro-endocrine bien défini permettant d'aborder le problème de la régulation de la sécrétion des corticotrophines chez les Poissons et ultérieurement chez d'autres Vertébrés.

La fixation des catécholamines exogènes soulève un problème de physiologie. Il s'avère que dans le complexe hypothalamo-hypophysaire les fibres aminergiques présentent les mêmes propriétés que les fibres du système sympathique. Elles fixent la noradrénaline exogène qui, dès lors, est susceptible d'intervenir dans les processus complexes du contrôle de l'activité des cellules hypophysaires. Il est permis de se demander dans quelle mesure l'intervention de la noradrénaline exogène est susceptible de moduler l'intervention des fibres aminergiques sur les différents effecteurs. Cette intervention ne semble d'ailleurs pas se limiter aux seules fibres nerveuses aminergiques. L'autoradiographie au microscope électronique a permis de montrer que certaines cellules hypophysaires dans la mésoadénohypophyse fixent la noradrénaline très rapidement (FOLLENIUS, 1967). Récemment WEISS et RUHLE (1969) ont d'ailleurs montré que chez la Truite (*Salmo trutta fario*), la Perche (*Perca fluviatilis*) et la Tanche (*Tinca tinca*) la mésoadénohypophyse renferme un certain nombre de cellules riches en catécholamines primaires. Pour l'instant, nous ne savons cependant pas si les cellules hypophysaires de l'Epinoche fixant la noradrénaline exogène correspondent aux cellules fluorescentes des autres espèces.

Quoi qu'il en soit, il ressort clairement des résultats apportés par l'autoradiographie de catécholamines marqués ou mis en évidence par les méthodes de fluorescence que ces substances sont susceptibles d'agir par deux voies différentes. Elles se fixent à la fois sur un certain nombre de fibres nerveuses allant sur des cellules du lobe intermédiaire et à un degré moindre sur celles de la mésoadénohypophyse, et d'autre part directement sur certaines cellules hypophysaires qui les absorbent sélectivement. Il conviendra de préciser dans quelle mesure la fixation de noradrénaline exogène correspond à un mécanisme d'action et quelle est son importance dans les régulations hypothalamo-hypophysaires et dans les régulations endocrines générales.

Il s'avère, par ailleurs, que l'innervation adrénergique de la métaadénohypophyse, c'est-à-dire du lobe intermédiaire est une caractéristique assez générale des relations hypothalamo-hypophysaires dans plusieurs groupes de Vertébrés. Aussi bien chez certains Poissons (ITURRIZA, 1967), que chez les Amphibiens (ENEMAR et coll., 1967), les Mammifères (Björklund, 1968), des fibres adrénergiques, allant dans ce lobe ont été décrites.

Chez certains Poissons, la mésoadénohypophyse reçoit également des fibres aminergiques alors que chez les Tétrapodes la pars distalis en est dépourvue. On note par contre une très riche innervation de ce type sur les capillaires du système porte. A ce point de vue il semble que la principale différence entre Poissons et Tétrapodes soit due à l'isolement de l'éminence médiane chez les Tétrapodes avec comme corrolaire la réalisation d'un système de liaison vasculaire, alors que chez les Poissons l'ensemble de la neurohypophyse est susceptible de réaliser des contacts nerveux directs avec certaines catégories de cellules hypophysaires.

## Résumé

L'autoradiographie au microscope électronique a permis de localiser les terminaisons nerveuses capables de fixer la D.L. Noradrénaline $H^3$, administrée par injection, au niveau des différentes zones de contact entre la neurohypophyse et les autres structures hypophysaires.

Dans la zone rostrale, face à la bandelette chromophobe, les nombreuses fibres nerveuses, à granulations fines, se terminant contre la basale, ne présentent pas de marquage. L'absence de marquage au-dessus des terminaisons à fines granulations semble indiquer qu'il ne s'agit pas de fibres adrénergiques.

Dans la mésoadenohypophyse, quelques fibres fixent la noradrénaline tritiée. Il n'est pas exclu qu'il s'agisse, au moins en partie, de fibres associées aux capillaires.

Les résultats positifs les plus démonstratifs concernent les terminaisons à granules fins, situées entre les cellules de la metaadénohypophyse. Un très important marquage, bien localisé au dessus des terminaisons, démontre leur très grande affinité pour la noradrénaline circulante. Dans la mesure où ce critère est spécifique des fibres adrénergiques, on peut admettre qu'il y a une innervation de ce type très importante dans ce secteur de l'hypophyse des Poissons.

Dans la pars nervosa proprement dite, par contre, aucune fixation de noradrénaline tritiée n'a été décelée.

### Bibliographie

Ball, J. N., Olivereau, M.: Experimental identification of ACTH cells in the pituitary of two teleosts Poecilia latipinna and Anguilla anguilla; correlated changes in the interrenal and in the pars distalis resulting from administration of metopirone. (S. u. 4885.) Gen. comp. Endocr. 6, 5–18 (1966).

Bargmann, W.: Über das Zwischenhirn-Hypophysensystem von Fischen. Z. Zellforsch. 38, 275–298 (1953).

— Knoop, A.: Über die morphologischen Beziehungen des neurosekretorischen Zwischenhirnsystems zum Zwischenlappen der Hypophyse. Z. Zellforsch. 52, 256–277 (1960).

— Lindner, E., Andres, K. H.: Über Synapsen an endokrinen Epithelzellen und die Definition sekretorischer Neurone. Untersuchungen am Zwischenlappen der Katzenhypophyse. Z. Zellforsch. 77, 282–298 (1967).

Billenstien, D. C.: The seasonal secretory cycle of the nucleus lateralis tuberis of the hypothalamus and its relation to reproduction in the eastern Brook Trout Salvelinus fontinalis. Gen. comp. Endocr. 2, 111–112 (1961).

BJÖRKLUND, A.: Monoamine containing fibres in the pituitary neuro-intermediate lobe of the pig and rat. Z. Zellforsch. **89**, 573–589 (1968).
— FALCK, B., LJUNGGREN, L.: Monoamines in the bird median eminence. Failure of cocaine to block the accumulation of exogenous amines. Z. Zellforsch. **89**, 193–200 (1968).
— — Pituitary monoamines of the cat with special reference to the presence of an unidentified monoamine-like substance in the adenohypophysis. Z. Zellforsch. **93**, 254–264 (1969).
BUGNON, C., LENYS, D.: Recherches sur les relations hypothalamo-préhypophysaires chez diverses espèces de poissons. 1er Congr. Européen d'Anatomie Strasbourg, Anat. Anz. Erg.-Bd. **109**, 520–529 (1960).
BURDMAN, J. A.: Uptake of (H³) catecholamines by chick embryo sympathetic ganglia in tissue culture. J. Neurochem. **15**, 1321–1323 (1968).
DA LAGE, CHR.: Recherches sur le complexe hypophysaire de l'Hippocampe. Arch. Anat. micr. Morph. exp. **47**, 401–405 (1958).
DIEPEN, R.: Über das Hypophysen-Hypothalamussystem bei Knochenfischen. Anat. Anz., Erg.-H. **100**, 111–122 (1953–1954).
DEVINE, C. E., SIMPSON, F. O.: Localization of tritiated norepinephrine in vascular sympathetic axons of the rat intestine and mesentery by electron microscope autoradiography. J. Cell Biol. **38**, 184–192 (1968).
ENEMAR, A., FALCK, B., ITURRIZA, F. C.: Adrenergic nerves in the pars intermedia of the pituitary in the toad *Bufo arenarum*. J. Zellforsch. **77**, 325–330 (1967).
EULER, U. S. V.: Aufnahme, Speicherung und Freisetzung von Katecholaminen in adrenergischen Neuronen. Z. Vitamin-, Hormon- u. Fermentforsch. **14**, 174–186 (1965).
FALCK, B., HILLARP, N. A., THIEME, G., TORP, A.: Fluorescence of catecholamines and related compounds condensed with formaldehyde. J. Histochem. Cytochem. **10**, 348–354 (1962).
FOLLENIUS, E.: Bases structurales et ultrastructurales des corrélations hypothalamo-hypophysaires chez quelques espèces de téléostéens. Thèse Es-sciences publiée dans Ann. Sci. Nat. Zool., Sér. XVIII, **7**, 1–150 (1965).
— Etude comparative de la cytologie fine du noyau préoptique (NPO) et du noyau latéral du tuber (NLT) chez la Truite (*Salmo irideus Gibb.*) et chez la Perche (*Perca fluviatilis*). Comparaison des deux types de neurosécrétion. Gen. comp. Endocr. **3**, 66–85 (1963).
— Cytologie des systèmes neurosécréteurs hypothalamo-hypophysaires des poissons téléostéens. In: Neurosecretion, IVè Symposium Internat. Strasbourg, p. 42–55. Berlin-Heidelberg-New York: Springer 1967a.
— Marquage séléctif des cellules acidophiles de la mésoadénohypophyse de *Gasterosteus aculeatus* après injection de D.L. noradrénaline 3 H 7. Etude autoradiographique au microscope électronique. C. R. Acad. Sci. (Paris) **265**, 358–361 (1967b).
— Innervation adrénergique de la métaadénohypophyse de l'Epinoche (*Gasterosteus aculeatus* L.). Mise en évidence par autoradiographie au microscope électronique. C. R. Acad. Sci. (Paris) **267**, 1208–1211 (1968).
GRANDBOULAN, P.: In: The use of radioautography in investigating protein synthesis, p. 43. Ed. by: Leblond et Warren — Acad. Press 1965.
GRILLO, M. A., PALAY, S. L.: Granule-containing vesicles in the autonomic nervous system. 5e Congr. Int. Micr. Electr. Philadelphia 2 u. 1 (1962).
ITURRIZA, F. C.: Monoamines in the neurointermediate lobe of the pituitary of the argentinian eel. Naturwissenschaften **54**, 565 (1967).
KNOWLES, Sir F.: Evidence for a dual control by neurosecretion of hormone synthesis and hormone release in the pituitary of the dogfish *Scylliorhinus stellaris*. Phil. Trans. B **249**, 435–456 (1965).
— VOLLRATH, L.: Neurosecretory innervation of the pituitary of the eels *Anguilla* and *Conger*. I. The structure and ultrastructure of the neurointermediate lobe under normal and experimental conditions. Phil. Trans. B **250**, 311–327 (1966a).
— — Neurosecretory innervation of the eels *Anguilla* and *Conger*. II. The structure and innervation of the pars distalis at different stages of the life cycle. Phil. Trans. B **250**, 329–342 (1966b).
KOBAYASHI, H., OOTA, J., UEMURA, H., HIRANO, T.: Electron microscopic and pharmacologic studies on the rat median eminence. Z. Zellforsch. **71**, 387–404 (1966).

16*

Lenys, D.: Etude morphologique des relations neurovasculaires hypothalamo-hypophysaires. Thèse Faculté de Médecine, Nancy (1962).

Matsui, T.: Fine structure of the posterior median eminence of the pigeon *Columba livia domestica*. J. Fac. Sci. Univ. Tokyo **4**, part 1 (1966).

Snipes, R. L., Thoenen, H., Tranzer, J. P.: Fine structural localization of exogenous 5 HT in vesicles of adrenergic nerve terminals. Experientia (Basel) **24**, 1026–1027 (1968).

Stahl, A.: La neurosécrétion chez les poissons téléostéens. Contribution à l'étude de la neurohypophyse chez les Mugilidés. C. R. Soc. Biol. (Paris) **147**, 841–843 (1953).

Stutinsky, F.: La neurosécrétion chez l'anguille normale et hypophysectomisée. Z. Zellforsch. **39**, 276–297 (1953).

Taxi, J.: Contribution à l'étude des connexions des neurones moteurs du système nerveux autonome. Ann. Sci. Nat. Zool. Sér. XII, **7**, 413–674 (1965).

— Droz, B.: Localisation d'amines biogènes dans le système neurovégétatif périphérique (Etude radioautographique en microscopie électronique après injection de noradrénaline H3 et de 5 hydroxytryptophane H3). In: Neurosecretion, p. 191–202. Berlin-Heidelberg-New York: Springer 1967.

Tranzer, J. P., Thoenen, H.: Electronmicroscopic localization of 5 hydroxydopamine (3, 4, 5 trihydroxy-ethylamine). A new "false" sympathetic transmitter. Experientia (Basel) **23**, 743 (1967).

Vollrath, L.: The ultrastructure of the eel pituitary at the elver stage with special reference to its neurosecretory innervation. Z. Zellforsch. **73**, 107–131 (1966).

— Über die neurosekretorische Innervation der Adenohypophyse von Teleostiern im besonderen von *Hippocampus cuda* und *Tinca tinca*. Z. Zellforsch. **78**, 237–260 (1967).

Weiss, J., Ruhle, H. J.: Nachweis katecholaminhaltiger Zellen in der Adenohypophyse von Knochenfischen. Acta biol. med. germ. **22**, 431–433 (1969).

Wood, J. G., Barrnett, R. J.: Histochemical demonstration of norepinephrine at a fine structural level. J. Histochem. Cytochem. **12**, 197–209 (1964).

# Recherches sur le rôle des monoamines infundibulaires dans le contrôle de la sécrétion gonadotrope chez le cobaye et la souris*

J. Barry

Laboratoire d'Histologie et Embryologie (Pr. Barry), Faculté de Médecine et Pharmacie
Lille (France)

**Key words:** Infundibulum — Monoamines — Gonadotropic function.

La mise au point d'une technique de détection des monoamines en fluorescence U.V. (Falck, 1962; Falck, Hillarp, Thieme et Thorp, 1962) a permis de révéler la présence, dans l'hypothalamus, d'une part de cellules principalement dopaminergiques, particulièrement abondantes dans la région du noyau arqué, d'autre part de terminaisons monoaminergique d'origine mésencéphalique (Fuxe, 1964; Dahlström et Fuxe, 1964).

Le problème du role des monoamines hypothalamiques dans le contrôle des activités hypophysaires (Fuxe et Hökfelt, 1967) se trouve, de ce fait, reposé dans des termes nouveaux.

Dans le présent travail nous nous sommes proposé de préciser la topographie des neurones monoaminergiques de l'hypothalamus chez le cobaye et la souris et d'étudier la destinée de leurs axones, ainsi que leurs modifications dans certaines circonstances physiologiques ou expérimentales interessant les axes hypothalamo-préhypophyso-gonadique et hypothalamo-préhypophyso-mammaire.

## Matériel et méthode

Nos animaux (cobayes et souris, des deux sexes) ont été sacrifiés par décapitation; chaque animal expérimenté a été comparé avec un témoin. Dans chaque couple «témoin-expérimenté» les dissections ont été faites à quelques dizaines de secondes l'une de l'autre et les fragments prélevés ont subi simultanément les mêmes manipulations: immersion dans du propane liquide refroidi par de l'azote liquide (30 secondes) puis dans l'azote liquide (1 à quelques minutes); lyophilisation (1 à 3 jours) à $-35°$C et $10^{-2}$ Torr dans un lyophilisateur type Speedivac Pearse (Edwards modèle I); traitement 1 à 3 heures à $80°$C par les vapeurs de formol (6 g de formaldéhyde Merck à 80% d'humidité); inclusion rapide (quelques minutes) sous vide à $50°$C (dans la paraffine dégazée); réfrigération pour accélérer la prise de la paraffine; coupes sériées à $10~\mu$; montage rapide à l'Entellan; examen en fluorescence U.V. (éventuellement associé au contraste de phase) avec le grand microscope de fluorescence Zeiss (lampe HBO 200; filtres d'excitation $BG_3$ ou $BG_{12}$, donnant une lumière de $\lambda$ max 410 m$\mu$). Les microphotographies ont été faites sur films Rayoscope (pose 15 secondes environ) et Anscochrome 500 (pose 45 secondes environ).

* Ce travail a été effectué dans le cadre d'une subvention de l'INSERM. Nous remercions le Dr. Corrodi et les Laboratoires A. B. Hassle (Göteborg) pour la fourniture gracieuse d'alpha-méthyl-métatyrosine. Le montage des préparations à l'Entellan a été fait par Mme Masse,

Table. *Conditions expérimentales et nombres d'animaux*

| Traitement | Doses en mg/g de poids corporel | Temps avant le sacrifice | Cobayes | Souris |
|---|---|---|---|---|
| Normaux | — | — | 28 | 28 |
| Castration | — | 5 jours à 14 mois | 15 | 15 |
| Gestation | — | 1 à 12 jours | — | 4 |
| Allaitement | — | 1 à 14 jours | — | 26 |
| Oestrus constant | — | 3 à 6 mois | 3 | — |
| Benzogynestryl retard s.c. | 0,0005/2 fois par semaine | 10 à 34 jours | 5 | 5 |
| Alpha-méthyl-metatyrosine i.p. | 0,5 à 1/2 fois | 6 heures | 6 | 7 |
| D.L. Métatyrosine i.p. | 0,5 à 1/3 fois | 8 heures | 6 | 6 |

# Resultats

## A. Données morphologiques

### 1. Cellules catécholaminergiques

Les cellules catécholaminergiques de l'hypothalamus occupent une aire très vaste; elles sont particulièrement abondantes dans la région du noyau arqué (groupe A12, Dahlström et Fuxe, 1964) et dans la région prémamillaire.

Des cellules légèrement plus volumineuses et d'aspect différent se rencontrent de part et d'autre du faisceau de Vicq d'Azyr, dans les régions hypothalamiques latérales et latérodorsales; ces cellules rappellent les cellules du groupe A11 des auteurs suédois, qu'elles prolongent vraisemblablement vers l'avant. Chez le cobaye surtout, certaines cellules volumineuses s'observent de part et d'autre de la région périventriculaire postérieure prémamillaire; elles semblent avoir un comportement particulier et forment notre groupe A13 (Barry, 1968c).

Dans la région hypothalamique antérieure enfin de petites cellules fluorescentes peuvent s'observer chez le cobaye et la souris; souvent difficiles à voir elles peuvent être assez nombreuses chez certains animaux et constituer un véritable noyau périventriculaire antérieur (notre groupe A14) dont le nombre de neurones peut atteindre 50% de celui des cellules du noyau infundibulaire (Barry, 1968c).

### 2. Fibres monoaminergiques du tractus hypothalamo-hypophysaire (THH)

Les fibres monoaminergiques du THH proviennent principalement des cellules du noyau arqué. Elles se terminent essentiellement au niveau de l'infundibulum (plexus intercalaire surtout, mais aussi anses intra-infundibulaires). Certaines d'entre elles se terminent autour des capillaires de la tige, du hile et de la périphérie du lobe nerveux, parfois même dans le lobe intermédiaire (rat). Il est vraisemblable que ces divers contingents exercent des fonctions distinctes.

### 3. Afférences monoaminergiques d'origine mésencéphalique

Ces fibres qui empruntent principalement la voie du faisceau médian du télencéphale et accessoirement celle du faisceau de Schütz contiennent : des composants catécholaminergiques, se distribuant aux NSO, NPV, NPV latéro-hypothalamiques, et dans les régions hypothalamique antérieure, postérieure, infundibulaire et périventriculaire : des fibres sérotoninergiques, difficiles à voir, se distribuant principalement aux noyaux supra-chiasmatiques.

Les neurones monoaminergiques de l'hypothalamus, qui présentent généralement une nette activité acétylcholinestérasique et sont situés par ailleurs dans des zones riches en afférences monoaminergiques, reçoivent probablement une double innervation, cholinergique et catécholaminergique (notamment noradrénergique).

## B. Données expérimentales

### 1. Castration

La castration détermine généralement chez le cobaye (BARRY et LEONARDELLI, 1968) et la souris mâle (BARRY, inédit) une diminution du matériel fluorescent péricapillaire de l'infundibulum ou une répartition plus hétérogène de ce matériel.

L'administration d'alpha-méthyl-métatyrosine accentue cette diminution (BARRY, 1968a) et entraine une vidange des petites cellules fluorescentes du noyau arqué. Par contre les grandes cellules fluorescentes (notre groupe A 13), souvent plus nombreuses chez le castré, demeurent visibles ; elles représentent donc probablement des éléments hypoactifs (BARRY, 1968a).

### 2. Oestrus constant

L'oestrus constant, par lésions stéréotaxiques de l'hypothalamus antérieur (cobayes stéréotaxés par notre collaborateur P. POULAIN) semble s'accompagner d'une diminution du matériel fluorescent infundibulaire, l'alpha-méthyl-métatyrosine accentuant cette diminution.

### 3. Benzogynoestryl retard

L'administration de benzogynoestryl retard chez la souris et le cobaye donne des modifications variables d'interprétation difficile (BARRY, 1969). Elle entraine, dans un certain nombre de cas, une augmentation de nombre des cellules fluorescentes du noyau arqué, et parfois, du matériel fluorescent infundibulaire, tandis qu'elle réduit le nombre des grandes cellules fluorescentes prémamillaires du cobaye (activation ?).

### 4. Gestation

Durant la première partie de la gestation les cellules fluorescentes du noyau arqué sont généralement nombreuses et la charge en matériel fluorescent moyenne ou forte. L'administration d'alphaméthyl-métatyrosine entraine une disparition presque complète de ce matériel au niveau de la zona externa et une vidange des cellules fluorescentes du noyau arqué. Les fibres sérotoninergiques des NSC sont parfois très apparentes (BARRY, inédit).

## 5. Allaitement

Au cours de l'allaitement la charge en matériel fluorescent est généralement notable ou forte. Le nombre des cellules fluorescentes du noyau infundibulaire est variable, parfois inférieur à celui observé au cours de la gestation (Barry, 1968 c). L'administration d'alpha méthyl-métatyrosine entraine une vidange cellulaire de degré variable et une diminution plus ou moins marquée du matériel fluorescent dans la zone externe de l'infundibulum.

Il existe peu de différences entre animaux sacrifiés quelques heures après enlèvement de leurs petits et aussitôt après la tétée. Toutefois lorsqu'on examine des hypothalamus de souris séparées de leurs petits depuis 24 heures et de souris ayant subi plusieurs heures de tétée, on constate que la vidange des cellules du noyau arqué après métatyrosine est plus marquée chez les animaux venant d'allaiter (Barry, inédit). Ce fait suggère que ces cellules sont plus actives chez ces animaux.

Il est à noter enfin que nous avons observé le plus grand nombre de petites cellules fluorescentes dans l'hypothalamus antérieur chez des souris en cours d'allaitement.

# Discussion

Nos observations morphologiques sont en parfait accord avec les données topographiques généralement admises (Dahlström et Fuxe, 1964; Dahlström, Fuxe et Larsson, 1965; Fuxe, 1964; Fuxe et Hökfelt, 1966; Fuxe, Hökfelt et Ungerstedt, 1969; Moore et Heller, 1967; Odake, 1967); de même en ce qui concerne la présence éventuelle de fibres catécholaminergiques au niveau du lobe intermédiaire et de la neurohypophyse (Björklund, 1968; Hermand, 1969). Les techniques stéréotaxiques devraient permettre de préciser davantage ces données (Barry, 1967) l'existence d'effets «transsynaptiques» (Moore et Heller, 1967) nous paraissant peu probable.

Par contre l'existence d'un groupe cellulaire particulier dans l'hypothalamus antérieur (notre groupe A 14) mérite de retenir l'attention, d'autant que ses cellules sont localisées précisément dans la région dont la destruction par stéréotaxie détermine l'apparition d'un état d'oestrus constant chez le cobaye (Poulain, 1968). Ces cellules pourraient peut-être représenter les neurones inhibiteurs des neurones qui élaborent le FRF.

Nos observations expérimentales conduisent à penser que la castration active les cellules dopaminergiques du noyau arqué, hypothèse en accord avec les observations d'Anton-Tay et Wurtmann (1968): accélération du taux de renouvellement de la noradrénaline; de Donoso et Stefano (1967): baisse du taux de noradrénaline et augmentation du taux de dopamine; de Zambrano et de Robertis (1968): augmentation du nombre des vésicules granuleuses dans la zone infundibulaire externe chez le rat.

L'administration d'oestrogènes semble entrainer une mise au repos relative des cellules dopaminergiques du noyau arqué, fait en accord avec les observations de Donoso et Cukier (1968) qui observent une élévation du taux de dopamine et une diminution du taux de noradrénaline dans l'hypothalamus antérieur, après administration d'oestradiol et de progestérone chez le rat castré.

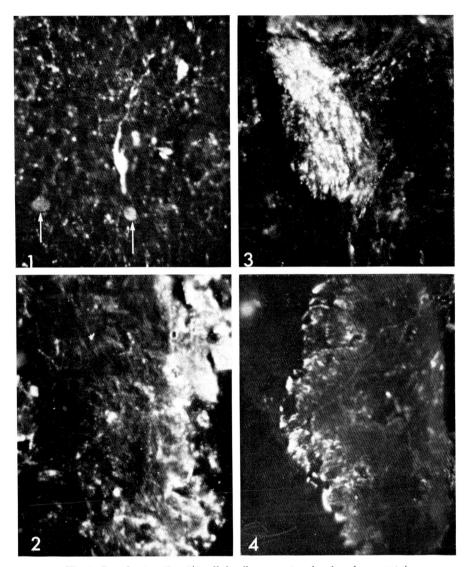

Fig. 1. Grande et petites (↑) cellules fluorescentes chez le cobaye castré

Fig. 2. Eminence médiane de cobaye témoin

Fig. 3. Eminence médiane de souris sous benzogynoestryl retard depuis 1 mois: forte charge en matériel fluorescent sous épendymaire

Fig. 4. Eminence médiane de cobaye castré: noter la faible charge en matériel fluorescent au niveau de la zona externa

Ces données et le fait que les cellules dopaminergiques du noyau arqué sont par ailleurs actives au cours de la gestation et de l'allaitement suggèrent qu'elles interviennent probablement dans le contrôle de la sécrétion gonadotrope préhypophysaire et, plus particulièrement, dans la cession de FRF et, également, de LRF.

Ces hypothèses concordent avec les observations de Leonardelli (1968 b): nombre
maximum de cellules fluorescentes infundibulaires en oestrus préovulatoire, activité
importante de ces cellules en oestrus; de Zambrano (1969): maximum préovulatoire de terminaisons infundibulaires à vésicules granuleuses; de Zolovick, Pearse,
Boehlke et Eleftheriou (1966): activité monoamino-oxydasique maximum en
oestrus; de Lichtensteiger (1969): fluorescence cellulaire maximum en oestrus
préovulatoire chez la ratte.

L'inhibition de l'ovulation par les dépléteurs de la noradrénaline chez le rat
(Coppola, Leonardi et Lippmann, 1966) ou par l'administration intrapéritonéale
d'alpha-méthyl-métatyrosine chez le rat (Lippmann, Leonardi, Ball et Coppola,
1967) et chez le hamster (Lippmann, 1968) concorde également avec les hypothèses
précédentes.

Le problème du rôle des monoamines hypothalamiques au cours de l'allaitement apparait plus complexe. L'administration systémique de réserpine ou d'alpha-
méthyl-métatyrosine entraine un état de pseudogestation chez le rat (Coppola,
Leonardi et Lippmann, 1966), de même que l'implantation locale de réserpine
dans l'éminence médiane (Maanen et Smelik, 1968), ces effects étant bloqués par
l'iproniazide, et les inhibiteurs de la monoamine oxydase, (d°), la pargyline et la
nialamide (Meyerson et Sawyer, 1968). Ces faits suggèrent que les monoamines
interviennent dans le côntrole de la sécrétion de prolactine, et même que la dopamine pourrait être identique au PIF (Maanen et Smelik, 1968). En réalité l'administration répétée de dopamine en intra-péritonéale ne semble pas perturber
appréciablement le déroulement de la lactation; par ailleurs les cellules dopaminergiques infundibulaires semblent actives au cours de la lactation et plus actives
chez les animaux ayant subi une tétée prolongée que chez ceux séparés de leurs
petits. Ces faits semblent peu favorables à l'hypothèse d'une identité du PIF et
de la dopamine, d'autant que le taux hypophysaire de prolactine (et probablement
le taux hypothalamique de PIF) semblent nettement diminués après une tétée de
3 heures, succèdant à 10–12 heures sans tétée (Sar et Meites, 1969). Si l'hypothèse d'une intervention des monoamines centrales dans le contrôle de l'activité
gonadotrope ne parait pas douteuse, les modalités de cette intervention restent à
préciser.

Il est en particulier difficile de faire la part des afférences monoaminergiques
à l'hypothalamus et des cellules dopaminergiques infundibulaires et de choisir
entre une action centrale et une action préhypophysaire, spécifique ou non, de la
dopamine. Il est possible enfin que le noyau arqué comprenne une population
cellulaire hétérogène.

Les grandes cellules fluorescentes de la région prémamillaire du cobaye, hypo-
actives chez le castré (Barry et Leonardelli, 1968), activées par la progestérone
(Barry, 1968a) et la testostérone (Leonardelli, 1968a), semblent avoir une
fonction différente de celle des cellules dopaminergiques «classiques» du noyau
arqué.

## Conclusions

Les cellules monoaminergiques du noyau arqué semblent intervenir principalement dans le contrôle de la sécrétion folliculotrope préhypophysaire, vraisemblablement en stimulant la cession de FSH et, ègalement, de LH. Elles semblent égale-

ment intervenir dans le contrôle de la sécrétion de prolactine. Les modalités et la nature (directe ou indirecte) de ces diverses actions restent à préciser.

## Résumé

Les neurones monoaminergiques de l'hypothalamus sont groupés dans diverses régions occupant une aire relativement importante. Ceux de ces neurones qui entrent dans la constitution du tractus hypothalamo-hypophysaire semblent avoir une double innervation, cholinergique et monoaminergique. Leurs axones se terminent principalement dans la région infundibulaire, à titre secondaire dans le lobe intermédiaire ou le lobe nerveux.

Les cellules dopaminergiques de la région ventrale du tuber semblent intervenir essentiellement dans le contrôle de l'activité folliculotrope préhypophysaire (stimulation) et probablement dans celui de la sécrétion de prolactine.

### Bibliographie

ANTON-TAY, F., WURTMAN, R. J.: Norepinephrine: turnover in rat brains after gonadectomy. Science **159**, 1245 (1968).

BARRY, J.: Mise en évidence par stéréotaxie du transport hypothalamique et télencéphalique des monoamines élaborées au niveau du mésencéphale. C. R. Soc. Biol. (Paris) **161**, 2182–2184 (1967).

— Etude en fluorescence U.V. des monoamines tubéro-infundibulaires chez le cobaye mâle normal ou castré, après injections de réserpine ou de α-méthyl-m-tyrosine. C. R. Soc. Biol. (Paris) **162**, 449–452 (1968a).

— Recherches sur l'origine et les sites de terminaison des fibres monoaminergiques du tractus hypothalamo-hypophysaire. C. R. Soc. Biol. (Paris) **162**, 1946–1948 (1968b),

— Recherches sur le rôle des monoamines infundibulaires au cours de l'allaitement chez la souris. C. R. Soc. Biol. (Paris) **162**, 1954–1955 (1968c).

— Etude en fluorescence U.V. des monoamines tubéro-infundibulaires chez le cobaye mâle et la souris oestrogénisés. C. R. Soc. Biol. (Paris) (à paraître).

— LEONARDELLI, J.: Etude de la topographie des neurones et des fibres monoaminergiques au niveau de l'hypothalamus chez la cobaye normal ou stéréotaxé. C. R. Acad. Sci. (Paris) **265**, 557–560 (1967).

— — Etude comparée des neurones et des fibres monoaminergiques de la région tubéro-infundibulaire chez le cobaye mâle normal ou castré. C. R. Acad. Sci. (Paris) **265**, 1141–1144 (1968).

BJÖRKLUND, A.: Monoamine containing fibres in the neuro-intermediate lobe of the pig and rat. Z. Zellforsch. **89**, 573–590 (1968).

— FALCK, B.: Pituitary monoamines of the cat with special reference to the presence of an unidentified monoamine like substance in the adenohypophysis. Z. Zellforsch. **93**, 254–264 (1969).

COPPOLA, J. A., LEONARDI, R. G., LIPPMANN, W.: Ovulatory failure in rats after treatment with brain norepinephrine depletors. Endocrinology **78**, 225–228 (1966).

DAHLSTRÖM, A., FUXE, K.: Evidence for the existence of monoamine containing neurons in the central nervous system. I. Demonstration of monoamines in the cell bodies of brain stem neurons. Acta physiol. scand. **62**, Suppl. 232, 1–55 (1964).

— — Monoamines in the pituitary gland. Acta endocr. (Kbh.) **51**, 301–314 (1966).

— — LARSSON, K.: Mapping out of catecholamine and 5-hydroxytryptamine neurons innervating the telencephalon and diencephalon. Life Sci. **4**, 1275–1279 (1965).

DONOSO, A. O., CUKIER, J. O.: Oestrogen as depressor of noradrenaline concentration in the anterior hypothalamus. Nature (Lond.) **218**, 969–970 (1968).

— STEFANO, F. J. E.: Sex hormones and concentration of noradrenaline and dopamine in the anterior hypothalamus of castrated rats. Experientia (Basel) **23**, 665–667 (1967).

— — BISCARDI, A. M., CUKIER, J.: Effects of castration on hypothalamic catecholamines. Amer. J. Physiol. **212**, 737–740 (1967).

Falck, B.: Observations on the possibilities of the cellular localization of monoamines by a fluorescence method. Acta physiol. scand. **56**, Suppl. 197 (1962).
— Hillarp, N. A., Thieme, G., Thorp, A.: Fluorescence of catecholamines and related compounds condensed with formaldehyde. J. Histochem. Cytochem. **10**, 348–354 (1962).
Fuxe, K.: Cellular localization of monoamines in the median eminence and the infundibular stem of some mammals. Z. Zellforsch. **61**, 710–724 (1964).
— Hökfelt, T.: Further evidence for the existence of tubero-infundibular dopamine neurons. Acta physiol. scand. **66**, 243–244 (1966).
— — Ungerstedt, U.: Distribution of monoamines in the mammalian central nervous system by histochemical studies. In: Metabolism of amines in the brain (G. Hooper, ed.), p. 10–22. Macmillan 1969.
Hermand, E.: Recherches sur le rôle des monoamines hypothalamiques dans le controle de l'activité gonadotrope chez le Hamster doré (*Mesocricetus auratus*). Thèse Med. Lille, 163 + XLVIII (1969).
Leonardelli, J.: Modifications des cellules et des fibres monoaminergiques de la région infundibulo-tubérienne du cobaye après injections de propionate de testostérone. C. R. Soc. Biol. (Paris) **162**, 452–455 (1968a).
— Modifications des fibres et des cellules monoaminergiques dela région infundibulo-tubérienne du cobaye au cours du cycle oestral. C. R. Soc. Biol. (Paris) **162**, 1937–1940 (1968b).
— Action de l'injection de m-tyrosine sur les monoamines infundibulo-tubériennes du cobaye femelle et du cobaye mâle traité par la progestérone. C. R. Soc. Biol. (Paris) **162**, 1956–1959 (1968c).
Lichtensteiger, W.: Cyclic variations of catecholamine content in hypothalamic nerve cells during the estrous cycle of the rat, with a concomitant study of the substantia nigra. J. Pharmacol. exp. Ther. **165**, 204–215 (1969).
Lippmann, W.: Relationship between hypothalamic norepinephrine and serotonin and gonadotrophin secretion in the hamster. Nature (Lond.) **218**, 173–174 (1968).
— Leonardi, R., Ball, J., Coppola, J. A.: Relationship between hypothalamic catecholamines and gonadotrophin secretion in rats. J. Pharmacol. exp. Ther. **156**, 258–266 (1967).
Maanen, J. H., Smelik, P. G.: Induction of pseudopregnancy in rats following local depletion of monoamines in the median eminence of the hypothalamus. Neuroendocrinology **3**, 177–187 (1968).
Maeda, T., Dresse, A.: Possibilités d'études des trajets des fibres cérébrales monoaminergiques chez le rat nouveau-né. C. R. Soc. Biol. (Paris) **162**, 1626–1629 (1968).
Meyerson, B. J., Sawyer, Ch. H.: Monoamines and ovulation in the rat. Endocrinology **83**, 170–177 (1968).
Moore, R. Y., Heller, A.: Monoamines levels and neuronal degeneration in rat brain following lateral hypothalamic lesions. J. Pharmacol. exp. Ther. **156**, 12–22 (1967).
Odake, G.: Fluorescence microscopy of the catecholamine containing neurons of the hypothalamo-hypophyseal system. Z. Zellforsch. **82**, 46–64 (1967).
Poulain, P.: Modifications de l'appareil génital du cobaye femelle après des lésions de l'hypothalamus antérieur. DEA Lille, 35 p., 6 planches, 1968.
Sar, M., Meites, J.: Effects of suckling on pituitary release of prolactin, GH and ISH in postpartum lactating rats. Neuroendocrinology 4, 25–31 (1969).
White, W. F., Cohen, A. I., Rippel, R. H., Story, J. C., Schally, A. V.: Some hypothalamic polyamines that deplete pituitary follicle stimulating hormone. Endocrinology **82**, 742–753 (1968).
Zambrano, D.: The arcuate complex of the female rat during the sexual cycle. Z. Zellforsch. **93**, 560–570 (1969).
— De Robertis, E.: The effect of castration upon the ultrastructure of the rat hypothalamus. II. Arcuate nucleus and outer zone of the median eminence. Z. Zellforsch. **87**, 409–421 (1968).
Zolovick, A. J., Pearse, R., Boehlke, K. W., Eleftheriou, B. E.: MAO activity in various parts of the rat brain during the oestrous cycle. Science **154**, 649–650 (1966).

# Zur Kontrolle der Gonadotropin-Sekretion bei *Zonotrichia leucophrys gambelii**

EBERHARD HAASE

Institut für Haustierkunde der Universität (Direktor: Prof. Dr. Dr. h.c. W. HERRE)
Kiel (Germany)

**Key words:** Gonadotropin secretion — Birds.

**Summary.** GTH-function of the AChE containing cells in the pars distalis of *Zonotrichia leucophrys gambelii* is indicated by the following observations:

1. Their appearance is correlated with the photoperiodically induced testicular growth. They are absent in photorefractory birds.

2. After castration of photosensitive birds and subsequent photoperiodic stimulation the AChE-cells change into castration cells.

3. Inhibition of thyroid or adrenal cortex activity in photorefractory males does not cause the appearance of AChE in their pituitary glands.

The electron microscopic localization of AChE suggests that the enzyme is related to the synthesis of GTH.

The observation that AChE-cells are present in highly photosensitive birds on short-day photoperiods that lack gonadal growth leads to the following conclusions concerning control of GTH-secretion:

a) Synthesis and release of GTH can be controlled separately, and

b) the hormone can be synthesized under short-day conditions, whereas long-days are necessary for its release.

The stimulation of GTH-synthesis by long-days in less photosensitive birds suggests the existence of a connexion between the GTH-release-centre and the GTH-synthesis-centre. The occurrence of castration cells in gonadectomized photosensitive, photostimulated animals is in favour of this connexion. Under short-day conditions castration does not cause change of AChE-cells into castration cells. Therefore the feed-back mechanism between hypothalamus, pituitary and gonads can be activated via the release-centre.

Da in einem Kontrollsystem cine funktionelle Abhängigkeit besteht, muß es prinzipiell möglich sein, aus dem Studium des kontrollierten Organs Rückschlüsse auf den Kontrollmodus zu ziehen. Die nordamerikanische Ammer *Zonotrichia leucophrys gambelii* ist ein geeignetes Objekt für die Untersuchung der Kontrolle der Gonadotropin-Sekretion, die bei ihr durch einfache Versuchsbedingungen beeinflußt werden kann. Diese Art hat nämlich einen jahresperiodischen Fortpflanzungscyclus, der, wie z.B. FARNER (1966), FARNER und FOLLETT (1966)

* Mit Unterstützung durch National Institutes of Health, Grant 5RO1 NBO6187, Principal Investigator Prof. Dr. D. S. FARNER, Seattle, dem ich für Förderung zu größtem Dank verpflichtet bin.

zeigen konnten, von Zahl und Verteilung der täglichen Licht-Dunkel-Stunden abhängt. Unter natürlichen Bedingungen stimuliert die steigende Lichtstundenzahl im Frühjahr bei diesen Vögeln die Gonadotropin-Sekretion und folglich das Gonadenwachstum. Setzt man solche Vögel künstlichen Kurztagen (8 L 16 D) aus, so kehren die Gonaden in das Ruhestadium zurück. Interessanterweise tritt unter natürlichen Bedingungen die Gonadenregression jedoch unter Langtagbedingungen ein, und selbst eine weitere Steigerung der täglichen Lichtstundenzahl kann dann ein erneutes Gonadenwachstum nicht auslösen. Die Vögel werden in diesem Zustand als „photorefraktär" bezeichnet. Um wieder „photosensitiv" zu werden, d. h. in den Zustand zu gelangen, in dem sie auf photoperiodische Stimulation mit Gonadenwachstum antworten können, benötigen sie Kurztage, wie sie ihnen der Winter ihres Verbreitungsareals bietet. Daß das photoperiodisch induzierte Gonadenwachstum und damit die GTH-Sekretion dieser Art über den Hypothalamus gesteuert werden, haben die Experimente von WILSON und FARNER (1965), WILSON (1967) und STETSON (1969) bewiesen.

In einer histologisch-histochemischen Studie konnten MATSUO, VITUMS, KING und FARNER (1969) in der Adenohypophyse von Z. l. gambelii zwei gonadotrope Zelltypen identifizieren und jahreszeitliche Änderungen an ihnen feststellen, die sich mit dem Hodenwachstum und dem Gonadotropin-Gehalt der Pars distalis (FARNER, FOLLETT, KING und MORTON, 1966) korrelieren lassen. Ein noch exakteres Bild von der gonadotropen Funktion der Pars distalis dieser Art liefert der Nachweis der Acetylcholinesterase in dieser Drüse. HAASE und FARNER (1969) konnten in der Adenohypophyse von Z. l. gambelii Männchen, die bis Anfang November unter natürlichen Lichtbedingungen und danach für einen Monat unter experimentellem Kurztag (8 L 16 D) gehalten wurden und dadurch die Photorefraktivität überwunden hatten, keine oder fast keine AChE histochemisch nachweisen. Wurden diese Vögel photoperiodisch unter Langtagbedingungen (20 L 4 D) stimuliert, so traten AChE-haltige Zellen in beiden Lobi der Pars distalis auf. Dabei nahmen die Zahl der AChE-Zellen, ihre Größe und ihr Enzymgehalt mit der Dauer der Stimulation zu bis zu einem Maximum, das zwischen Tag 31 und Tag 52 lag. Danach sank die AChE-Aktivität wieder, und am Tag 80 war sie annähernd verschwunden. Die Hodengewichte der Vögel dieses Experiments zeigten eine Abhängigkeit von der Dauer der Stimulationsperiode, die der des AChE-Gehalts der Pars distalis weitgehend glich. Von Minimalgröße am Tag 0 ausgehend, erreichten sie ihr Maximum am Tag 45 und waren am Tag 80 fast auf das Ausgangsstadium zurückgekehrt. Zu diesem Zeitpunkt waren die Vögel also photorefraktär.

Die Korrelation zwischen Hodengröße und AChE-Gehalt der Pars distalis legte die Produktion gonadotropen Hormons durch die AChE-Zellen nahe. Dafür spricht auch, daß diese Zellen die gleiche Verbreitung in der Adenohypophyse aufweisen wie die von MATSUO et al. (1969) und von MIKAMI, VITUMS und FARNER (1969) identifizierten GTH-Zellen dieser Art. Darüber hinaus ist der positive Ausfall der PAS-Reaktion den AChE-Zellen und den von MATSUO et al. beschriebenen GTH-Zellen gemein.

Doch bemerkenswerterweise enthalten nicht alle GTH-Zellen AChE; andererseits war es aber auch nicht möglich, die AChE-Zellen mit nur einem der beiden von MATSUO et al. charakterisierten GTH-Zelltypen zu identifizieren. Das könnte bedeuten, daß die AChE-Zellen ein bestimmtes Aktivitätsstadium der GTH-Zellen repräsentieren.

Doch zunächst galt es, die GTH-Produktion in den AChE-Zellen experimentell zu beweisen. Obwohl Ergebnisse verschiedener Autoren bereits gegen eine TSH-Bildung in den AChE-Zellen sprechen (vgl. HAASE und FARNER, 1969), haben HAASE und FARNER (1970) die Schilddrüsen- bzw. Nebennierenrindentätigkeit

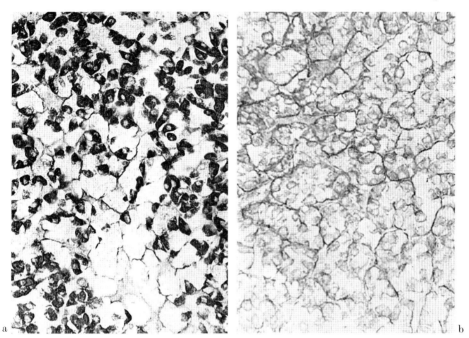

a                                                                                      b

Abb. 1a u. b. Darstellung der Acetylcholinesterase in der Pars distalis; a einer intakten photosensitiven männlichen *Z. l. gambelii* nach 31 Tagen photoperiodischer Stimulation; b einer am Tag 0 der Stimulationsperiode kastrierten männlichen photosensitiven *Z. l. gambelii* nach 28 Tagen photoperiodischer Stimulation. Die AChE-haltigen Zellen sind bei b in Kastrationszellen verwandelt

photorefraktärer Vögel blockiert, um dadurch TSH- bzw. ACTH-Zellen der Pars distalis zu aktivieren. Das führte jedoch nicht zum Auftreten AChE-haltiger Zellen in der Adenohypophyse. Auch die Kastration photorefraktärer Vögel änderte trotz stimulatorischer Photoperiode am Fehlen solcher Zellen während der Refraktärzeit nichts.

Einen positiven Beweis für die GTH-Produktion in den AChE-Zellen erbrachte die Kastration photosensitiver Männchen und die anschließende photoperiodische Stimulation. Bei diesen Tieren verwandelten sich die AChE-Zellen frühzeitig in hypertrophierte, vacuolisierte sog. Kastrationszellen, die nach 3 und 4 Wochen die ganze Pars distalis überschwemmten (Abb. 1).

Die bisherigen Untersuchungen haben also gezeigt, daß bei *Z. l. gambelii* die AChE-Zellen mit der GTH-Sekretion in Zusammenhang stehen.

Aufschluß über die Kontrolle dieser Sekretion lieferte ein weiteres Experiment. *Z. l. gambelii*-Männchen, die bis dahin in Freiluftvolieren gelebt hatten, wurden

am 15. Januar in Klimakammern auf experimentelle Kurztagbedingungen (8 L
16 D) überführt. Am 23. Januar (Tag 0) wurden 2 von ihnen getötet. Ihre Adeno-
hypophysen waren frei von AChE-haltigen Zellen. Sechs weitere Männchen wurden
an diesem Tag kastriert und verblieben mit 2 intakten Männchen unter Kurztagbedingungen. Nach 10, 20 und 30 Tagen wurden je 2 von ihnen getötet, mit der
letzten Gruppe kamen auch die beiden intakten Kontrolltiere zur Untersuchung.

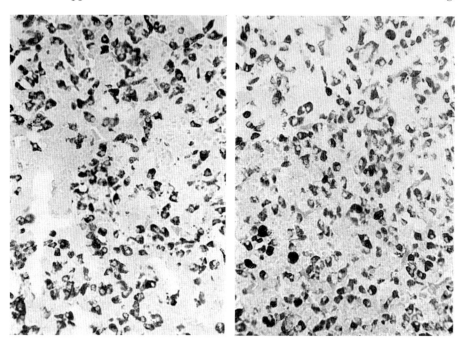

Abb. 2. Darstellung der Acetylcholinesterase in der Pars distalis stark photosensitiver *Z. l.
gambelii*-Männchen. Die AChE-Zellen haben sich unter Kurztagbedingungen entwickelt; bei
Tier b, das 30 Tage vor seinem Tod kastriert worden war, sind keine Kastrationszellen
aufgetreten

In den Hypophysen der kastrierten Vögel traten bereits nach 10 Tagen AChE-
haltige Zellen auf, und ihre Zahl nahm mit der Versuchsdauer zu. Doch über-
raschenderweise wandelten sich diese AChE-Zellen nicht wie bei kastrierten,
photosensitiven, photostimulierten Tieren in Kastrationszellen um. Auch die
Hypophysen der am Tag 30 getöteten intakten Kontrollen, deren Hoden Minimalgröße aufwiesen, enthielten AChE-Zellen und unterschieden sich im histochemi-
schen Präparat nicht von denen der kastrierten Vögel (Abb. 2).

Die Befunde über den AChE-Gehalt der Hypophysen intakter *Z. l. gambelii*-
Männchen stehen mit RUSSELLs (1968) quantitativen biochemischen Cholin-
esterasebestimmungen am gleichen Objekt in Einklang.

Da die AChE in der Adenohypophyse dieser Art auf GTH-Zellen beschränkt
ist, muß geschlossen werden, daß bei stark photosensitiven *Z. l. gambelii*-Männchen
GTH-Zellen auch ohne photoperiodische Stimulation auftreten können. Weil die
Hoden der betreffenden Vögel aber inaktiv blieben, kann keine Hormonabgabe

stattgefunden haben. Daraus folgt, daß bei dieser Art Hormonbereitung und Hormonausschüttung getrennt kontrolliert werden können.

Morphologische Beobachtungen veranlaßten BARGMANN (1964), den Sekretionsablauf in die Vorgänge der Synthese und der Extrusion zu unterteilen. Gleichzeitig wandte er sich gegen den Vergleich des Sekretionsprozesses mit einer Kettenreaktion. Die elektronenmikroskopische Lokalisation der AChE in der Adenohypophyse des Stars (*Sturnus vulgaris*) ergab (HAASE und WELSCH, in Vorbereitung), daß dieses Enzym hauptsächlich im ribosomenbesetzten endoplasmatischen Reticulum, im Golgi-Apparat und auf der Kernmembran vorkommt und läßt daher an eine Beteiligung an Syntheseprozessen denken.

Aus dem letzten Experiment geht damit hervor, daß für die GTH-Synthese Kurztage, die noch kein Gonadenwachstum stimulieren, ausreichen. Dagegen ist für die Sekretabgabe (Release) und folglich das Gonadenwachstum die photoperiodische Stimulation unter Langtagbedingungen erforderlich.

Das erste Experiment mit verhältnismäßig schwach photosensitiven Vögeln zeigt darüber hinaus, daß der Langtag auch auf die Synthese stimulierend einwirken kann. Möglicherweise geschieht das über eine Querverbindung von einem Gonadotropin-Release-Zentrum zu einem Gonadotropin-Synthese-Zentrum. Auch das Auftreten von Kastrationszellen läßt sich im Sinne einer solchen Querverbindung deuten.

Weiterhin tragen die genannten Befunde zu einer Klärung des Begriffes ,,Photorefraktivität'' bei. Sie beinhaltet das Unvermögen zur Gonadotropin-Synthese. Eventuell wird das Synthese-Zentrum durch eine Vielzahl von Langtagen inhibiert und durch zahlreiche Kurztage wieder regeneriert und stimuliert. Der letzte Versuch schließt auch nicht aus, daß der Synthese ein endogener Jahresrhythmus zugrunde liegt, der allerdings nur zur Wirkung kommen kann, nachdem die inhibitorische Aktion des Langtages aufgehoben wurde. Schließlich veranlassen die verschiedenen Kastrationsexperimente zu dem Schluß, daß der Rückkoppelungsmechanismus zwischen Gonaden, Hypothalamus und Hypophyse über das Release-Zentrum zur Aktion kommt. Unter Kurztagbedingungen, als lediglich die Synthese des Hormons ablief, war kein Einfluß der Kastration auf die GTH-Zellen festzustellen, die sich aber in Kastrationszellen umwandelten, als die Hormonausschüttung durch Langtage angeregt wurde. Das schließt nicht aus, daß Testosteron außerdem auch direkt auf das Synthese-Zentrum wirken könnte, wie GOGAN (1968) es nach Implantationsversuchen vermutet.

Über die Lokalisation des Synthese-Zentrums sind noch keine genauen Angaben möglich. Obwohl es unwahrscheinlich ist, daß diese Kontrollstation in den GTH-Zellen selbst liegt, bedarf diese Annahme der experimentellen Bestätigung durch Transplantationsversuche, die bereits in Angriff genommen sind. Eher wird man das Synthese-Zentrum im Hypothalamus suchen müssen. GOGAN (1968) fand bei der Hausente zwei Regionen, in denen Testosteronimplantate den GTH-Gehalt der Pars distalis vermindern und eine Reduktion des Gonadenwachstums bewirken. Bisher ist auch nicht entschieden, ob die von WILSON und FARNER (1965), WILSON (1967) und STETSON (1969) beschriebenen hypothalamischen Gebiete, deren elektrolytische Zerstörung das photoperiodisch induzierte Gonadenwachstum blockiert, die Synthese oder die Extrusion gonadotropen Hormons oder beide kontrollieren.

Anzeichen für eine separate Kontrolle der Bereitung und Ausschüttung von Luteinisierungshormon (LH) sind bei Säugern u. a. von Kanematsu und Sawyer (1963, 1964, Kaninchen) und Samli und Geschwind (1967, 1968, Ratte) gefunden worden. Bei Vögeln liegen entsprechende Angaben für gonadotropes Hormon von Gogan (1968) bei der Ente und von Farner und Follett (1966) sowie Follett, Farner und Morton (1967) bei *Z. l. gambelii* vor. Follett und Farner (1966) stützen sich dabei auf die Beobachtung, daß bei längerem Halten unter Kurztagbedingungen der Gonadotropin-Gehalt der Hypophyse zusammen mit der Photoresponsibilität anstiegen, ohne daß eine bemerkenswerte Gewichtszunahme der Hoden festzustellen war. Dieser Befund, der mit den hier beschriebenen Ergebnissen völlig übereinstimmt, wurde allerdings an Vögeln gewonnen, die von natürlichen Lichtbedingungen auf experimentellen Kurztag erst am Anfang des Monats (Februar) überführt wurden, in dessen Verlauf unter natürlichen Verhältnissen eine Entwicklung ihrer Hoden einsetzt. Die Resultate von Follett, Farner und Morton (1967), die nach Experimenten mit wiederholten Cyclen regelmäßig alternierender stimulatorischer und nicht-stimulatorischer Photoperioden eine lineare Beziehung zwischen gespeichertem Gonadotropin und der Zahl der nicht-stimulatorischen Photoperioden aufdeckten, und daraus auf eine getrennte, wenn vielleicht auch nicht völlig unabhängige Kontrolle für Synthese und Release gonadotropen Hormons schlossen, stehen mit den hier vorgetragenen in Einklang und lassen sich leicht im Sinn der hier genannten Interpretationen deuten.

## Literatur

Bargmann, W.: Exokrine und endokrine Sekretionsmechanismen auf Grund elektronenmikroskopischer Untersuchungen. Arch. Biol. **75**, 419–436 (1964).

Farner, D. S.: Über die photoperiodische Steuerung der Jahreszyklen bei Zugvögeln. Biol. Rdsch. **4**, 228–241 (1966).

— Follett, B. K.: Light and other environmental factors affecting avian reproduction. J. animal Sci. **25** (Suppl.), 90–115 (1966).

— — King, J. R., Morton, M. L.: A quantitative examination of ovarian growth in the White-crowned Sparrow. Biol. Bull. **130**, 67–75 (1966).

Follett, B. K., Farner, D. S., Morton, M. L.: The effects of alternating long and short daily photoperiods on gonadal growth and pituitary gonadotropins in the White-crowned Sparrow, *Zonotrichia leucophrys gambelii*. Biol. Bull. **133**, 330–342 (1967).

Gogan, F.: Sensibilité hypothalamique à la testostérone chez le Canard. Gen. comp. Endocr. **11**, 316–327 (1968).

Haase, E., Farner, D. S.: Acetylcholinesterase in der Pars distalis von *Zonotrichia leucophrys gambelii* (Aves). Z. Zellforsch. **93**, 356–368 (1969).

— — The function of the acetylcholinesterase cells of the pars distalis of the White-crowned Sparrow, *Zonotrichia leucophrys gambelii*. Acta Zool. **51**, 99–106 (1970).

— Welsch, U.: Licht- und elektronenmikroskopische Untersuchungen an den AChE-Zellen in der Adenohypophyse des Stars (*Sturnus vulgaris*). (In Vorbereitung.)

Kanematsu, S., Sawyer, C. H.: Effects of hypothalamic estrogen implants on pituitary LH and prolactin in rabbits. Amer. J. Physiol. **205**, 1073–1076 (1963).

— — Effects of hypothalamic and hypophysial estrogen implants on pituitary and plasma LH in ovariectomized rabbits. Endocrinology **75**, 579–585 (1964).

Matsuo, S., Vitums, A., King, J. R., Farner, D. S.: Light microscopic studies of the cytology of the adenohypophysis of the White-crowned Sparrow, *Zonotrichia leucophrys gambelii*. Z. Zellforsch. **95**, 143–176 (1969).

Mikami, S., Vitums, A., Farner, D. S.: Electron microscopic studies of the adenohypophysis of the White-crowned Sparrow, *Zonotrichia leucophrys gambelii*. Z. Zellforsch. **97**, 1–27 (1969).

RUSSELL, D. H.: Acetylcholinesterase in the hypothalamo-hypophyseal axis of the White-crowned Sparrow, *Zonotrichia leucophrys gambelii*. Gen. comp. Endocr. **11**, 51–63 (1968).

SALMI, M. H., GESCHWIND, I. I.: Some effects of hypothalamic luteinizing hormone releasing factor on the biosynthesis and release of luteinizing hormone. Endocrinology **81**, 835–848 (1967).

— — Some effect of energy transfer inhibitors and of Ca$^{++}$-free or K$^{+}$-free enhanced media on the release of luteinizing hormone (LH) from the rat pituitary gland in vitro. Endocrinology **82**, 225–231 (1968).

STETSON, M. H.: The role of the median eminence in control of photoperiodically induced testicular growth in the White-crowned Sparrow, *Zonotrichia leucophrys gambelii*. Z. Zellforsch. **93**, 369–394 (1969).

WILSON, F. E.: The tubero-infundibular neuron system: A component of the photoperiodic control mechanism of the White-crowned Sparrow, *Zonotrichia leucophrys gambelii*. Z. Zellforsch. **82**, 1–24 (1967).

— FARNER, D. S.: Effects of hypothalamic lesions on testicular growth. Fed. Proc. **24**, 129 (1965).

# Inhibitory Hypothalamic Control of Thyroid Gland Activity in the Goldfish, *Carrassius auratus**

RICHARD E. PETER**

Department of Zoology, University of Washington, Seattle (U.S.A.)

**Key words:** Hypothalamus — Thyroid — Inhibitory control.

BALL *et al.* (1963, 1965) found that *Poecilia formosa* with an ectopic pituitary homotransplant were hyperthyroid, which suggests that the hypothalamus normally inhibits the secretion of thyroid stimulating hormone (TSH). JOHANSEN (1967) also found that goldfish, *Carassius auratus*, with an autotransplanted pituitary were hyperthyroid.

In the present studies goldfish, *Carassius auratus*, were electrolytically lesioned in the hypothalamus in an attempt to acquire evidence on the mechanism of hypothalamic control of thyroid gland activity. Electrode placement was by a stereotaxic method developed for the goldfish. Thyroid glandular activity was measured by the conversion ratio, and the follicular cell height of the pronephric thyroid or the percent uptake of radioiodine, at 30 days postoperatively.

Lesion of the nucleus lateralis tuberis (NLT) pars posterior and the NLT pars anterior made the animals hyperthyroid. Destruction of the nucleus praeopticus, or bilateral destruction of the nucleus praeopticus tracts, had no effect on thyroid activity. Lesions in the posterior hypothalamus, and the dorsal hypothalamus had no effect on thyroid activity.

Viewed together the lesions isolate the NLT pars anterior and NLT pars posterior as the region of the hypothalamus that controls thyroid activity. The results provide direct evidence for hypothalamic control of thyroid activity, and indicate that the control is by a factor that inhibits the secretion of TSH. This factor is called the thyrotropin inhibitory factor.

*Acknowledgements:* I wish to thank Dr. AUBREY GORBMAN for his guidance and advice throughout the study.

## References

BALL, J. N., OLIVEREAU, M., KALLMAN, K. D.: Secretion of thyrotrophic hormone by pituitary transplants in a teleost fish. Nature (Lond.) **199**, 618–620 (1963).
— — SLICKER, A. M., KALLMAN, K. D.: Functional capacity of ectopic pituitary transplants in the teleost *Poecilia formosa*, with a comparative discussion on the transplanted pituitary. Phil. Trans. B **249**, 69–99 (1965).
JOHANSEN, P. H.: The role of the pituitary in the resistance of the goldfish (*Carassius auratus* L.) to a high temperature. Canad. J. Zool. **45**, 329–345 (1967).

\* To be published in detail elsewhere.
\*\* Postgraduate fellow of the National Research Council of Canada.

# Weitere Befunde zur Struktur und Funktion des Zwischenhirn-Hypophysensystems der Vögel

A. Oksche*, H.-J. Oehmke* und D. S. Farner**

Anatomisches Institut (Lehrstuhl I) der Universität Gießen (Germany) und
Department of Zoology, University of Washington, Seattle (U.S.A.)

Key words: Hypothalamo-hypophysial system — Birds — Structure — Function.

Summary. Our electron-microscopic studies (Oksche, 1965; Oehmke et al., 1969) on *Passer domesticus* have shown that the granules (diameters up to 1,000 Å) of the tubero-infundibular tract are formed in the Golgi zone of the neurons of the infundibular nucleus (Fig. 5A). Except for the size of the granules, this process is cytologically indistinguishable from the formation of secretion in the supraoptic nucleus. If one applies electron-microscopic criteria, the neurons of the infundibular nucleus of birds have all of the characteristics of neurosecretory cells; the secretory product is not selectively stainable but fluoresces on application of the technique of Falck (1962), and Falck and Owman (1965). The avian hypothalamus, therefore, in addition to the classical neurosecretory system of the supraoptic and paraventricular nucleus, contains at least a further, aminergic neurosecretory system involving the infundibular and ventromedial nucleus. With the introduction of the questions concerning the origin of the "Gomori-positive"[1] neurosecretory material in fibers leading to the rostral division of the median eminence and concerning the significance of the non-fluorescing neurones associated with the infundibular nucleus, the problem becomes substantially more complex. The infundibular nucleus consists of a mosaic of small cell groups which cytologically are conspicuously differentiated. Also, the rostral region of the avian hypothalamus in the vicinity of the optic recess may contain additional neuroendocrinologically active cell types. Still completely puzzling are the "Gomori-positive" nerve cells that are scattered in the optic tract and in the entopeduncular tract.

The experiments of Wilson and Stetson with stereotaxically placed lesions should be viewed within the framework of this anatomical picture. The results of these experiments have already brought considerable verification concerning the components of the avian hypothalamus involved in the photoperiodically controlled development of the gonads. Without the infundibular nucleus photoperiodically induced testicular growth does not occur whereas the rostral division of the median eminence with its "Gomori-positive" material appears to have no

---

\* Mit Unterstützung durch die Deutsche Forschungsgemeinschaft.

\*\* Investigations supported by the National Institutes of Health through a grant to D. S. Farner.

1 Stainable with chrome-alum hematoxylin, paraldehyde-fuchsin, alcian-blue, pseudo-isocyanine.

essential role in this process. There is still no explanation for the fluctuations in "Gomori-positive" material as observed during the annual cycle and under various functional conditions. It should not be overlooked that in mammals (*e.g.* rat), certain manipulations such as adrenalectomy (and hypophysectomy), are followed by the appearance of "Gomori-positive" material in the otherwise non-stainable median eminence (Bock and Goslar, 1969).

The following working hypothesis provides from our point of view the frame-work for further experimental and cytological studies: It is proposed that the avian hypothalamus contains, in addition to the classical neurosecretory system and the aminergic tuberal system, still further (peptidergic) neuroendocrine centers which produce releasing factors. The differentiation of portal vessels into anterior and posterior groups, as observed in *Zonotrichia leucophrys gambelii* (Vitums et al., 1964) and in *Coturnix coturnix japonica* (Sharp and Follett, 1969), lead to the assumption that the neuroendocrine pathway may have point to point relation-ships. Since the giant portal capillaries (portal "vessels") of fringillid species have neither epithelioid cell pads nor muscle sphincters the site of active circulatory control must be sought primarily in the innervation of the arterioles leading to the portal vessel system. The possibility of tumefying ability by the capillary endo-thelial cells (direct action by a hypothalamic agent?) and the inclusion of these vessels in a characteristic encasement by the pars tuberalis, which is surrounded by reticular fibers, must not be overlooked.

For the future we might recommend the following with respect to investigations of the avian hypothalamo-hypophysial system: (1) The use of still more discrete stereotaxic lesions based on the cytoarchitectonic map of the hypothalamus showing especially the mosaic-like arrangement of cell groups. (2) Fluorescence-microscopic detection of monoamines after microlesions in individual tuberal nuclei and their associated tracts. (As in the classical neurosecretory system the fluorescing material should then accumulate in the section of the fiber proximal from the site of the lesion). (3) A search for the cells that produce releasing factors using light- and electron-microscopic autoradiography and immunohistochemistry. These procedures may make possible the differential diagnosis of the various nerve endings in the median eminence since size of granule is not a sufficiently useful criterion. (4) Stereotaxic and electrophysiological studies to clarify the signi-ficance of the numerous synapses, as observed in electron-microscopy, on the neurones and in the neuropile of the supraoptic and infundibular nucleus of birds. (5) Clarification of the possible mutual nervous and humoral functional relation-ships of the various nerve-fiber and ependymal endings in the median eminence (Kobayashi and Farner, 1969). This problem is closely related to the question as to whether or not the biogenic amines of the tuberal nuclei have a direct function as releasing factors.

We are of the opinion that the anatomical arrangement of the neuroendocrine centers of birds provides an especially favorable basis for such studies.

## Ergebnisse

Seit dem 3. Symposium über Neurosekretion (Bristol, 1961) ist es für uns zur Tradition geworden, einen Tagungsbericht über das neurosekretorische System der Vögel vorzulegen. Auf eine allgemeine Beschreibung dieses neurovasculären Komplexes kann mit Hinweis auf die Schemata von OKSCHE (1962, 1963, 1965) und auf die ausgestellte Demonstration (vgl. OKSCHE, MÖLLER und LANGBEIN, 1969) verzichtet werden. 1961 stand noch das klassische neurosekretorische System Nucleus supraopticus — Nucleus paraventricularis — Pars nervosa der Hypophyse im Vordergrund unserer Überlegungen (FARNER, OKSCHE und LORENZEN; OKSCHE, 1962); es wurde aber schon auf die tubero-infundibulare Verknüpfung[2] hingewiesen (Abbildungen s. OKSCHE, 1962, vgl. hierzu OKSCHE, 1960, 1963). 1966 (s. OKSCHE, 1967) lag bereits der elektronenmikroskopische Befund vor, daß im Golgi-Apparat der Nervenzellen des Nucleus infundibularis Sekretgranula mit einem Durchmesser um 1000 Å gebildet werden. Dieses Material fand sich auch im Verlauf des Tractus tubero-infundibularis und in der Außenzone (Palisadenschicht) der Eminentia mediana. Eigene fluorescenzmikroskopische Befunde (Monoaminnachweis) konnten aber zu diesem Zeitpunkt noch nicht vorgelegt werden. Offen blieben vor allem die folgenden Fragen: 1. Herkunft der elektiv färbbaren Substanz im rostralen Teil der Eminentia mediana, 2. Bedeutung des innerhalb der neurosekretorischen Hauptbahn nachweisbaren kleingranulären Materials.

Die Ergebnisse der stereotaktischen Operationen von WILSON (1967), WILSON und HANDS (1968) und STETSON (1969) haben gezeigt, daß bei den von uns vorwiegend untersuchten Passeriformes die lichtabhängige Gonadenreaktion (Gewichtszunahme) nur dann ausbleibt, wenn entweder die neurovasculäre Kontaktzone der Eminentia mediana oder das Gebiet des Infundibularkerns ausgeschaltet werden. Eine Unterbrechung der elektiv färbbaren neurosekretorischen Bahn in Höhe der Sehnervenkreuzung hat dagegen keinen Einfluß auf die lichtbedingte Hodenvergrößerung. Diese Ergebnisse zwingen uns, das theoretische Konzept des neurosekretorischen Zwischenhirn-Hypophysensystems der Vögel erneut zu durchdenken (vgl. FARNER und FOLLETT, 1966). Wichtige neue Angaben über seine Struktur und Funktion sind den von KOBAYASHI und FARNER (1969) herausgegebenen Verhandlungen über neuroendokrine Funktionen der Vögel zu entnehmen.

Im Mittelpunkt unserer Studien steht nach wie vor der nordamerikanische Ammernfink *Zonotrichia leucophrys gambelii*. Bei dieser Art wurden nach neurohistologischen Präparaten photographische Rekonstruktionen des Zwischenhirn-Hypophysensystems angefertigt (OKSCHE, MÖLLER und LANGBEIN, 1969) und cytoarchitektonische Analysen der Tuberkerne durchgeführt (OEHMKE, 1968, 1969; unveröffentlicht). Aus technischen Gründen war es aber notwendig, auch noch andere Vogelarten in die Untersuchungen einzubeziehen. So wurde der fluorescenzmikroskopische Aminnachweis vor allem am Zwischenhirn-Hypophysensystem von *Passer domesticus* und *Carduelis chloris* (Passeriformes) durchgeführt (zur Methodik s. OEHMKE u.a., 1969, und OEHMKE, 1969) und damit die bei *Zonotrichia leucophrys gambelii* erzielten Ergebnisse (WARREN, 1968) erweitert.

Die kleinzelligen Tuberkerne der Vögel nehmen ein ausgedehntes Gebiet ein, das sich von der Sehnervenkreuzung bis zur caudalen Begrenzung des Infundi-

---

2 Unsere Studien (seit OKSCHE, 1960) knüpften hier an eine Beschreibung von WINGSTRAND (1951) an, die besagt, daß in der Eminentia mediana der Vögel neben dem von BENOIT und ASSENMACHER (1953/1959) analysierten, elektiv färbbaren neurosekretorischen System auch eine tubero-infundibulare Komponente vorhanden ist.

bulums erstreckt. Innerhalb dieser Kernmasse lassen sich — im Sinne der am Säugerhypothalamus gebräuchlichen Untergliederung — die Areale eines Nucleus infundibularis (= Nucl. arcuatus) und Nucleus ventromedialis (= Nucl. principalis) unterscheiden, die allerdings fließend ineinander übergehen. Dem besonders stark ausgebildeten basalen Abschnitt des Nucl. infundibularis, der auch die stärkste Aminfluorescenz zeigt, sind dorsal zwei weitere Kernabschnitte aufgelagert. Feine marklose Nervenfasern dringen aus den topographisch am engsten benachbarten Teilen des Infundibularkerns in den rostralen und — unter zunehmender Verdichtung des Tr. tubero-infundibularis — in den caudalen Abschnitt der Eminentia mediana ein (Oksche, Möller und Langbein, 1969). Am caudalen Abhang des Hypothalamus stellt sich der Tr. tubero-infundibularis als ein vom Tuberkomplex bis zur Außenschicht der Eminentia mediana durchgehender Faserstrang dar, der auch eine besonders kräftige Aminfluorescenz zeigt (Abb.1—3). Funktionell wichtig ist die Frage, ob der aus dem Nucl. ventromedialis stammende Faserstrang im Nucl. infundibularis synaptisch umgeschaltet wird. Mit dem Elektronenmikroskop lassen sich in dem varicösen Neuropil des Nucl. infundibularis zwar zahlreiche axo-dendritische und axo-somatische Synapsen mit elektronendichten präsynaptischen Granula darstellen, der genaue Ursprungsort dieser präsynaptischen aminergen Fasern konnte aber bisher nicht ermittelt werden (vgl. Abb. 5A).

Neue cytoarchitektonische Studien an den Tuberkernen von Z. l. gambelii und anderen Spatzenvögeln haben gezeigt (Oehmke, 1969), daß die obengenannten größeren Kerngebiete wieder mosaikartig aus kleineren Zellverbänden zusammengesetzt sind. Der sog. Basiskern des Nucleus infundibularis läßt in seinem mittleren und caudalen Abschnitt zwei dichter gelagerte und durch feine Neuropilstreifen getrennte Zellkomplexe erkennen. In seiner ersten dorsalen Auflagerung sind 3 und in der zweiten 2 weitere deutlich abgrenzbare Unterabteilungen auszumachen (Abb. 4a, b). Solche Untereinheiten der Tuberkerne bestehen aus verschieden großen, unterschiedlich basophilen multipolaren Neuronen. Diese Gliederung, die im Prinzip der von Grünthal (1930) aufgezeichneten feineren Kerntopographie des Säugerhypothalamus entspricht, findet sich also auch in den Abschnitten des Infundibularkerns, die von Stetson (1969) als besonders wesentlich für den normalen Ablauf der lichtabhängigen Hodengewichtszunahme erkannt wurden. Mit der Methode nach Falck zeigt nur ein Teil dieser Perikaryen eine positive Monoaminfluorescenz. War hier bei *Carduelis chloris* und *Anas platyrhynchos* eine Unterscheidung zwischen Noradrenalin und Dopamin noch nicht möglich (Oehmke, 1969)[3], so scheint bei *Coturnix coturnix japonica* diese Frage bereits zugunsten von Noradrenalin entschieden zu sein (Sharp und Follett, 1969a).

Obwohl die Faserzüge des Tr. tubero-infundibularis in neurohistologischen Präparaten bis zur Außenzone der Eminentia mediana zu verfolgen sind, leuchten ihre Palisaden im Fluorescenzmikroskop nur noch schwach. Dieses steht in einem gewissen Gegensatz zu den zahlreichen, mit elektronendichten Granula gefüllten Nervenendigungen der Zona externa (Abb. 5 B). Bei *Passer domesticus* (Oehmke u. a., 1969), Ente (Assenmacher und Calas, 1969) und Taube (Matsui, 1969) dominiert hier ein Endigungstyp mit einem Granuladurchmesser bis zu 1000 Å. 1200—1600 Å

---

3 Warren (1968) gelangte bei *Zonotrichia leucophrys gambelii* zum gleichen Schluß.

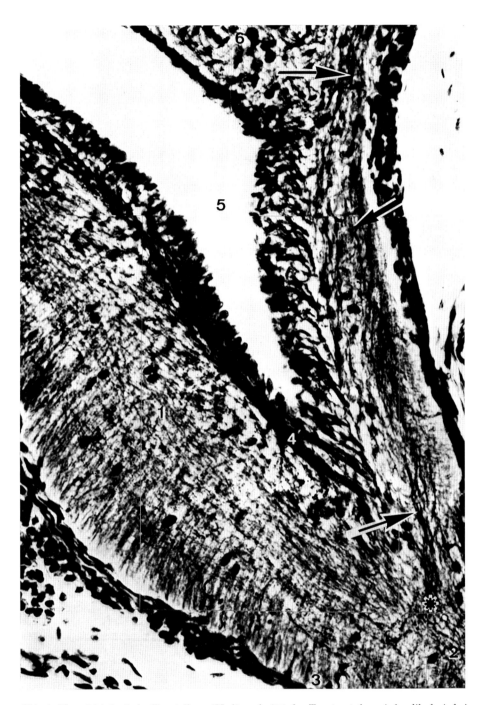

Abb. 1. Neurohistologische Darstellung (Medianschnitt) des Tractus tubero-infundibularis bei *Zonotrichia leucophrys gambelii*. Caudaler Abschnitt des Systems. Formalin. Bodian-Ziesmer. Montage aus 520fach vergrößerten Einzelaufnahmen (Teil einer Hirnkarte). Ein starker Zug des Tr. tubero-infundibularis (↑) biegt an der Grenze (*) der caudalen Eminentia mediana (*1*) und des Infundibularstamms (*2*) in die Zona externa (*3*) ein. Tr. supraoptico-paraventriculo-hypophyseus (*4*). Recessus infundibuli (*5*). Nucleus infundibularis (*6*)

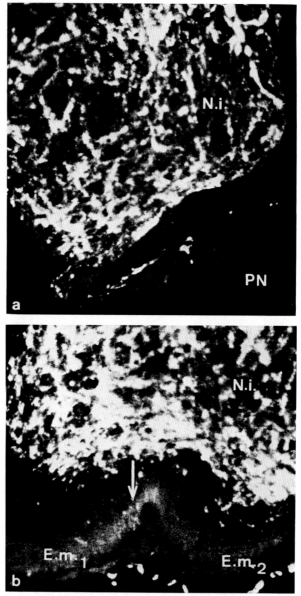

Abb. 2a u. b. *Carduelis chloris.* Paraformaldehyd-Methode zur Monoamindarstellung. a Medianschnitt durch den caudalen Hypothalamus. Nucleus infundibularis (*N.i.*). *PN* Pars nervosa der Hypophyse. Vergr. 140fach. b Paramedianschnitt. *N.i.* Nucleus infundibularis. Beachte den stärkeren Monoamingehalt im Basiskern. Eminentia mediana (*E.m.*) mit ihrer Pars anterior (*E.m.*$_1$) und Pars posterior (*E.m.*$_2$). ↑ Deutlich fluorescierender Saum in der Pars anterior. Vergr. 200fach

große Granula scheinen in dem elektiv färbbaren rostralen Abschnitt der Eminentia mediana häufiger zu sein als in ihrem caudalen Teil. Bei *Carduelis chloris* und *Anas platyrhynchos* ist aber die Monoaminfluorescenz der rostralen Eminentia mediana

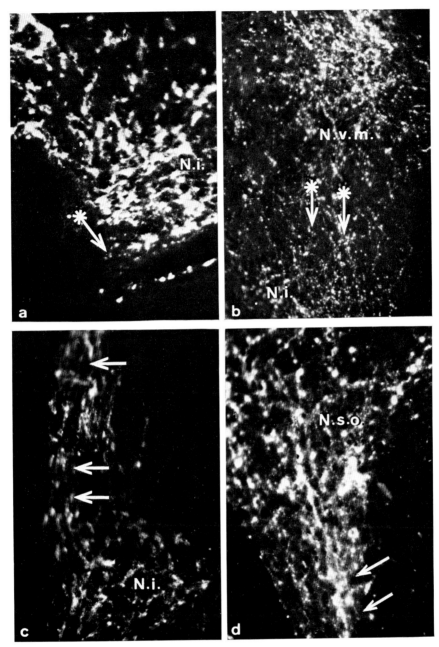

Abb. 3a—d. *Carduelis chloris*. a Mediansehnitt durch den Nucleus infundibularis (etwas weiter seitlich als in Abb. 2a). Starke Monoaminfluorescenz (*) der auf die rostrale Eminentia mediana gerichteten Züge des Tractus tubero-infundibularis (↑). Vergr. 120fach. b Mediansehnitt durch den Hypothalamus. Amindarstellung (*) im Nucleus ventromedialis (*N.v.m.*). ↑ Fluorescierende Faserzüge des Tractus tubero-infundibularis. *N.i.* Nucleus infundibularis. Vergr. 80fach. c Paramedianschnitt. ↑ Fluorescierende Faserzüge im Verlauf der neurosekretorischen Bahn in Höhe der Sehnervenkreuzung. *N.i.* Nucleus infundibularis. Vergr. 120fach. d Fluorescierende Neuropilstrukturen in einer lateralen Zellgruppe des Nucleus supraopticus (*N.s.o.*). Beachte die abgehenden leuchtenden Faserzüge (↑). Vergr. 220fach

stärker als die der caudalen (Oehmke, 1969), ein Befund, der zuerst überrascht, da die Faserzüge des Tractus tubero-infundibularis in caudaler Richtung zunehmend stärker werden. Allerdings hat Kobayashi (1965) in beiden Protrusionen der Vogeleminentia eine kräftige Monoaminoxydase-Reaktion beobachtet.

Woher kommen die fluorescierenden monoaminhaltigen Fasern der rostralen Eminentia mediana? Die Züge, die vom Komplex des Infundibularkerns senkrecht in die rostrale Eminentia mediana eindringen, sind relativ schwach. Von der

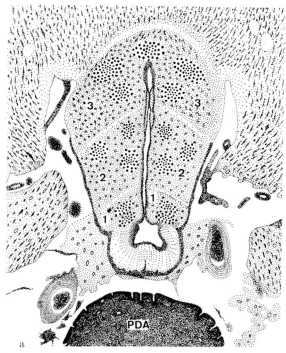

a

Abb. 4a u. b. Schematische Darstellung einzelner Kernabschnitte des Tuber cinereum von *Zonotrichia leucophrys gambelii* im *Frontal-* (a) und *Paramedianschnitt* (b). Nucleus infundibularis mit Basalkern (*1*) und der ersten (*2*) und zweiten (*3*) dorsalen Auflagerung, sowie ihren Unterabteilungen[4]. *PDA* Pars distalis adenohypophyseos; *PN* Pars nervosa; *Ch.o.* Chiasma opticum. (Gezeichnet D. Vaihinger)

intensiv leuchtenden retikulären Schicht dieser Protrusion lassen sich aber Faserformationen in ein stark leuchtendes Bündel zurückverfolgen, das, dicht der Sehnervenkreuzung angeschmiegt, mit dem Haupttrakt der neurosekretorischen Bahn verläuft. Bei Grünfink und Ente (Oehmke, 1969) war diese Faserformation noch deutlicher als beim Sperling (Oehmke u.a., 1969) oder bei der japanischen Wachtel (Sharp und Follett, 1968). Auf Grund ihrer Lage und Verteilung ist es sehr unwahrscheinlich, daß sie aus der Medulla oblongata aufsteigt (vgl. Fuxe

---

[4] Beachte die starke Ausbildung des Infundibularkerns. Der mit der Falck-Hillarp-Methode ebenfalls fluorescierende Ventromedialkern liegt *dorsal* von der mit (**3**) gekennzeichneten zweiten Auflagerung des Infundibularkerns. Die Lage des *Ventromedialkerns* muß vergleichend auf die Höhenposition des Nucl. supraopticus bezogen werden. Bei allen Betrachtungen der unteren (basalen) Tuberetage sind grundsätzliche Unterschiede in der Konfiguration des Vogel- und Säugerhypothalamus zu beachten (s. Oehmke, in Vorbereitung).

und Hökfelt, 1967). Dieses Bündel steht in einem räumlichen Zusammenhang mit der großen lateralen Zellansammlung des Nucl. supraopticus.

Zwei Befunde erscheinen in diesem Zusammenhang von Bedeutung: 1. Um den Recessus opticus, in der Nähe der Lamina terminalis, finden sich zwischen typischen Nervenzellen des Nucleus supraopticus (Granuladurchmesser um 2000 Å) Neurone mit einem wesentlich kleineren Granulatyp (Durchmesser um 1000 Å, Oehmke u.a., 1969). Dieses Gebiet weist eine mäßig starke Monoaminfluorescenz auf (Oehmke). 2. Das mit der rostralen Eminentia mediana zusammenhängende leuchtende Bündel entspricht räumlich dem Verlauf des mit Paraldehydfuchsin und Pseudoisocyanin elektiv färbbaren, in die rostrale Eminentia mediana eindringenden Faserstranges.

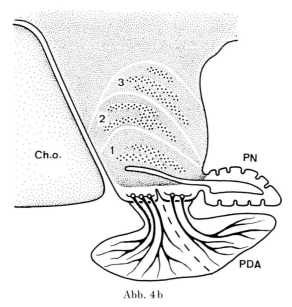

Abb. 4 b

Noch unbeantwortet bleibt die Frage, ob das zuerst beschriebene fluorescierende und das zuletzt geschilderte elektiv färbbare (im Sinne der klassischen Definition „neurosekretorische") System identisch sind. Es müßte dann bewiesen werden, daß auch bestimmte aminerge Faserzüge ein mit den typischen Neurosekretfarbstoffen färbbares Material enthalten. Die andere Möglichkeit ist aber, daß die zum Hinterlappen gerichtete, 2000 Å-Granula führende neurosekretorische Bahn bis zur rostralen Eminentia mediana sowohl von aminergen als auch von elektiv färbbaren peptidergen Faserzügen begleitet wird; beide enthalten Granula vom 1000 Å-Typ, die sich nicht mit der elektronenmikroskopischen Routinemethodik voneinander unterscheiden lassen. Dasselbe Problem könnte auch an der caudalen Eminentia mediana bestehen. Es wurde bereits darauf hingewiesen, daß nicht alle Neurone des Nucl. infundibularis fluorescieren. Sollten hier zwischen den aminergen Nervenzellen kleingranuläre, nicht elektiv färbbare peptiderge Neurone eingestreut sein, dann wäre die Unterscheidung der beiden Fasersysteme in der Palisadenschicht der Eminentia mediana mit der üblichen elektronenmikroskopischen Methodik nicht möglich.

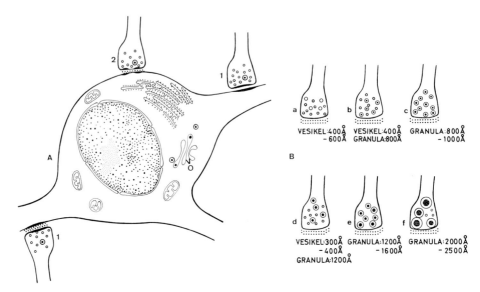

Abb. 5A u. B. *Passer domesticus.* A Schematische Darstellung der Sekretbildung in Nerven-
zellen des Nucleus infundibularis. o Golgi-Zone; *1* axo-dendritische; *2* axo-somatische Syn-
apsen. B Nervenendigungen in der Eminentia mediana (*a—e*) und in der Pars nervosa der
Hypophyse (*f*) mit verschiedenartigen granulären und vesiculären Einschlüssen (nach
Oehmke, Priedkalns, Vaupel-von Harnack und Oksche, 1969). Im Schema sind mit
„Granula" stets granulierte Vesikel gemeint

## Ausblick

Unsere elektronenmikroskopischen Studien (Oksche, 1967; Oehmke u.a.,
1969) haben bei *Passer domesticus* gezeigt, daß die Granula des Tr. tubero-infundibularis (Durchmesser bis zu 1000 Å) im Golgi-Apparat der Nervenzellen des
Nucl. infundibularis gebildet werden (Abb. 5A). Abgesehen von dem Granulakaliber unterscheidet sich dieser Vorgang cytologisch nicht von der Sekretbildung
im Nucl. supraopticus. Verwendet man elektronenmikroskopische Kriterien, so
finden sich am Nucl. infundibularis der Vögel alle für neurosekretorische Zellen
geforderten Merkmale; das Sekretionsprodukt läßt sich zwar nicht elektiv an-
färben, dafür fluoresciert es nach Anwendung des Verfahrens von Falck (1962),
Falck und Owman (1965). Somit beherbergt der Vogelhypothalamus neben dem
klassischen neurosekretorischen System des Nucl. supraopticus und Nucl. paraventricularis zumindest noch einen weiteren, aminergen neurosekretorischen
Apparat des Nucl. infundibularis — Nucl. ventromedialis. Fragt man aber nach
der Herkunft der mit Neurosekretfarbstoffen elektiv färbbaren, in die rostrale
Protuberanz der Eminentia mediana gerichteten Faserzüge und nach der Bedeutung der nicht fluorescierenden Neurone im Verband des Infundibularkerns, so
stellt sich das Problem noch komplexer dar. Nucl. infundibularis besteht aus einem
Mosaik kleiner Zellgruppen, die cytologisch verschieden ausgeprägt sind. Auch die
rostrale, um den Recessus opticus gelegene Region des Vogelhypothalamus dürfte
mehrere neuroendokrin aktive Zelltypen enthalten. Ganz rätselhaft sind auch
noch die mit Neurosekretfarbstoffen färbbaren, in den Verlauf des Tr. opticus und
des Tr. entopeduncularis eingestreuten Nervenzellen.

Auf diesem anatomischen Hintergrund sind die nachfolgenden stereotaktischen Beiträge von WILSON und STETSON zu sehen. Diese Eingriffe haben bereits einige Klarheit über die an der Steuerung der lichtabhängigen Gonadenreaktion beteiligten Komponenten des Vogelhypothalamus gebracht. Ohne den Nucl. infundibularis ist diese Reaktion nicht auslösbar, wogegen das mit Neurosekretfarbstoffen färbbare Material der rostralen Eminentia mediana für die Stimulierung der Hodenvergrößerung keine essentielle Bedeutung zu haben scheint. Damit liegt aber noch keine Erklärung für die im Jahrescyclus und unter funktionellen Bedingungen beobachtete Fluktuation des elektiv färbbaren Materials der Eminentia mediana vor. Es darf nicht übersehen werden, daß nach bestimmten Eingriffen auch in der sonst nicht spezifisch färbbaren Eminentia mediana der Säuger solche Substanzen auftreten können, z.B. bei der Ratte nach Adrenalektomie und Hypophysektomie (BOCK und GOSLAR, 1969).

Die folgende Arbeitshypothese umreißt nach unserer Ansicht den Rahmen für weitere experimentelle und cytologische Studien. Es wird vermutet, daß der Vogelhypothalamus neben dem klassischen neurosekretorischen und dem aminergen tuberalen System noch weitere (peptiderge) neuroendokrine Zentren beherbergt, die verschiedene "releasing factors" produzieren. Die bei *Zonotrichia leucophrys gambelii* (VITUMS u.a., 1964) und bei *Coturnix coturnix japonica* (SHARP und FOLLETT, 1969[5]) beobachtete differenzierte Bündelung der portalen Gefäße legt die Annahme nahe, daß hier in der neuroendokrinen Kette Punkt-zu-Punkt-Verbindungen vorliegen könnten. Da die portalen Riesencapillaren weder mit Epitheloidzellpolstern noch mit Muskelsphincteren ausgestattet sind, muß der Ort der aktiven Kreislaufregulation in erster Linie an den innervierten zuführenden Arteriolen des portalen Gefäßsystems gesucht werden. Man darf aber nicht die Quellungsmöglichkeit von Capillarendothelien (direkte Wirkungen hypothalamischer Wirkstoffe?) und den Einbau dieser Gefäße in einen eigentümlichen, von Gitterfasern umsponnenen Zellverband der Pars tuberalis übersehen.

Für die Zukunft möchten wir am Zwischenhirn-Hypophysensystem der Vögel das folgende Vorgehen empfehlen: 1. Noch enger umschriebene stereotaktische Läsionen, die der mosaikartigen cytoarchitektonischen Karte des Hypothalamus Rechnung tragen; 2. Fluorescenzmikroskopischen Aminnachweis nach Mikroläsionen an einzelnen Tuberkernen und ihren Bahnkomponenten. (Ähnlich wie im klassischen neurosekretorischen System müßte sich dann proximal von der Läsionsstelle das fluorescierende Material stauen.) 3. Fahndung nach "releasing factors" produzierenden Zellen mit den Methoden der licht- und elektronenmikroskopischen Autoradiographie und Immunhistochemie. Diese Verfahren dürften die Differentialdiagnostik der verschiedenartigen Nervenendigungen in der Eminentia mediana ermöglichen; Granulakaliber sind kein ausreichendes Kriterium; 4. Stereotaktische und elektrophysiologische Studien zur Aufklärung der im elektronenmikroskopischen Bild so zahlreichen Synapsen an den Neuronen und im Neuropil des Nucl. supraopticus und Nucl. infundibularis der Vögel; 5. Klärung der gegenseitigen nervösen und humoralen Beeinflussungsmöglichkeiten der verschiedenartigen Nerven- und Ependymendigungen in der Eminentia mediana (vgl. KOBAYASHI u. FARNER, 1969). Dieses Problem ist eng mit der Frage verknüpft, ob die

---

[5] J. Anat. **104**, 227–232 (1969).

biogenen Amine der Tuberkerne *unmittelbar* Eigenschaften von "releasing factors" besitzen.

Wir sind der Meinung, daß die anatomische Untergliederung der neuroendokrinen Zentren der Vögel eine besonders günstige Basis für solche Studien darstellt.

## Literatur

Assenmacher, I., Calas, A.: Fine structure of the median eminence of the duck. In: Seminar on hypothalamic and endocrine functions in birds (Tokyo, May 19–24, 1969). Abstracts, p. 22, 1969.

Benoit, J., Assenmacher: Rapport entre la stimulation sexuelle préhypophysaire et la neurosécrétion chez l'Oiseau. Arch. Anat. micr. Morph. exp. **42**, 334–386 (1953).

— — The control by visible radiations of the gonadotropic activity of the duck hypophysis. Recent Progr. Hormone Res. **15**, 143–164 (1959).

Bock, R., Goslar, H.-G.: Enzymhistochemische Untersuchungen an Infundibulum und Hypophysenhinterlappen der normalen und beidseitig adrenalektomierten Ratte. Z. Zellforsch. **95**, 415–428 (1969).

Falck, B.: Observations on the possibilities of the cellular localization of monoamines by a fluorescence method. Acta physiol. scand., Suppl. **197**, 1–26 (1962).

— Owman, Ch.: A detailed methodological description of the fluorescence method for the cellular demonstration of biogenic monoamines. Acta Univ. Lund. **2**, No. 7, 5–23 (1965).

Farner, D. S., Oksche, A., Lorenzen, L.: Hypothalamic neurosecretion and the photoperiodic testicular response in the White-crowned Sparrow, *Zonotrichia leucophrys gambelii*. Neurosecretion. Memoirs of the Society for Endocrinology No 12 (ed. H. Heller and R. B. Clark), p. 187–197. London and New York: Academic Press 1962.

— Follett, B. K.: Light and other environmental factors affecting avian reproduction. J. animal Sci. **25**, 90–118 (1966).

— Wilson, F. E., Oksche, A.: Neuroendocrine mechanisms in birds. In: Neuroendocrinology (L. Martini and W. F. Ganong, eds.), vol. 2, p. 529–582. New York and London: Academic Press 1967.

Fuxe, K., Hökfelt, T.: The influence of central catecholamine neurons on the hormone secretion from the anterior and posterior pituitary. IV. Internat. Symp. Neurosecretion in Strasbourg 1966, p. 165–177. Berlin-Heidelberg-New York: Springer 1967.

Grünthal, E.: Vergleichend anatomische und entwicklungsgeschichtliche Untersuchungen über die Zentren des Hypothalamus der Säuger und des Menschen. Arch. Psychiat. Nervenkr. **90**, 216–267 (1930).

Kobayashi, H.: Histochemical, electron microscopic and pharmacologic studies on the median eminence. In: Proc. II. World Congr. Endocr. (S. Taylor, ed.), p. 570–576. Amsterdam: Excerpta Medica Foundation 1965.

— Farner, D. S.: Seminar on hypothalamic and endocrine functions in birds. (Abstracts.) Tokyo 1969.

Matsui, T.: Fine structural difference between the anterior and posterior divisions in the pigeon median eminence. In: Seminar on hypothalamic and endocrine functions in birds (Tokyo, May 19–24, 1969). Abstracts, p. 19–20 (1969).

Mikami, S.-I., Oksche, A., Farner, D. S., Vitums, A.: Fine structure of the vessels of the hypophysial portal system of the White-crowned Sparrow, *Zonotrichia leucophrys gambelii*. Z. Zellforsch. **106**, 155–174 (1970).

Oehmke, H.-J.: Unveröffentlichte Befunde.

— Regionale Strukturunterschiede im Nucleus infundibularis der Vögel (Passeriformes). Z. Zellforsch. **92**, 406–421 (1968).

— Topographische Verteilung der Monoaminfluoreszenz im Zwischenhirn-Hypophysensystem von *Carduelis chloris* und *Anas platyrhynchos*. Z. Zellforsch. **101**, 266–284 (1969).

— Priedkalns, J., Vaupel-von Harnack, M., Oksche, A.: Fluoreszenz- und elektronenmikroskopische Untersuchungen am Zwischenhirn-Hypophysensystem von *Passer domesticus*. Z. Zellforsch. **95**, 109–133 (1969).

— Weitere Untersuchungen an den portalen Hypophysengefäßen von *Zonotrichia leucophrys gambelii*. Z. Zellforsch. **106**, 175–188 (1970).

OKSCHE, A.: Optico-vegetative regulatory mechanisms of the diencephalon. Anat. Anz. **108**, 320–329 (1960).
— The fine nervous, neurosecretory, and glial structure of the median eminence in the White-crowned Sparrow. Neurosecretion. Memoirs of the Society for Endocrinology, No 12 (ed. H. HELLER and R. B. CLARK), p. 199–208. London and New York: Academic Press 1962.
— Über die anatomische Verknüpfung des Vogelhypothalamus mit der Hypophyse. Verh. d. Anat. Ges. 57 (Hamburg, 1961), 236–244 (1963).
— The fine structure of the neurosecretory system of birds in relation to its functional aspects. In: Proc. II. World Congr. Endocr. (S. TAYLOR, ed.), p. 167–171. Amsterdam: Excerpta Medica Foundation 1965.
— Eine licht- und elektronenmikroskopische Analyse des neuroendokrinen Zwischenhirn-Vorderlappen-Komplexes der Vögel. In: Neurosecretion (F. STUTINSKY, ed.), p. 75–88. Berlin-Heidelberg-New York: Springer 1967.
— MÖLLER, G., LANGBEIN, M.: Nervenbahnen und neurohämale Kontaktflächen des Zwischenhirn-Hypophysensystems von *Zonotrichia leucophrys gambelii* (Aves, Passeriformes). Anat. Anz. Erg.-Bd. **126** (1970), Verh. Anat. Ges. (64. Verslg. Homburg/Saar, 1969), S. 593–595.
PRIEDKALNS, J., OKSCHE, A.: Ultrastructure of synaptic terminals in Nucleus infundibularis and Nucleus supraopticus of *Passer domesticus*. Z. Zellforsch. **98**, 135–147 (1969).
SHARP, P. J., FOLLETT, B. K.: The distribution of monoamines in the hypothalamus of the japanese quail, *Coturnix coturnix japonica*. Z. Zellforsch. **90**, 245–262 (1968).
— — The localization of monoamines, monoamine oxidase and acetyl-cholinesterase in the quail hypothalamo-hypophysial system. In: Seminar on hypothalamic and endocrine functions in birds (Tokyo, May 19–24, 1969). Abstracts, p. 18, 1969a.
— — Hypothalamic centres controlling gonadotrophin release in quail. In: Seminar on hypothalamic and endocrine functions in birds (Tokyo, May 19–24, 1969). Abstracts, p. 41–42, 1969b.
— — The effect of reserpine on the pituitary-gonadal axis in quail. In: Seminar on hypothalamic and endocrine functions in birds (Tokyo, May 19–24, 1969). Abstracts, p. 43, 1969c.
STETSON, M. H.: The role of the median eminence in control of photoperiodically induced testicular growth in the White-crowned Sparrow, *Zonotrichia leucophrys gambelii*. Z. Zellforsch. **93**, 369–394 (1969).
VITUMS, A., MIKAMI, S., OKSCHE, A., FARNER, D. S.: Vascularization of the hypothalamo-hypophysial-complex in the White-crowned Sparrow, *Zonotrichia leucophrys gambelii*. Z. Zellforsch. **64**, 541–569 (1964).
WARREN, S. P.: Primary-catecholamine fibers in the ventral hypothalamus of the White-crowned Sparrow. Master's Thesis. University of Washington, Seattle 1968.
WILSON, F. E.: The tubero-infundibular neuron system: A component of the photoperiodic control mechanism of the White-crowned Sparrow, *Zonotrichia leucophrys gambelii*. Z. Zellforsch. **82**, 1–24 (1967).
— HANDS, F. E.: Hypothalamic neurosecretion and photoinduced testicular growth in the Tree Sparrow, *Spizella arborea*. Z. Zellforsch. **89**, 303–319 (1968).
WINGSTRAND, K. G.: The structure and development of the avian pituitary. Lund: C. W. K. Gleerup 1951.

# The Tubero-Infundibular Region of the Hypothalamus: A Focus of Testosterone Sensitivity in Male Tree Sparrows (*Spizella arborea*)*

Fred E. Wilson

Division of Biology, Kansas State University, Manhattan, Kansas (U.S.A.)

**Key words:** Tubero-infundibular region — Male birds — Testosterone sensitivity.

The tubero-infundibular region of the mammalian hypothalamus, implicated in the control of pituitary gonadotropin secretion by ablative and implantation techniques (Halász *et al.*, 1962, 1965; Szentágothai *et al.*, 1962; Davidson, 1966; Donovan, 1966; Everett, 1969) and shown by bioassay to have FSH-releasing activity (Watanabe and McCann, 1968), appears capable of reducing gonadotropic function in response to increased local concentrations of sex steroid hormones (Lisk, 1960, 1962; Davidson and Sawyer, 1961; Davidson and Smith, 1967). Although several studies suggest the existence of negative feedback relations between gonadal steroids and pituitary gonadotropin(s) in birds (Kobayashi, 1954; Hohlweg and Daume, 1959; Benoit, 1961; Lofts, 1962, 1968; Tixier-Vidal *et al.*, 1962, 1968; Uemura and Kobayashi, 1963; Gogan and Kordon, 1964; Uemura, 1964; Kobayashi and Farner, 1966; Matsuo *et al.*, 1969; Mikami *et al.*, 1969), evidence for the central nervous system as intermediary is, for the most part, fragmentary and inconclusive. Recently, however, testosterone sensitivity of neural substrates, as revealed by reduced pituitary gonadotropic function, has been demonstrated in the domestic mallard (Kordon and Gogan, 1964; Gogan, 1968). The more posterior of two hypothalamic areas sensitive to testosterone in that species roughly corresponds to the basal tuberal region known to play an important role in the photoperiodic testicular response of the White-crowned Sparrow (Wilson, 1967; Stetson, 1969) and in the control of tonic release of pituitary gonadotropin(s) in male domestic fowl (Lepkovsky and Yasuda, 1966; Graber *et al.*, 1967; Koike and Lepkovsky, 1967; Snapir *et al.*, 1969). Although scattered and incomplete, these recent observations suggest conformance with the pattern of neuroendocrine control that has emerged from more extensive studies on male mammals, and with the observations of Lisk (1967) on the desert iguana, raise the possibility of utilization by widely divergent species of

* Contribution No. 1060, Division of Biology, Kansas Agricultural Experiment Station, Manhattan 66502. I am grateful to Richard S. Donham and J. Kenneth Boon for technical assistance. French's Pet Bird Laboratory, Rochester, N.Y., kindly provided the parakeet foods, and Berlin Laboratories, Inc., New York, N.Y., the cyproterone. Gerald W. Peterson prepared the drawing, and Don Pihlaja assisted with the photomicrography.

similar kinds of afferent hormonal information in the control of pituitary gonadotropic function.

The present investigation was designed to confirm the potential for negative
feedback control of pituitary gonadotropin secretion in the Tree Sparrow (*Spizella
arborea*) and had as its principal objective identification of substrate(s) through
which gonadal feedback might operate. Accordingly, minute amounts of solid
androgen were implanted stereotaxically into the hypothalamus-pituitary region
in photosensitive males; testicular weight after three weeks of photostimulation
was the endpoint. This report presents evidence consistent with the concept of
tubero-infundibular control of photoperiodic testicular responses (WILSON, 1967;
STETSON, 1969) and provides a base from which investigations on the mechanism
of seasonal testicular regression may proceed.

## Materials and Methods

Tree Sparrows (*Spizella arborea*) for this study were captured with mist nets from wintering
flocks near Manhattan, Kansas, between 11 November 1967 and 31 January 1968. Captive
birds were held on 8-hr daily photoperiods (0830–1630 CST) until midsummer when the
experiment began. Sex was determined by laparotomy under Nembutal anesthesia (DONOVAN,
1958); only photosensitive males were used.

Stainless steel tubes (27- or 30-gage), either empty or containing a minute amount of solid
testosterone propionate or cholesterol (for method of preparation, see KANEMATSU and SAW-
YER, 1963), were implanted stereotaxically (WILSON, 1965, 1967) into the hypothalamus-
pituitary region in 88 birds and fixed in place with dental cement between 17 June and 12 July
1968. Five intact birds sacrificed at the beginning of that period, five sacrificed at the end,
and nine that died during surgery or were killed on the first postoperative day because prog-
nosis for recovery was dubious constituted groups of initial controls. Five additional intact
birds served as photostimulated terminal controls.

Birds were transferred from 8- to 20-hr daily photoperiods (0830–0430 CST) on the day
after implantation. During the 3-week period of photostimulation, they were retained, usually
two to four per cage, in small cages (23×25×41 cm) housed in an air-conditioned room.
Lighting was provided by fluorescent lamps at an intensity of at least 300 lux; daylight and
extraneous light were excluded. Water and food (a vitamin- and mineral-enriched chick-
starter crumble supplemented with parakeet foods) were freely available. Birds were handled
three times weekly when body weights were taken.

Birds were killed by decapitation. Brains were fixed for three to four days in BOUIN's fluid,
dissected, and embedded in Paraplast through dioxane. Parallel sagittal sections (10 μ) were
stained with paraldehyde-fuchsin for localization of implantation sites.

Testes were removed at sacrifice and fixed for five days in an aqueous mixture of acetic
acid, formalin, and ethanol. After five additional days in 70% ethanol, they were debrided
and weighed on a torsion balance.

## Results

As noted before, implantations were performed between 17 June and 12 July in
birds held on 8-hr daily photoperiods since capture. Testicular weights of birds
sacrificed on 17 June (Group ICBB) were not significantly different from those
of birds sacrificed on 12 July (Group ICBE) or from those of birds that died
during surgery or were killed on the first postoperative day (Goup ICBK) (Table 1).
Therefore, for subsequent purposes of comparison, groups of initial controls were
combined. Testicular weights of birds in the group so formed (Group ICB) were
essentially identical to those of birds sacrificed at capture several months earlier

(Group BFS) (Table 1). Thus, at the time of implantation, testicular weight was at the midwinter level.

Table 1. *Testicular weights of initial control birds and of birds sacrificed at capture*

| Group[a] | Date of sacrifice | Photoperiod at sacrifice | Weight of two testes (mg)[b] | Range (mg) |
|---|---|---|---|---|
| ICBB | 17 June 1968 | 8 L–16 D | 1.29 ± 0.34 (5) | 0.51–2.49 |
| ICBE | 12 July 1968 | 8 L–16 D | 1.41 ± 0.23 (5) | 0.84–1.91 |
| ICBK | 20 June to 4 July 1968 | 8 L–16 D | 1.44 ± 0.28 (9) | 0.61–3.04 |
| ICB | 17 June to 12 July 1968 | 8 L–16 D | 1.39 ± 0.16 (19) | 0.51–3.04 |
| BFS | 11 Nov. 1967 to 31 Jan. 1968 | NDL[c] | 1.42 ± 0.23 (14) | 0.30–3.39 |

  [a] See text for explanation of group designation.
  [b] Mean ± SE. Number of birds in each sample is indicated in parentheses.
  [c] Natural day length.

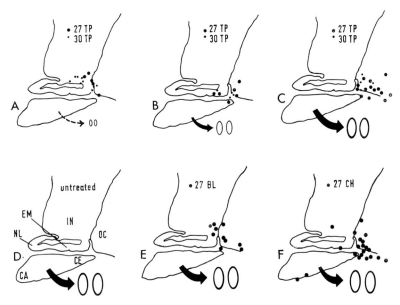

Fig. 1 A–F. Summary of results: schematic parasagittal sections through the hypothalamus-pituitary region showing locations (dots) of steroid and blank implants and their effects on the photoperiodic testicular response of the Tree Sparrow. Size of arrows and ellipses reflects relative intensity of gonadotropin release. *27 T P* testosterone propionate in 27-gage tubing; *30 T P* testosterone propionate in 30-gage tubing; *27 BL* 27-gage tubing (empty); *27 CH* cholesterol in 27-gage tubing. A Testosterone implants: severe gonadosuppression (14 birds; combined testicular weights, 0.52–9.93 mg). B Testosterone implants: moderate gonadosuppression (10 birds; combined testicular weights, 20.27–45.5 mg). C Testosterone implants: no gonadosuppression (23 birds; combined testicular weights, 51.0–285.5 mg). Some dots represent more than one implant. D Photostimulated untreated controls: normal testicular response (5 birds; combined testicular weights, 86.5–354.9 mg). *IN* infundibular nucleus; *EM* median eminence; *NL* neural lobe; *OC* optic chiasm; *CE* cephalic lobe of anterior pituitary; *CA* caudal lobe of anterior pituitary. E Blank implants: no gonadosuppression (10 birds; combined testicular weights, 96.3–220.7 mg). F Cholesterol implants: no gonadosuppression (21 birds; combined testicular weights, 49.8–341.5 mg)

Testicular weight was maintained at or near the midwinter level in photo-stimulated birds with testosterone implants in the anterobasal region of the infundibular nucleus (Fig. 1 A; Table 2). Testosterone implants along the rostral border of the median eminence or in that region of the optic chiasm or tract adjacent thereto were equally effective in some birds (Fig. 1 A), but in other birds with testosterone implants in roughly comparable regions the photoperiodic testicular response was less severely suppressed (Fig. 1 B) or unaltered (Fig. 1 C). Implants in

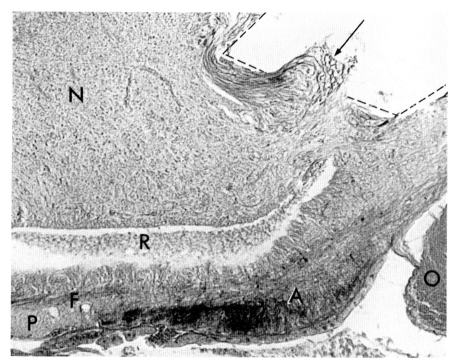

Fig. 2. Implantation site in the infundibular nucleus (*N*) of a 30-gage tube that contained solid testosterone propionate. Tissue-steroid contact occurred in the anterobasal portion (at arrow). Outline of tube track is superimposed. 0485. Weight of two testes after 21 days on 20-hr daily photoperiods: 0.52 mg. *R* infundibular recess of the third ventricle; *A* anterior division of the median eminence; *P* posterior division of the median eminence; *F* fiber layer; *O* optic chiasm.
Bouin. Parasagittal section (0.05 mm left of midline). Paraldehyde-fuchsin. ×183

more rostral regions of the optic chiasm or in the space below were always ineffective (Fig. 1 C). Testicular growth was retarded, but not prevented, in birds with testosterone implants *in* the median eminence (Fig. 1 B). That was also true for some birds with testosterone implants in or near the cephalic lobe of the anterior pituitary (Fig. 1 B). Without exception, testicular growth was induced photoperiodically in untreated birds (Fig. 1 D) and in birds with blank (Fig. 1 E; Table 3) or cholesterol (Fig. 1 F; Table 4) implants, irrespective of site (Table 5).

Centers of testosterone implants in the infundibular nucleus extended from 0.04 to 0.13 mm left of the midline (Table 2), from the base of the nucleus to about 0.5 mm above the floor of the median eminence, and from the caudal margin of the

F. E. WILSON:

Table 2. *Locations of testosterone implants in photostimulated Tree Sparrows*[a]

| Bird No. | Gage | Direction and distance of implant center from midline (mm) | Location of implant center | | | | | Region[b] | Weight of two testes (mg) |
|---|---|---|---|---|---|---|---|---|---|
| | | | IN | EM | OCT | APC | APCa | | |
| 0485 | 30[c] | L 0.04 | * | | | | | A | 0.52 |
| 1045 | 30 | L 0.11 | * | | | | | | 1.49 |
| 0414 | 27[d] | L 0.06 | * | | | | | | 1.57 |
| 1041 | 30 | L 0.04 | * | | | | | | 1.61 |
| 1049 | 30 | L 0.10 | * | | | | | | 2.59 |
| 0491 | 30 | L 0.07 | * | | | | | | 3.11 |
| 0451 | 30 | L 0.13 | * | | | | | | 4.12 |
| 0478 | 27 | L 0.06 | * | | | | | | 7.23 |
| 1004 | 27 | L 0.10 | † | † | † | | | B | 2.40 |
| 0472 | 27 | L 0.02 | | † | † | | | | 1.20 |
| 0584 | 30 | L 0.16 | | † | † | | | | 1.37 |
| 1025 | 30 | R 0.01 | | † | † | | | | 3.84 |
| 0456 | 27 | L 0.01 | | † | † | | | | 190.3 |
| 1047 | 30 | L 0.18 | | | * | | | C | 4.12 |
| 0582 | 30 | L 0.01 | | | * | | | | 20.27 |
| 0404 | 27 | L 0.19 | | | * | | | | 31.4 |
| 1010 | 30 | L 0.08 | | | * | | | | 33.0 |
| 0421 | 27 | L 0.17 | | | * | | | | 39.9 |
| 0581 | 27 | L 0.14 | | | * | | | | 41.2 |
| 0482 | 30 | L 0.22 | | | * | | | | 61.1 |
| 0407 | 27 | L 0.39 | | | * | | | | 76.0 |
| 1051 | 30 | L 0.28 | | | * | | | | 106.8 |
| 0484 | 27 | L 0.11 | | | * | | | | 159.8 |
| 0550 | 27 | L 0.09 | | | * | | | | 250.4 |
| 1008 | 27 | L 0.10 | | | * | | | D | 56.4 |
| 0437 | 27 | L 0.24 | | | * | | | | 80.9 |
| 0431 | 27 | L 0.02 | | | * | | | | 85.6 |
| 0445 | 27 | R 0.01 | | | * | | | | 91.9 |
| 0448 | 27 | L 0.19 | | | * | | | | 110.5 |
| 0464 | 27 | L 0.05 | | | * | | | | 133.5 |
| 1034 | 30 | L 0.19 | | | * | | | | 135.3 |
| 0412 | 27 | L 0.21 | | | * | | | | 167.6 |
| 0409 | 27 | L 0.32 | | | * | | | | 182.2 |
| 0559 | 27 | L 0.09 | | | §§ | | | | 197.5 |
| 0438 | 30 | 0 | | * | | | | E | 20.50 |
| 0512 | 27 | L 0.12 | | * | | | | | 28.8 |
| 0508 | 27 | L 0.20 | | * | | | | | 37.9 |
| 1009 | 27 | L 0.09 | | | † | † | | F | 9.93 |
| 0480 | 30 | L 0.12 | | | † | † | | | 25.4 |
| 0430 | 27 | L 0.26 | | | † | † | | | 70.7 |
| 0517 | 27 | L 0.02 | | | † | † | | | 188.2 |
| 1007 | 30 | 0 | | | † | † | | | 285.5 |

Table 2 (continued)

| Bird No. | Gage | Direction and distance of implant center from midline (mm) | Location of implant center | | | | | Region[b] | Weight of two testes (mg) |
|---|---|---|---|---|---|---|---|---|---|
| | | | IN | EM | OCT | APC | APCa | | |
| 0520 | 27 | R 0.02 | | | | * | | G | 45.5 |
| 0562 | 27 | L 0.25 | | | | § | | | 51.0 |
| 0551 | 27 | L 0.01 | | | | § | | | 57.8 |
| 0515 | 27 | L 0.10 | | | | § | | | 83.4 |
| 0552 | 27 | L 0.32 | | | | §§ | | | 58.6 |

IN = infundibular nucleus; EM = median eminence; OCT = optic chiasm-optic tract; APC = anterior pituitary, cephalic lobe; APCa = anterior pituitary, caudal lobe.

* = Implant within structure specified. †...† = Implant at common borders of structures specified. § = Implant at border of structure specified. §§ = Implant near, but displaced from, structure specified.

[a] One bird in which carrier tube became dislodged and was lost is not included in this analysis.

[b] For comparisons among Tables 2, 3, and 4. C = posteroventral; D = anteroventral.

[c] Inside diameter, 0.15 mm.

[d] Inside diameter, 0.20 mm.

Table 3. *Locations of blank implants in photostimulated Tree Sparrows*

| Bird No. | Gage | Direction and distance of implant center from midline (mm) | Location of implant center | | | | | Region | Weight of two testes (mg) |
|---|---|---|---|---|---|---|---|---|---|
| | | | IN | EM | OCT | APC | APCa | | |
| 1033 | 27 | L 0.11 | * | | | | | A | 192.2 |
| 0460 | 27 | L 0.17 | * | | | | | | 203.0 |
| 1029 | 27 | L 0.23 | * | | | | | | 220.7 |
| 0487 | 27 | R 0.06 | † | † | | | | | 166.1 |
| 1059 | 27 | L 0.22 | † | | † | | | B | 145.1 |
| 0458 | 27 | L 0.38 | | | * | | | C | 96.3 |
| 1036 | 27 | L 0.05 | | | * | | | | 117.5 |
| 1062 | 27 | L 0.26 | | | * | | | D | 108.5 |
| 1022 | 27 | R 0.06 | | | * | | | | 136.1 |
| 1048 | 27 | L 0.27 | | | † | † | | F | 125.3 |

Designations and symbols as in Table 2.

optic chiasm to about 0.5 mm posterior thereto (Fig. 1 A). The two least effective implants were along the dorsolateral boundary of that region. Although implants usually terminated in the main mass of the nucleus, as illustrated in Fig. 2, one implant terminated on the ependyma overlying the infundibular recess. In some birds implants extended medially into the third ventricle. Blank (Fig. 1 E; Table 3) or cholesterol (Fig. 1 F; Table 4) implants in or near the testosterone-sensitive region did not affect the photoperiodic testicular response.

Table 4. *Locations of cholesterol implants in photostimulated Tree Sparrows*

| Bird No. | Gage | Direction and distance of implant center from midline (mm) | IN | EM | OCT | APC | APCa | Region | Weight of two testes (mg) |
|---|---|---|---|---|---|---|---|---|---|
| 1023 | 27 | 0 | * | | | | | A | 69.7 |
| 0471 | 27 | L 0.23 | † | | † | | | B | 180.4 |
| 0597 | 27 | R 0.04 | † | | † | | | | 204.7 |
| 0476 | 27 | L 0.13 | | | * | | | C | 68.0 |
| 0579 | 27 | L 0.14 | | | * | | | | 68.9 |
| 0429 | 27 | L 0.12 | | | * | | | | 157.2 |
| 0587 | 27 | L 0.04 | | | * | | | | 211.0 |
| 0593 | 27 | R 0.01 | | | * | | | | 318.4 |
| 1044 | 27 | R 0.01 | | | § | | | | 167.6 |
| 0461 | 27 | L 0.33 | | | * | | | D | 101.2 |
| 0402 | 27 | L 0.29 | | | §§ | | | | 49.9 |
| 0583 | 27 | R 0.25 | | | §§ | | | | 143.9 |
| 0549 | 27 | 0 | | | §§ | §§ | | | 99.9 |
| 0449 | 27 | L 0.04 | | † | | † | | E | 52.8 |
| 0465 | 27 | R 0.10 | | | † | † | | F | 341.5 |
| 0546 | 27 | R 0.03 | | | | * | | G | 121.2 |
| 0543 | 27 | L 0.22 | | | | § | | | 177.2 |
| 0547 | 27 | L 0.31 | | | | §§ | | | 117.4 |
| 0545 | 27 | L 0.21 | | | | §§ | | | 139.0 |
| 0574 | 27 | L 0.20 | | | | | * | H | 49.8 |
| 0524 | 27 | L 0.17 | | | | | § | | 63.9 |

Designations and symbols as in Table 2.

Table 5. *Testicular weights of terminal control birds*

| Group[a] | Days on 20-hr daily photoperiods | Weight of two testes[b] (mg) | Range (mg) |
|---|---|---|---|
| PSL | 21 | $191.4 \pm 44.52$ (5) | 86.5–354.9 |
| 27-BL | 21 | $151.1 \pm 13.47$ (10) | 96.3–220.7 |
| 27-CH | 21 | $138.3 \pm 17.89$ (21) | 49.8–341.5 |

[a] PSL, untreated birds; 27-BL, birds with blank implants; 27-CH, birds with cholesterol implants.

[b] Mean $\pm$ SE. Number of birds in each sample is indicated in parentheses.

Four of five testosterone implants along the median eminence-optic chiasm border caused severe gonadosuppression (Fig. 1A, C; Table 2), but the fifth, surrounded by a clot that probably retarded, if not prevented, spread of hormone from the implantation site, did not block the photoperiodic testicular response.

Testosterone implants *in* the median eminence also inhibited testicular growth, but much less effectively than those along its anterodorsal border or those in the infundibular nucleus (Fig. 1B; Table 2). The most dorsomedial of three implants was the most effective while the most posterolateral was the least effective.

Although the median eminence was always locally hypotrophic, those parts not in contact with the carrier tube were practically normal in appearance.

There was no consistent effect of testosterone implants in the immediate vicinity of the anterior pituitary. Testicular growth was slightly retarded in one bird with testosterone in the cephalic lobe (Fig. 1 B), but in three others with testosterone at its rostral tip testicular growth was apparently unaffected (Fig. 1 C; Table 2). Similarly, testosterone implants closely apposed to the anterodorsal border of the cephalic lobe, but separated from that border by compressed optic fibers, had varied effects; the photoperiodic testicular response was severely to moderately impaired in some birds (Fig. 1 A, B), but definitely unaffected in others (Fig. 1 C; Table 2).

## Discussion

This study shows that a minute amount of solid testosterone propionate implanted unilaterally into the tubero-infundibular region of the hypothalamus can prevent or retard testicular growth in the Tree Sparrow. The possibility that testosterone implants in the tubero-infundibular region were effective because of tissue elimination or damage or because of a nonspecific effect of steroid is unlikely since blank or cholesterol implants in or near that region did not inhibit photoperiodic testicular growth. That testosterone implants in the tubero-infundibular region were effective *only* because they yielded a uniform distribution of hormone to the pars distalis also seems unlikely. Implants in the infundibular nucleus were considerably more effective than those in the median eminence even though the latter were nearer the anterior pituitary, including its afferent vascular supply. Thus, prevention of photoperiodic testicular growth by testosterone implants in the tubero-infundibular region is probably best explained as a specific effect of testosterone on testosterone-sensitive structures within or near that region.

The posterior limit of testosterone sensitivity in the basal infundibular nucleus (*der Grundkern* of OEHMKE, 1968) cannot be defined since the caudalmost implant, terminating above the rostral margin of the posterior median eminence, abolished the photoperiodic testicular response. The finding that implants along the antero-dorsal border of the median eminence inhibited testicular growth more effectively than those *in* the median eminence may indicate that testosterone-sensitive structures are localized along that border or, alternatively, that a better distribution of hormone to sensitive structures throughout the median eminence is achieved when implants appose the median eminence than when implants are buried in it. The observation that the most dorsomedial of three implants in the median eminence was the most effective is consistent with the latter suggestion. Spread of hormone into the median eminence probably also occurred from implants in the basal infundibular nucleus. The data of PALKA et al. (1966), applied to this study, suggest that 10% or more of the quantity of hormone at implantation sites in the infundibular nucleus may have been present in the median eminence. Because implants were even closer to the third ventricle or its infundibular recess, spread of hormone into cerebrospinal fluid cannot be excluded.

GOGAN (1968) demonstrated in the domestic mallard that, although testosterone implants in the median eminence were ineffective, testosterone implants in the dorsomedian-ventromedian nuclear complex (see also KORDON and GOGAN,

1964) or in the mediobasal region of the middle hypothalamus prevented photo-periodic testicular growth. Despite differences in terminology, regions of testosterone sensitivity in the Tree Sparrow and the domestic mallard appear to be roughly comparable, the sensitive region in the infundibular nucleus of the former probably corresponding to the ventral portion of the sensitive region in the middle hypothalamus of the latter. Whether more dorsal portions of the parvicellular tuberal complex in the Tree Sparrow are sensitive to testosterone remains to be established. Testosterone implants *in* the median eminence of the Tree Sparrow, while never ineffective, were always less effective than those in the basal infundibular nucleus. Although not in complete agreement, observations on both species are consistent in that they identify as a focus of testosterone sensitivity a parvicellular nuclear region dorsal to the median eminence.

Studies of Wilson (1967) and of Stetson (1969), based on ablative techniques, emphasize the importance of the infundibular nucleus-median eminence region in the mechanism of photoperiodic testicular growth in the White-crowned Sparrow. Selective destruction of the anterobasal region of the infundibular nucleus has not yet been achieved, but destruction of the entire nucleus or its median basal portion (Wilson, 1967) prevents testicular growth as does destruction of the entire median eminence (Wilson, 1967; Stetson, 1969) or its posterior division (Stetson, 1969). Lesions in the basal tuberal region in male domestic fowl also impair gonadotropic function (Lepkovsky and Yasuda, 1966; Graber *et al.*, 1967; Snapir *et al.*, 1969). Regions shown by ablation to control gonadotropin release and by implantation to be sensitive to testosterone seem to correspond inasmuch as the anterobasal region of the infundibular nucleus is within or near zones of damage that block pituitary gonadotropin secretion. Results of this study are not necessarily inconsistent with Stetson's suggestion that control of testicular growth in the White-crowned Sparrow is mediated through the posterior division of the median eminence. As noted before, the tubero-infundibular region sensitive to testosterone in the Tree Sparrow must be regarded as open-ended posteriorly. Moreover, it is possible that the posterior division was impregnated by testosterone from implants in the basal infundibular nucleus or along the anterodorsal border of the median eminence.

It is unlikely that the gonadosuppressive effect of testosterone is mediated by the eminential component of the hypothalamic neurosecretory system since almost complete interruption of the paraldehyde-fuchsin-stainable innervation of the anterior median eminence neither prevents photoperiodic testicular growth in Tree (Wilson and Hands, 1968) or White-crowned (Wilson, 1967; Stetson, 1969) Sparrows nor causes testicular regression in domestic fowl (Graber *et al.*, 1967). A more plausible suggestion—consistent with results of lesion studies (Graber *et al.*, 1967; Wilson, 1967; Stetson, 1969)—is that ganglionic cells of the basal infundibular nucleus and/or tubero-infundibular fibers that terminate in the median eminence mediate the effect of the hormone. Although testosterone sensitivity of ependymal and extraependymal glial cells cannot be excluded, little functional significance can be attached to that possibility at this time.

The present study does not permit a firm conclusion regarding sensitivity of the pars distalis to testosterone. As noted above, effects of testosterone implants in the immediate vicinity of the cephalic lobe ranged from none to rather severe suppression of the photoperiodic testicular response; in one bird in which an implant of testosterone ended in the pars distalis, testicular growth was slightly retarded. LISK (1967) noted retardation of seasonal testicular development in two desert iguanas with intrapituitary implants of testosterone propionate, but similar implants in mammals appear to have little or no inhibitory effect on the testes (DAVIDSON and SAWYER, 1961; LISK, 1962). Because a direct effect cannot be excluded, the anterior pituitary of the Tree Sparrow must tentatively be considered a focus of testosterone sensitivity. The limited effectiveness of some testosterone implants in the posteroventral portion of the optic chiasm or tract is probably due to diffusion of hormone to sensitive structures in the tubero-infundibular region or in the pars distalis. The occurrence of testosterone-sensitive structures in the optic chiasm or tract seems unlikely.

The data presented here, confirming the potential for negative feedback control of pituitary gonadotropin secretion in the Tree Sparrow, raise the question of whether feedback of androgen plays a role in the onset of seasonal testicular regression. In an initial attack on that question, 30-gage tubing containing a minute amount of the free alcohol of cyproterone (6-chloro-17-hydroxy-1$\alpha$,2$\alpha$-methylenepregna-4,6-diene-3,20-dione) was implanted into the hypothalamus-pituitary region in photosensitive males on the day prior to transfer from 8- to 20-hr daily photoperiods. Testes of birds with blank or ineffective cyproterone implants weighed $\sim$2–4 mg at autopsy, 15 weeks after transfer to long days, but *in one bird* regression was prevented by chronic implantation of cyproterone; the testes weighed 599.0 mg. The single effective implant terminated in an indentation created by the carrier tube in the rostral tip of the cephalic lobe of the anterior pituitary. At the base of that indentation, an apparently functional vascular channel separated the tube from the cephalic lobe. Histological evidence suggests that both cyproterone and cephalic lobe were in direct contact with the vascular channel, but whether the channel, which probably developed secondary to implantation, was associated with the afferent vascular supply of the anterior pituitary or its efferent vascular drainage could not be determined. The latter possibility seems more likely in view of the proximity of the cavernous sinus to the implantation site, but because the portal vessels may have been disrupted by displacement of the anterior pituitary during implantation, the possibility that the vascular channel could have developed in a regenerative process cannot be excluded. On the basis of location of implantation site alone, a pituitary focus of cyproterone action is suggested. The peculiar vascularization of the implantation site raises the alternative possibility of an effect of cyproterone outside the pituitary, possibly on the hypothalamus, but that is weakened by the observation that cyproterone implants in the tubero-infundibular region did not prevent testicular regression. In view of the minute amount of cyproterone implanted, the possibility of an effect peripheral to the hypothalamo-pituitary axis seems remote.

Cyproterone, a testosterone antagonist (BLOCH and DAVIDSON, 1967; VON BERSWORDT-WALLRABE and NEUMANN, 1967, 1968), is believed to be a competitive inhibitor of androgen-sensitive receptors. If that is true, then the evidence cited here leads to the tenuous and unconfirmed conclusion that feedback of androgen may play an important role in the initiation of seasonal testicular regression in the Tree Sparrow.

# Summary

Photoperiodic testicular growth was prevented or severely retarded in the Tree Sparrow (*Spizella arborea*) when minute amounts of solid testosterone propionate were implanted into the anterobasal region of the infundibular nucleus or along the anterodorsal border of the median eminence. Implants of testosterone propionate *in* the median eminence caused only moderate gonadosuppression. Similar implants in the middle part of the optic chiasm or blank or cholesterol implants, irrespective of site, did not impair photoperiodic testicular growth. These observations, confirming the potential for negative feedback control of pituitary gonadotropin secretion, suggest that the gonadosuppressive effect of testosterone is mediated through the tubero-infundibular region of the hypothalamus. Since interruption of the paraldehyde-fuchsin-stainable innervation of the anterior median eminence fails to modify the photoperiodic testicular response (Wilson and Hands, 1968), they suggest in addition that ganglionic cells of the basal infundibular nucleus and/or tubero-infundibular fibers that terminate in the median eminence may be foci of testosterone action. Because implants of testosterone propionate in or near the anterior pituitary sometimes suppressed photoperiodic testicular growth, that gland must tentatively be considered a focus of testosterone sensitivity. Preliminary evidence based on chronic implantation of cyproterone suggests that feedback of androgen may play an important role in the initiation of seasonal testicular regression in the Tree Sparrow.

## References

Benoit, J.: Opto-sexual reflex in the duck: physiological and histological aspects. Yale J. Biol. Med. **34**, 97–116 (1961).

Berswordt-Wallrabe, R. von, Neumann, F.: Influence of a testosterone antagonist (cyproterone) on pituitary and serum FSH-content in juvenile male rats. Neuroendocrinology **2**, 107–112 (1967).

— — Influence of a testosterone antagonist (cyproterone) on pituitary and serum ICSH content in juvenile male rats. Neuroendocrinology **3**, 332–336 (1968).

Bloch, G. J., Davidson, J. M.: Antiandrogen implanted in brain stimulates male reproductive system. Science **155**, 593–595 (1967).

Davidson, J. M.: Control of gonadotropin secretion in the male. In: Neuroendocrinology, ed. by L. Martini and W. F. Ganong, vol. I, p. 565–611. New York: Academic Press 1966.

— Sawyer, C. H.: Evidence for an hypothalamic focus of inhibition of gonadotropin by androgen in the male. Proc. Soc. exp. Biol. (N.Y.) **107**, 4–7 (1961).

— Smith, E. R.: Testosterone feedback in the control of somatic and behavioral aspects of male reproduction. In: Proceedings of the Second Internat. Congr. on Hormonal Steroids, Milan 1966, p. 805–813. Amsterdam: Excerpta Medica Foundation 1967.

Donovan, B. T.: The regulation of the secretion of follicle-stimulating hormone. In: The pituitary gland, ed. by G. W. Harris and B. T. Donovan, vol. II, p. 49–98. Berkeley and Los Angeles: University of California Press 1966.

Donovan, C. A.: Restraint and anesthesia of caged birds. Vet. Med. **53**, 541–543 (1958).

Everett, J. W.: Neuroendocrine aspects of mammalian reproduction. Ann. Rev. Physiol. **31**, 383–416 (1969).

Gogan, F.: Sensibilité hypothalamique à la testostérone chez le Canard. Gen. comp. Endocr. **11**, 316–327 (1968).

— Kordon, C.: Influence du feed-back par la testostérone sur la gonadostimulation induite par la lumière chez le Canard. J. Physiol. (Paris) **56**, 364–365 (1964).

Graber, J. W., Frankel, A. I., Nalbandov, A. V.: Hypothalamic center influencing the release of LH in the cockerel. Gen. comp. Endocr. **9**, 187–192 (1967).

HALÁSZ, B., PUPP, L., UHLARIK, S.: Hypophysiotrophic area in the hypothalamus. J. Endocr. **25**, 147–154 (1962).

— — — TIMA, L.: Further studies on the hormone secretion of the anterior pituitary transplanted into the hypophysiotrophic area of the rat hypothalamus. Endocrinology **77**, 343–355 (1965).

HOHLWEG, W., DAUME, E.: Lokale hormonelle Beeinflussung des Hypophysen-Zwischenhirnsystems bei Hähnen. Endokrinologie **37**, 95–104 (1959).

KANEMATSU, S., SAWYER, C. H.: Effects of hypothalamic estrogen implants on pituitary LH and prolactin in rabbits. Amer. J. Physiol. **205**, 1073–1076 (1963).

KOBAYASHI, H.: Inhibition by sex steroids and thyroid substance of light-induced gonadal development in the passerine bird, *Zosterops palpebrosa japonica*. Endocr. jap. **1**, 51–55 (1954).

— FARNER, D. S.: Evidence of a negative feedback on photoperiodically induced gonadal development in the White-crowned Sparrow, *Zonotrichia leucophrys gambelii*. Gen. comp. Endocr. **6**, 443–452 (1966).

KOIKE, T., LEPKOVSKY, S.: Hypothalamic lesions producing polyuria in chickens. Gen. comp. Endocr. **8**, 397–402 (1967).

KORDON, C., GOGAN, F.: Localisation par une technique de microimplantation de structures hypothalamiques responsables du feed-back par la testostérone chez le Canard. C. R. Soc. Biol. (Paris) **158**, 1795–1798 (1964).

LEPKOVSKY, S., YASUDA, M.: Hypothalamic lesions, growth and body composition of male chickens. Poultry Sci. **45**, 582–588 (1966).

LISK, R. D.: Estrogen-sensitive centers in the hypothalamus of the rat. J. exp. Zool. **145**, 197–205 (1960).

— Testosterone-sensitive centers in the hypothalamus of the rat. Acta endocr. (Kbh.) **41**, 195–204 (1962).

— Neural control of gonad size by hormone feedback in the desert iguana *Dipsosaurus dorsalis dorsalis*. Gen. comp. Endocr. **8**, 258–266 (1967).

LOFTS, B.: The effects of exogenous androgen on the testicular cycle of the Weaver-Finch *Quelea quelea*. Gen. comp. Endocr. **2**, 394–406 (1962).

— Patterns of testicular activity. In: Perspectives in endocrinology—Hormones in the lives of lower vertebrates, ed. by E. J. W. BARRINGTON and C. B. JØRGENSEN, p. 239–304. New York: Academic Press 1968.

MATSUO, S., VITUMS, A., KING, J. R., FARNER, D. S.: Light-microscope studies of the cytology of the adenohypophysis of the White-crowned Sparrow, *Zonotrichia leucophrys gambelii*. Z. Zellforsch. **95**, 143–176 (1969).

MIKAMI, S., VITUMS, A., FARNER, D. S.: Electron microscopic studies on the adenohypophysis of the White-crowned Sparrow, *Zonotrichia leucophrys gambelii*. Z. Zellforsch. **97**, 1–29 (1969).

OEHMKE, H.-J.: Regionale Strukturunterschiede im Nucleus infundibularis der Vögel (Passeriformes). Z. Zellforsch. **92**, 406–421 (1968).

PALKA, Y. S., RAMIREZ, V. D., SAWYER, C. H.: Distribution and biological effects of tritiated estradiol implanted in the hypothalamo-hypophysial region of female rats. Endocrinology **78**, 487–499 (1966).

SNAPIR, N., NIR, I., FURUTA, F., LEPKOVSKY, S.: Effect of administered testosterone propionate on cocks functionally castrated by hypothalamic lesions. Endocrinology **84**, 611–618 (1969).

STETSON, M. H.: The role of the median eminence in control of photoperiodically induced testicular growth in the White-crowned Sparrow, *Zonotrichia leucophrys gambelii*. Z. Zellforsch. **93**, 369–394 (1969).

SZENTÁGOTHAI, J., FLERKÓ, B., MESS, B., HALÁSZ, B.: Hypothalamic control of the anterior pituitary. Budapest: Akadémiai Kiadó 1962.

TIXIER-VIDAL, A., FOLLETT, B. K., FARNER, D. S.: The anterior pituitary of the Japanese Quail, *Coturnix coturnix japonica*. The cytological effects of photoperiodic stimulation. Z. Zellforsch. **92**, 610–635 (1968).

— HERLANT, M., BENOIT, J.: La préhypophyse du Canard Pékin mâle au cours du cycle annuel. Arch. Biol. (Liège) **73**, 318–368 (1962).

Uemura, H.: Effects of gonadectomy and sex steroids on the acid phosphatase activity of the hypothalamo-hypophysial system in the bird, *Emberiza rustica latifascia*. Endocr. jap. **11**, 185–203 (1964).

— Kobayashi, H.: Effects of prolonged daily photoperiods and estrogen on the hypothalamic neurosecretory system of the passerine bird, *Zosterops palpebrosa japonica*. Gen. comp. Endocr. **3**, 253–264 (1963).

Watanabe, S., McCann, S. M.: Localization of FSH-releasing factor in the hypothalamus and neurohypophysis as determined by *in vitro* assay. Endocrinology **82**, 664–673 (1968).

Wilson, F. E.: The effects of hypothalamic lesions on the photoperiodic testicular response in White-crowned Sparrows, *Zonotrichia leucophrys gambelii*. Doctoral Diss. Washington State University, Pullman 1965.

— The tubero-infundibular neuron system: a component of the photoperiodic control mechanism of the White-crowned Sparrow, *Zonotrichia leucophrys gambelii*. Z. Zellforsch. **82**, 1–24 (1967).

— Hands, G. R.: Hypothalamic neurosecretion and photoinduced testicular growth in the Tree Sparrow, *Spizella arborea*. Z. Zellforsch. **89**, 303–319 (1968).

# Various Problems of Neurosecretion

## Distribution of Peptidergic Neurons in Mammalian Brain

G. Zetler

Institut für Pharmakologie, Medizinische Akademie Lübeck, Lübeck (Germany)

Key words: Peptidergic neurons — Polypeptides — Substance P — Brain peptides.

The term "peptidergic neuron" was coined by Bargmann, Lindner and Andres (1967) and thought to be valid only for those hypothalamic neurons which synthesize octapeptides such as oxytocin and vasopressin, and belong functionally and morphologically to a neurosecretory system. The authors pointed out that these neurons not only release hormones into the blood stream, but also form "peptidergic synapses" on the surfaces of epithelial cells. The latter would mean that, as postulated by Knowles and Bern (1966), neurosecretory fibres performing "peptide neurosecretion" transmit impulses or other influences to target cells by means of a polypeptide released at a "neurosecretomotor junction". In this case the peptide would not function as a hormone but as a transmitter of nerve action. This possibility and our knowledge of the existence and distribution of other pharmacologically active polypeptides throughout the brain and especially in many nervous tissues not showing morphological signs of neurosecretory activity, make it necessary to consider whether the term "peptidergic neurons" should be extended to include all neurons containing active polypeptides and not confined to neurosecretory neurons only. One basis for these considerations is the "unitary concept of neurohumoral mechanisms" of de Robertis (1964) who wrote: "It can now be safely postulated that all neurons in addition to generating and spreading electrical phenomena have secretory functions by which active substances are synthesized and released."

## Facts and Findings

### 1. Oxytocin and Antidiuretic Hormone

(Review: Ginsburg, 1968)

A very large body of evidence now supports the view that the oxytocic and antidiuretic octapeptides are produced in the hypothalamus by the neurons of the nucleus supraopticus and of the nucleus paraventricularis. It was not difficult to demonstrate that the hormones are present only in these structures and in the tissues containing the nerve fibres which connect both nuclei with the neurohypophysis and transport the products of neurosecretion downwards (Hild and Zetler, 1951, 1953). Depending on the kind of stimulus, both hormones can be released separately (Beleslin, Bisset, Haldar and Polak, 1967; Bisset, Hilton and Poisner, 1967), which indicates but does not prove that oxytocin and vasopressin are produced, stored, and secreted by two different types of neurones. This possibility is suggested also in other neurological and pharmacological studies (cf. GINSBURG, 1968), and is strengthened by the fact that, in the posterior pituitary lobe, both hormones are stored in different neurosecretory granules (LA BELLA, REIFFENSTEIN and BEAULIEU, 1963; BARER, HELLER and LEDERIS, 1963; DEAN, HOPE and KAŽIĆ, 1968). In these granules, the hormones are bound to the carrier protein "neurophysin" (cf. ACHER, 1968; HOPE and HOLLENBERG, 1968), but it is not known whether neurophysin exists also in the hypothalamic nuclei which produce the hormones. Brain tissue as such, however, in contrast to many other organs, does not contain a neurophysin-like protein (GINSBURG and JAYA-SENA, 1968).

## 2. Hypothalamic Neurohormones Influencing the Adenohypophysis
(Reviews: GUILLEMIN, 1967; MARTINI, FRASCHINI and MOTTA, 1968; SCHALLY et al., 1968)

A factor which releases corticotropin from the adenohypophysis was detected in extracts made from hypothalamic tissue (SAFFRAN and SCHALLY, 1955). Since then, six more neurohormones were shown to be present in hypothalamus extracts, and to modify the secretion of anterior pituitary hormones. The (at least) seven hypothalamic neurohormones are: 1. the corticotropin-releasing hormones (CRH); 2. the thyreotropin-releasing hormone (TRH); 3. the growth hormone-releasing hormone (GH-RH); 4. the hormone releasing the follicle stimulating hormone (FSH-RH); 5. the luteinizing hormone-releasing hormone (LH-RH); 6. a hormone which inhibits the prolactine secretion (PRIH); and 7. a hormone which inhibits the release of the melanocyte-stimulating hormone (MRIH). It seems now clear that these compounds are transported within hypothalamic neurons downwards to the portal vessels, and secreted by the nerve endings into the blood stream which then flows through the anterior lobe. Present knowledge indicates that perhaps only CRH, TRH, and GH-RH are polypeptides which are possibly produced, transported, and secreted by three different types of neurons. These neurons exist only in the hypothalamus; extracts made from other brain parts were inactive in this respect.

Consequently, the hypothalamus could contain at least two groups of peptidergic neurons: neurons producing oxytocin and vasopressin, and neurons producing the releasing hormones CRH, TRH and GH-RH. A common property of both groups is the secretion into the blood stream.

## 3. Substance P-Polypeptides
(Reviews: HAEFELY and HÜRLIMANN, 1962; LEMBECK and ZETLER, 1962; ZETLER, 1970)

Substance P (SP) is a long-known tissue extract (EULER and GADDUM, 1931) which owes its gut-contracting and blood-pressure lowering activity to polypeptides. Unexpected difficulties prevented until now a complete purification of the peptides and the elucidation of their chemical structure, as is also true for the hypothalamic releasing hormones. Nevertheless, it is clear that the SP peptides in their pure state have tremendous pharmacological activity. In the context of this article, however, distribution within the brain is of greater importance.

Earlier studies revealed an uneven distribution of SP in the brain of man, the cow, and the dog. These investigations, based on the assumption that only one active SP peptide exists in brain extracts, were hampered by interfering impurities. We know now that crude SP preparations contain three active polypeptides (ZETLER, 1961, 1963) which can easily be separated by aluminium oxide column chromatography as shown in Fig. 1. The peptide in the fractions Fa is, in contrast with the peptides Fb and Fc, not adsorbed by the aluminium oxide; Fb is eluted

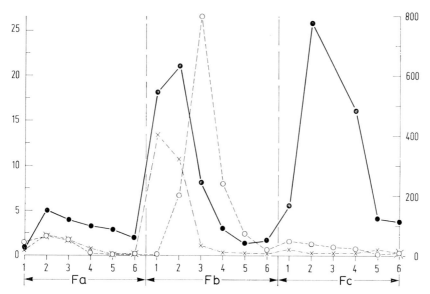

Fig. 1. Aluminium oxide column chromatography of substance P preparations made from human precentral gyrus ($\cdot$———$\cdot$; $\cong$ 115 g tissue), substantia nigra (o------o; $\cong$ 19.5 g tissue), and globus pallidus ($\times\cdots\cdots\times$; $\cong$ 33.3 g tissue). Abscissa: Number of 5 ml-fractions; Fa = 70% methanol, Fb = distilled water, Fc = 0.1 N sodium hydroxide. Ordinates indicate concentration of gut-contracting activity as Euler-units per fraction, the left ordinate refers to cortex, the right ordinate to substantia nigra and globus pallidus (condensed from BALDAUF, HARNACKE and ZETLER, 1968)

by distilled water, and Fc by 0.1 N sodium hydroxide. Fa is the SP peptide in the strict sense, loosely bound to an unknown carrier to form Fb which is transformed into Fa by repeated chromatography on, or shaking with, aluminium oxide. Fa and Fb are basic and destroyed by chymotrypsin and trypsin; Fc is acidic and destroyed by chymotrypsin but resistant to trypsin. In contrast with Fa and Fb, Fc stimulates isolated guts in an indirect way by releasing acetylcholine from the nerve endings of intramural plexuses (ZETLER, 1966). Therefore, the gut-contracting action of Fc is greatly diminished by morphine and atropine. Fig. 1 shows furthermore the most important fact that Fc was obtained only from cortical grey matter but not from globus pallidus and substantia nigra. This finding is strengthened by those summarized in Table 1.

In the experiments leading to this table, interference of impurities was greatly eliminated by preparing from each part a semi-purified SP preparation of EULER (1942). The second column shows practically the same difference between brain

Table 1. *Yields of substance P extraction from human brain areas, and of column chromatography on aluminium oxide* (condensed from Baldauf, Iven and Zetler, 1969)

| Human brain area | $N$[a] | Substance P[b] $U/g$[c] | NaOH phase of Aluminium oxide column | |
|---|---|---|---|---|
| | | | yield[d] | nature[e] |
| Frontal cortex | 5 | 4 | 63 | Fc-peptide |
| Occipital cortex | 2 | 6 | 95 | Fc-peptide |
| Precentral gyrus | 6 | 3 | 55 | Fc-peptide |
| Cingulate gyrus | 35 | 8 | 60 | Fc-peptide |
| Amygdaloid nucleus | 55 | 18 | 12 | Fc-like peptide |
| Putamen | 35 | 36 | 5 | Fb-tail |
| Caudate nucleus | 26 | 24 | 8 | Fb-tail |
| Globus pallidus | 7 | 28 | 5 | Fb-tail |
| Substantia nigra | 40 | 145 | 10 | Fb-tail |
| Red nucleus | 57 | 8 | 10 | Fc-like peptide |
| Thalamus | 26 | 6 | 8 | Fb-tail |
| Hypothalamus | 38 | 16 | 6 | Fc-like peptide |
| Medulla oblongata | 15 | 5 | 3 | Fb-tail |

[a] Number of brains.

[b] Dry powder prepared after Euler (1942).

[c] Gut-contracting activity, Euler-units per gram wet tissue.

[d] Active material eluted by 0.1 N NaOH; figures indicate percentages of total activity achieved by elution with 70% methanol, distilled water, and 0.1 N NaOH.

[e] See text.

parts already known from the biological evaluation of much cruder brain extracts. The high concentration in substantia nigra, and the great differences in concentration between adjacent or functionally connected areas is evident.

The SP preparation of each brain part was chromatographed on an aluminium oxide column to obtain results of the kind shown in Fig. 1. In this way we found that the peptide Fc was present only in cortical, but not in subcortical, grey matter. The same result was obtained when grey matter of cortex and subcortex was grosso modo extracted and analyzed (Baldauf and Zetler, 1968; Baldauf, Iven and Zetler, 1969; Baldauf, Dobek and Zetler, 1969). Peptides Fa and Fb were however present in SP made from all brain areas of Table 1. The relation of Fc to Fa + Fb differs: in occipital cortex practically all activity stemmed from Fc, but in other cortical tissues only 50–60% of total yield.

Only traces of SP (i.e. Fa), no Fc, or other peptides with comparable pharmacological activity were found in the cerebellum of man or animal.

In amygdaloid nucleus, red nucleus and hypothalamus we found small amounts of polypeptides (named Fc') which, like Fc, have acidic nature and indirect action on guts, but, in contrast with Fc, are destroyed by trypsin. Work on further biochemical characterization of these peptides is in progress and shows that they are perhaps not identical.

Polypeptides can be artifacts originating from proteins during aggressive steps of extraction and purification. Such steps leading to protein denaturation exist indeed in the usual SP preparing procedure of Euler (1942). We extracted therefore grey matter of bovine cortex and subcortex by hyposmotic shock at pH 3.5 and ultrafiltration through protein-tight filters and from the residues we made SP powder. About 30% of total yield was obtained by ultrafiltration (Fig. 2) which means that these polypeptides are very probably not artifacts and exist in the tissue partly in free form. The greater part of Fb and Fc was, however, obtained from the residues and is therefore bound to tissue particles; Fc was again present only in cortex extracts. These results strenghthen the view that Fa, Fb, and Fc may be different compounds.

It now appears that Fa is the SP peptide in the strict sense and exists in brain tissue to the greater part in the free form. Fb is Fa bound not only to a carrier but also to tissue particles. Fc is not strictly an SP peptide; it is cortex-specific and completely tissue-bound.

The kind of distribution and other findings (see reviews) indicate that these polypeptides are located in nerve cells and not in glia cells. Consequently, there

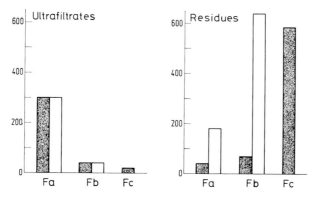

Fig. 2. Results of aluminium oxide chromatography of ultrafiltrates (left) and substance P preparations made from the residues (right) of 100 g cortical and 100 g subcortical grey matter of cattle brain. Black columns: Cortex. White columns: Subcortex. Ordinates: Biological activity as units (condensed from BALDAUF, DOBEK and ZETLER, 1969)

exist in all brain parts, except cerebellum, neurons containing SP (i.e. Fa + Fb); Fc neurons exist only in cortex. A third group of neurons containing the Fc-like peptides Fc' are located in amygdala, red nucleus, and hypothalamus.

In addition to gut-contracting and hypotensive polypeptides, crude SP preparations contain a component with sedative and anticonvulsive (e.g. anti-strychnine) activity which is destroyed by proteases and therefore bound to a polypeptide structure (ZETLER, 1956, 1959; for all subsequent references see ZETLER, 1970). This anticonvulsive polypeptide was isolated by chromatographic means and found to be without gut-contracting activity. It was obtained from bovine cortex, brain stem, cerebellum, and ventral and dorsal halves of spinal cord. Concentration was highest in cortex, but there was no parallelism with gut-contracting SP activity. Obviously, this anticonvulsive factor is another specific brain polypeptide.

## 4. Information-Transferring Polypeptides

Nothing is known about distribution in brain of a polypeptide which appears in the brain of morphine-tolerant rats and transfers tolerance when injected into normal animals (UNGAR and COHEN, 1966; UNGAR and GALVAN, 1969). This material is probably not identical with SP. Furthermore, polypeptides were also found to be essential constituents of brain extracts which transferred acquired information from trained rats to untrained rats (Rosenblatt, Farrow and Herblin, 1966; Ungar and Irwin, 1966; Ungar, Galvan and Clark, 1968). It was even found that four different brain polypeptides induced, in normal animals (rats), specifically four different types of behaviour (Ungar, 1969). However, distribution in brain of all these peptides is not known.

## Discussion

At least nine pharmacologically active polypeptides (Table 2) are present in brain tissue. The information transferring peptides must probably be added to this number, which can be expected to increase further by still unknown polypeptides and by a splitting of the group of Fc′ peptides into two or three compounds. While the presence of oxytocin and vasopressin in the posterior lobe teaches that the site of presence is not necessarily identical with that of production, nevertheless, as far as Table 2 is concerned, it is reasonable to accept, for the sake

Table 2. *Pharmacologically active brain polypeptides, and their location in brain*

| No. | Polypeptides | Location in brain |
|-----|--------------|-------------------|
| 1 | Oxytocin | Hypothalamus |
| 2 | Vasopressin (Antidiuretic hormone) | Hypothalamus |
| 3 | Corticotropin-releasing hormones[a] | Hypothalamus |
| 4 | Thyreotropin-releasing hormone | Hypothalamus |
| 5 | Growth hormone-releasing hormone | Hypothalamus |
| 6 | Substance P (peptides Fa and Fb) | Brain except cerebellum |
| 7 | Peptide Fc | Cortex of brain except cerebellum |
| 8 | Fc-like peptides (Fc′) | Hypothalamus, Nucleus amygdalae, Nucleus ruber |
| 9 | Anti-strychnine factor | Cortex, brain stem, cerebellum |

[a] $\alpha_1$, $\alpha_2$, $\beta$.

of discussion, that a polypeptide is produced where it is found in brain tissue. This means that the hypothalamus synthesizes seven to eight polypeptides, namely all those mentioned in Table 2 except peptide Fc. It is not probable that one type of nerve cell produces seven or eight active polypeptides. Therefore it may be hypothesized that each peptide is synthesized by a specific neuron. This may not be true in all cases, but it is supported by the knowledge about peptides No. 1–5 of Table 2, by the presence of peptide Fc′ in the red nucleus and its absence in the closely located and very SP-rich substantia nigra, and finally by the existence of Fc only in cortical grey matter. The latter fact means that peptide Fc is present in neurons which do not leave the cortex. The lack of active polypeptides in the cerebellum strengthens the view that presence and distribution of peptides in brain indicate a functional role. On the other hand, it shows that the cerebellum certainly deserves a closer pharmacological, biochemical, and histological investigation. Visible structures which indicate peptide synthesis (cf. Sewing, 1969) may be missing or at least less prominent in the cerebellum than in brain parts rich in active peptides, e.g. substantia nigra or hypothalamus.

It seems now to be justified and fruitful to postulate that peptidergic neurons of different character are widely distributed in the nervous system. Consequently, the principle of peptidergic action cannot be restricted to the hypothalamic neurosecretory system as thought by BARGMANN, LINDNER and ANDRES (1967). From the new point of view which fits into the "unitary concept of neurohumoral mechanisms" of DE ROBERTIS (1964), the hypothalamic neurons producing peptides No. 1–5 of Table 2 are special cases since the targets of their actions are located outside the brain.

The physiological role of the polypeptides No. 6–9 (Table 2) is not known. It is not necessary to postulate a transmitter function; an action as modulators of neuronal activity is more probable. FLOREY (1967) discussed extensively sources, chemical identity, and possible actions of modulator substances "that reach excitable cells by humoral pathways and originate in nerve cells, gland cells, neurosecretory cells, or ependyma (glia) cells". He mentioned eleven parameters of neuronal activity as possible targets of modulating influences, and made clear that there exists a wealth of functional possibilities. A viewpoint important with respect to polypeptides is that modulator substances "can be expected to be present for longer periods of time and to affect membrane regions outside the specific synaptic areas" (FLOREY, 1967). The behavioural actions exerted by the information transferring polypeptides could rather be the result of a specific or localized modulator influence than the realization of a complicated instruction which probably cannot be stored in a relatively simple small-sized polypeptide molecule. However, less sophisticated peptide functions are also possible, as for SP a neurone-triggered change of local circulation and vascular permeability (LEMBECK and STARKE, 1963).

## Summary

At least nine pharmacologically active polypeptides are present in brain tissue. According to present knowledge, distribution of the polypeptides is uneven; one peptide is, indeed, present only in cortical grey matter.

It is postulated that there exist peptidergic neurons which are, in addition to cholinergic and aminergic neurons, widely distributed in brain tissues. Special types of peptidergic neurons are those with targets of function outside the brain: neurons of the hypothalamic neurosecretory system, and neurons producing releasing hormones which stimulate the adenohypophysis.

The products of peptidergic neurons could act within nervous tissue as specific modulators of neuronal activity.

## References

ACHER, R.: Neurophysin and neurohypophysial hormones. Proc. roy. Soc. B 170, 7–16 (1968).
BALDAUF, J., DOBEK, W., ZETLER, G.: Freie und gebundene Substanz P-Peptide in Cortex und Subcortex des Rinderhirns. Naunyn-Schmiedebergs Arch. Pharmak. 264, 354–362 (1969).
— HARNACKE, P., ZETLER, G.: Aktive Peptide in Substanz P-Präparaten aus Cortex, Globus pallidus und Substantia nigra des menschlichen Gehirns. Naunyn-Schmiedebergs Arch. Pharmak. exp. Path. 260, 231–241 (1968).
— IVEN, H., ZETLER, G.: Verteilung von darmkontrahierenden Peptiden im menschlichen Gehirn. Naunyn-Schmiedebergs Arch. Pharmak. exp. Path. 262, 453–462 (1969).
— ZETLER, G.: Darmkontrahierende Hirnpeptide in Cortex und Subcortex. Naunyn-Schmiedebergs Arch. Pharmak. exp. Path. 260, 242–253 (1968).

Barer, R., Heller, H., Lederis, K.: The isolation, identification and properties of the hormone granules of the neurohypophysis. Proc. roy. Soc. B 158, 388–416 (1963).

Bargmann, W., Lindner, E., Andres, K. H.: Über Synapsen an endokrinen Epithelzellen und die Definition sekretorischer Neurone. Untersuchungen am Zwischenlappen der Katzenhypophyse. Z. Zellforsch. 77, 282–298 (1967).

Beleslin, D., Bisset, G. W., Haldar, J., Polak, R. L.: The release of vasopressin without oxytocin in response to haemorrhage. Proc. roy. Soc. B 166, 443–458 (1967).

Bisset, G. W., Hilton, S. M., Poisner, A. M.: Hypothalamic pathways for independent release of vasopressin and oxytocin. Proc. roy. Soc. B 166, 422–442 (1967).

Dean, C. R., Hope, D. B., Kažić, T.: Evidence for the storage of oxytocin with neurophysin-I and vasopressin with neurophysin-II in separate neurosecretory granules. Brit. J. Pharmacol. 34, 192P–193P (1968).

De Robertis, E.: Histophysiology of synapses and neurosecretion. Oxford-New York-Frankfurt: Pergamon Press 1964.

Euler, U. S. v.: Herstellung und Eigenschaften von Substanz P. Acta physiol. scand. 4, 373–375 (1942).

— Gaddum, J. H.: An unidentified depressor substance in certain tissue extracts. J. Physiol. (Lond.) 72, 74–87 (1931).

Florey, E.: Neurotransmitters and modulators in the animal kingdom. Fed. Proc. 26, 1164–1178 (1967).

Ginsburg, M.: Production, release, transportation and elimination of the neurohypophysial hormones, p. 286–371, in: B. Berde (ed.), Neurohypophyseal hormones and similar polypeptides, Handbuch der experimentellen Pharmakologie, vol. XXII. Berlin-Heidelberg-New York: Springer 1968.

— Jayasena, K.: The distribution of proteins that bind neurohypophysial hormones. J. Physiol. (Lond.) 197, 65–76 (1968).

Guillemin, R.: The adenohypophysis and its hypothalamic control. Ann. Rev. Physiol. 29, 313–348 (1967).

Haefely, W., Hürlimann, A.: Substance P, a highly active naturally occurring polypeptide. Experientia (Basel) 18, 297–303 (1962).

Hild, W., Zetler, G.: Über das Vorkommen der Hypophysenhinterlappenhormone im Zwischenhirn. Naunyn-Schmiedebergs Arch. exp. Path. Pharmak. 213, 139–153 (1951).

— — Experimenteller Beweis für die Entstehung der sog. Hypophysenhinterlappenwirkstoffe im Hypothalamus. Pflügers Arch. ges. Physiol. 257, 169–201 (1953).

Hope, D. B., Hollenberg, M. D.: Crystallization of complexes of neurophysins with vasopressin and oxytocin. Proc. roy. Soc. B 170, 37–47 (1968).

Knowles, Fr., Bern, H. A.: The function of neurosecretion in endocrine regulation. Nature (Lond.) 210, 271–272 (1966).

La Bella, F. S., Reiffenstein, R. J., Beaulieu, G.: Subcellular fractionation of bovine posterior pituitary glands by centrifugation. Arch. Biochem. 100, 399–408 (1963).

Lembeck, F., Starke, K.: Substance P content and effect on capillary permeability of extracts of various parts of human brain. Nature (Lond.) 199, 1295–1296 (1963).

— Zetler, G.: Substance P: A polypeptide of possible physiological significance, especially within the nervous system. Int. Rev. Neurobiol. 4, 159–215 (1962).

Martini, L., Fraschini, F., Motta, M.: Neural control of anterior pituitary functions. Recent Progr. Hormone Res. 24, 439–485 (1968).

Rosenblatt, F., Farrow, J. T., Herblin, W. F.: Transfer of conditioned responses from trained rats to untrained rats by means of a brain extract. Nature (Lond.) 209, 46–48 (1966).

Saffran, M., Schally, A. V.: Release of corticotrophin by anterior pituitary tissue in vitro. Canad. J. Biochem. 33, 408–415 (1955).

Schally, A. V., Arimura, A., Bowers, C. Y., Kastin, A. J., Sawano, S., Redding, T. W.: Hypothalamic neurohormones regulating anterior pituitary function. Recent Progr. Hormone Res. 24, 497–581 (1968).

Sewing, K.-Fr.: Das Zellsystem für die Synthese von Peptidhormonen. Dtsch. med. Wschr. 94, 502–504 (1969).

UNGAR, G.: Induction of specific behavior by peptides, p. 300, in: Abstracts Fourth Internat. Congr. on Pharmacol., July 14–18, Basel 1969.
— COHEN, M.: Induction of morphine tolerance by material extracted from brain of tolerant animals. Int. J. Neuropharmacol. **5**, 183–192 (1966).
— GALVAN, L.: Conditions of transfer of morphine tolerance by brain extracts. Proc. Soc. exp. Biol. (N.Y.) **130**, 287–290 (1969).
— — CLARK, R. H.: Chemical transfer of learned fear. Nature (Lond.) **217**, 1259–1261 (1968).
— IRWIN, L. N.: Transfer of acquired information by brain extracts. Nature (Lond.) **214**, 453–455 (1967).
ZETLER, G.: Substanz P, ein Polypeptid aus Darm und Gehirn mit depressiven, hyperalge-tischen und Morphin-antagonistischen Wirkungen auf das Zentralnervensystem. Naunyn-Schmiedebergs Arch. exp. Path. Pharmak. **228**, 513–538 (1956).
— Versuche zur anticonvulsiven Wirksamkeit des Polypeptids Substanz P. Naunyn-Schmie-debergs Arch. exp. Path. Pharmak. **237**, 11–16 (1959).
— Zwei neue pharmakologisch aktive Polypeptide in einem Substanz P-haltigen Hirnextrakt. Naunyn-Schmiedebergs Arch. exp. Path. Pharmak. **242**, 330–352 (1961).
— New pharmacologically active polypeptides present in impure preparations of substance P. Ann. N.Y. Acad. Sci. **104**, 416–435 (1963).
— The role of release of acetylcholine in the gut-contracting action of a brain polypeptide. In: ERDÖS, E. G., N. BACK, and F. SICUTERI (eds.), Hypotensive peptides, p. 621–630. Berlin-Heidelberg-New York: Springer 1966.
— Biologically active peptides (Substance P). In: A. LAJTHA (ed.), Handbook of Neuro-chemistry, vol. 4. New York: Plenum Press 1970.

# Qualitative and Quantitative Histochemistry of Mammalian Neurosecretory Centers

J. F. Jongkind and D. F. Swaab

Netherlands Central Institute for Brain Research, Amsterdam (The Netherlands)

**Key words:** Hypothalamus — TPP-ase — Histochemistry.

In the mammalian nervous system, the efferent neurons of a reflex-arc share a common physiological item, that a convergence of all input takes place at the receptive surface. They may be regarded as the final common path of central integration. These neurons can be divided into two groups. The first group consists of neurons which directly innervate their target-organ by means of a transmitter-substance liberated from the axon terminals. The second group of neurons —neurosecretory neurons—indirectly innervate their target organ by neuronal products (neurohormones) released in the bloodstream. Both groups share a common characteristic, that the neuronal products are stored in the axon endings. They should differ, however, as a consequence of their way of innervating their target organ, in the amount of neuronal products which are released during a steady state or upon stimulation. Therefore the hormone synthetizing machinery of the neurosecretory cell—adaequately tuned to the high demand—should operate at a higher level than its transmitter producing partner.

During stimulation of the supraoptic nucleus relatively large amounts of hormones are released from the neurohypophysis. These products are quickly repleted by the supraoptic cell bodies, which are synthetizing the hormone at an increased rate (TAKABATAKE and SACHS, 1964). The coupling of release and synthesis—probably by means of a feedback mechanism but not necessarily so—is also suggested by morphological studies (ORTMANN, 1960).

In addition to the supraoptic and paraventricular nucleus, the hypothalamus contains other neurons which produce releasing factors. The exact hypothalamic localization of these neurons however, although roughly indicated (SZENTÁGOTHAI, FLERKÓ, MESS, HALÁSZ, 1962), presents many difficulties due to the fact that the production sites of the specific releasing factors do not seem to be restricted by the borders of the hypothalamic nuclei.

Our investigations to localize the releasing factor neurons consisted of 2 different series of experiments. Firstly a biochemical parameter for neurosecretion was analysed and secondly this parameter was applied to the releasing factor neurons (RF-neurons).

## A Biochemical Parameter for Neurosecretory Activity

As judged from ultrastructural findings the synthesis of neurohormones and the formation of neurosecretory vesicles seem to follow the same pattern as the

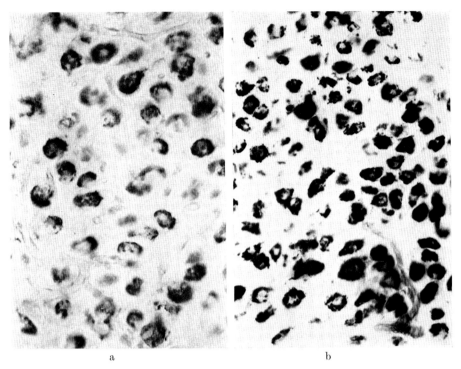

a                                                      b

Fig. 1 a and b. TPP-ase activity in the supraoptic nucleus of a control rat (a) and of one which
was subjected to a thirsting period of 6 days (b). Glyoxal fixation; Incubation time in TPP-ase
medium of Novikoff and Goldfischer (1961): 10 minutes at room temperature

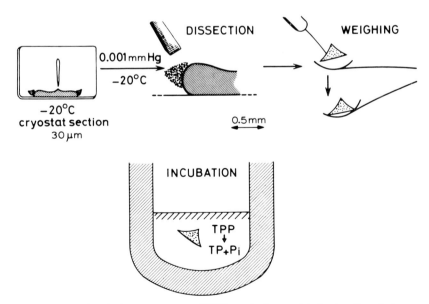

Fig. 2. Biochemical measurement of TPP-ase in frozen-dried microdissected
supraoptic nucleus

formation and packing of secretory material in any glandular system. The actual
formation of the neurosecretory vesicle takes place in the Golgi apparatus (Osinchak, 1964). In this connection it is likely to assume that the increased functional
demand during activation of the system, results in a stimulatory effect upon the
enzymatic equipment of this cellular organelle.

Since thiamine pyrophosphatase (TPP-ase) and nucleoside diphosphatase are
considered to be specific enzymes of the neuronal Golgi apparatus (Novikoff and
Goldfischer, 1961), we determined with histochemical and cytochemical methods
the changes in enzyme activity and distribution in the supraoptic nucleus upon
stimulation.

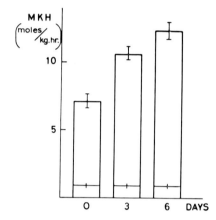

Fig. 3. Effect of a thirsting period of 3 and 6 days on the TPP-ase activities in supraoptic
nucleus (thick columns) and adjacent anterior hypothalamic tissue (thin horizontal lines).
Vertical lines indicate ± standard error of the mean ($n = 6$; three determinations per animal)

It could be demonstrated that the histochemical reaction product of TPP-ase
in the supraoptic nucleus covered a larger area of the activated cell bodies, indicating an increased functional involvement of the Golgi apparatus (Jongkind and
Swaab, 1967) (Fig. 1a, b).

The biochemical measurement of TPP-ase in frozendried microdissected material with quantitative cytochemical methods (Fig.2), demonstrated that the TPP-
ase activity increased some 40% after 3 days thirsting, while 3 more days of thirsting
resulted in a still further increase of TPP-ase activity (Jongkind, 1969) (Fig. 3).

Subsequently this enzymatic parameter for neurosecretory activity was used
to assay the activity of the RF-neurons in the hypothalamus.

## TPP-ase in Activated RF-Neurons

### a) The Thyrotropin Releasing Factor (TRF) System

Although the pituitary adjusts its TSH secretion autonomously to changing
levels of thyroid hormones, the existence of an additional hypothalamic influence
by way of the TRF system seems to be established. This hypothalamic influence
apparently maintains an independent tonic stimulation of the base-line of

pituitary-thyroid function, over which the pituitary responses to elevated and depressed blood levels of thyroid hormones are superimposed (REICHLIN, 1966). Results of determination of TRF in hypothalamic extracts after thyroidectomy suggest that after prolonged thyroid hypofunction the production of hypothalamic TRF is stimulated (SINHA and MEITES, 1966).

With the qualitative histochemical method for TPP-ase we studied 40 rats, thyroidectomized from 9 to 68 days; 12 hypothalamic nuclei were photographed and compared with those of sham operated controls.

It has not been possible to detect any difference in TPP-ase activity between the hypothalamus of thyroidectomized animals and those of control rats.

These results suggest that the stimulation of hypothalamic TRF synthesis was not sufficient to bring about the enzymatic signs of hyperactivity which we did observe in the above mentioned observations on magnocellular nuclei.

### b) The Gonadotropin-Releasing Factor (GRF) System

After gonadectomy the serum LH concentration in the rat increases 50 times above the control level (GAY and MIDGLEY, 1969). The same phenomenon has been observed regarding FSH after gonadectomy (PARLOW, 1964). The high gonado-tropin levels in gonadectomized animals are caused by an increased release from the pituitary. It has been calculated (GAY and MIDGLEY, 1969) that the release of LH in a castrated animal is about 21 µg per day, while a normal male will release about 0.6 µg per day. Since the gonadotropin release is under direct control of the hypothalamic neurohormones LHRF and FSHRF (FLERKÓ, 1966), the increase in gonadotropin release after gonadectomy points to an enhanced release and pro-duction of hypothalamic GRF.

We studied up till now qualitatively the TPP-ase in hypothalamic nuclei of 20 rats gonadectomized from 0 up to 130 days.

After gonadectomy the supraoptic and paraventricular nuclei showed an in-crease in TPP-ase activity already after 14 days of gonadectomy (SWAAB and JONGKIND, in press). The activation of the magnocellular nuclei lasted for at least 130 days after gonadectomy.

In analogy with the effect of osmotic stress in the magnocellular nuclei this result might suggest an increased production of LHRF and FSHRF. However the injection of human chorionic gonadotropin (HCG) (dose: 30 I.U. d.d. for 2 days), in 4 day gonadectomized animals resulted in a further increase in TPP-ase activity in the supraoptic and paraventricular nuclei (SWAAB, in preparation), indicating a participation of the magnocellular nuclei in a pituitary—gonadotropin—hypo-thalamic feedback loop.

So far no other nuclear area has been investigated after castration.

## Conclusions

The enzymatic parameter to determine the synthetic activity of the supra-optic cell bodies under osmotic stress conditions, presents an opportunity to analyse the secretory activity in other neurosecretory neurons.

Thyroidectomy, which increased the TRF content of the hypothalamus, did not lead to an increased TPP-ase activity.

Neurons of the supraoptic and paraventricular nucleus clearly reacted with an increase in TPP-ase activity after gonadectomy. These nuclei responded also to the elevated levels of human chorionic gonadotropin, and are probably not directly involved in the GRF production.

## References

FLERKÓ, B.: Control of gonadotropin secretion in the female. In: L. MARTINI and W. F. GANONG (eds.), Neuroendocrinology, vol. 1, p. 613–668. New York-London: Academic Press 1966.

GAY, V. L., MIDGLEY, A. R., JR.: Response of the adult rat to orchidectomy and ovariectomy as determined by LH radioimmunoassay. Endocrinology 84, 1359–1364 (1969).

JONGKIND, J. F.: Quantitative histochemistry of hypothalamus. II. Thiamine pyrophosphatase, nucleoside diphosphatase and acid phosphatase in the activated supraoptic nucleus of the rat. J. Histochem. Cytochem. 15, 23–29 (1969).

— SWAAB, D. F.: The distribution of thiamine diphosphate-phosphohydrolase in the neurosecretory nuclei of the rat following osmotic stress. Histochemie 11, 319–324 (1967).

NOVIKOFF, A. B., GOLDFISCHER, S.: Nucleosidediphosphatase activity in the Golgi apparatus and its usefulness for cytologic studies. Proc. nat. Acad. Sci. (Wash.) 47, 802–810 (1961).

ORTMANN, R.: Neurosecretion. In: J. FIELD (ed.), Handbook of physiology, sect. 1, vol. 2, p. 1039–1065. Washington, D.C., American Physiological Society 1960.

OSINCHAK, J.: Electron microscopical localization of acid phosphatase and thiamine pyrophosphatase activity in hypothalamic neurosecretory cells of the rat. J. Cell Biol. 21, 35–47 (1964).

PARLOW, A. F.: Differential actions of small doses of estradiol on gonadotrophins in the rat. Endocrinology 75, 1–8 (1964).

REICHLIN, S.: Control of thyrotropic hormone secretion. In: L. MARTINI and W. F. GANONG (eds.), Neuroendocrinology, vol. 1, p. 445–536. New York-London: Academic Press 1966.

SINHA, D., MEITES, J.: Effects of thyroidectomy and thyroxine on hypothalamic concentration of "thyrotropin releasing factor" and pituitary content of thyrotropin in rats. Neuroendocrinology 1, 4–14 (1965/66).

SZENTÁGOTHAI, J., FLERKÓ, B., MESS, B., HALÁSZ, B.: In: Hypothalamic control of the anterior pituitary, p. 289–308. Budapest: Akadémiai Kiado 1962.

TAKABATAKE, Y., SACHS, H.: Vasopressin biosynthesis. III. In vitro studies. Endocrinology 75, 934–942 (1964).

# Hypothalamic Neurosecretion in the Bat, *Myotis myotis* Borkhausen, during the Period of Hibernation and Activity*

Andrzej Jasiński

Department of Comparative Anatomy, Jagellonian University, Kraków (Poland)

Key words: Hypothalamus — neurosecretion — bats.

## Introduction

The mouse-eared bat (*Myotis myotis* Borkhausen) belongs to the hibernating mammals. During hibernation the ability of thermo-regulation is temporarily suspended. The optimum temperature of hibernation for this species is around 7—8°C (Brosset, 1966) although some specimens were found in the state of torpidity at a significantly lower temperature (0—2°C; Kowalski, 1953; Krzanowski, 1959), as well as at temperatures markedly above optimum values (Harmata, 1969). The body temperature of hibernating bats approaches ambient temperatures, and in the case of *Myotis velifer* it varies between 1 and 10°C (Tinkle and Patterson, 1965). The metabolic rate during torpidity is markedly decreased, and lowering of body temperature is followed by drastic reduction of respiratory movements, but these facts do not prevent the loss of body weight which in *Myotis myotis* exceeds 20% (Krzanowski, 1961).

A long period of hibernation entails a danger of desiccation and hence a special water retention mechanism is required. Biological adaptations to the hibernation period only partially prevent water loss. *Myotis myotis* requires high humidity of the air (approximately 75%) in a hibernaculum (Brosset, 1966). Specimens of this species often "... hibernate in such damp places that their fur may be beaded with drops of dew" (Allen, 1962). Moreover, the compactness of a bat colony reduces the contact of flight membranes with the air and decreases not only the loss of heat but also probably the evaporation of water (Kowalski, 1953). Quite often spontaneous awakening creates an opportunity for intake of water. *Myotis myotis* belongs, however, to the long torpidity species (Gaisler, 1966), hence this form of defence against desiccation is less important. Unfortunately information on the amount and concentration of urine passed during hibernation is still lacking.

Water retention depends on the activity of neurosecretory centres of the hypothalamus, mainly the nucleus supraopticus, and on the quantity of antidiuretic factor released by the pars nervosa (processus infundibularis) of the hypophysis. The neurosecretory substance staining with the Gomori methods is prob-

* Supported by a research grant from the Zoological Committee of the Polish Academy of Sciences.

ably related to, but not identical with, antidiuretic hormone (Bargmann and
Scharrer, 1951), since its release is accompanied by a rise in the blood level of
ADH (for references see: Jasiński et al., 1967). On this assumption the hypothalamo-hypophysial neurosecretory system was studied in the mouse-eared bat
during hibernation and summer activity. It was expected that metabolic differences
during these periods should be associated with marked changes in the activity of
the secretory centres of the hypothalamus. Similar problems concerning bats and
other hibernating mammals were studied by Azzali (1953, 1954, 1955), Barry
(1954), Suomalainen (1960), Troyer (1965, 1968) and Shapiro et al. (1966).

## Material and Methods

Observations were carried out on 30 male specimens of the mouse-eared bat (Myotis
myotis Borkhausen) captured in the Bat Cave near Ojców at the beginning of March (1st group,
15 specimens) and at the end of June (2nd group, 15 specimens).

The animals were anaesthetized with ether and killed by decapitation. After prompt and
broad exposure of the brain the preparation was immersed in Bouin's solution for a few
minutes. Then a block of tissue containing the diencephalon and adjoining structures of the
brain was excised; it was covered by bone only on the ventral side. The material was kept in
Bouin solution for six days; then the bones surrounding the hypophysis were removed and the
tissue bloc embedded in paraffin. Series of longitudinal or transverse sections, 7 μ thick, were
divided and mounted alternatingly so that from each brain two comparable series were obtained. One of them was stained with aldehyde fuchsine (AF), and orange G, light green FCF
and chromotrope 2 R as counterstain, while the other was stained with chrome-alum-hemat-
oxylin-phloxine (CHP).

By using an Abbe apparatus the nuclei of secretory cells in the n. paraventricularis (NPV)
and n. supraopticus (NSO) were drawn; only those were selected which contained well marked
nucleoli and where the cytoplasm contained a varying number of "Gomori-positive" granules.
In the NPV 100 nuclei per specimen were drawn and measured, whereas in the NSO 300 nuclei
were thus analyzed. Then the volume of the cellular nuclei was calculated (Rapola et al., 1965).
For the NPV this value was computed in 10 specimens of the first and second groups. Similar
calculations were made for cell nuclei in the NSO in 5 specimens of each group, but in every
case the determinations were carried out in three regions of the NSO: anterior, medialis and
posterior. Altogether the volume of 4,800 nuclei was estimated. Finally Student's t-test was
employed but in all cases differences between the mean values of the groups compared were
statistically insignificant ($p > 0.05$). The average nuclear volumes in cells of the NPV were
compared within the first and second group as well as between these groups. A similar
procedure was employed in the case of the NSO but the number of calculations was larger
since the measurements were made in three different regions of this nucleus in each of 10 specimens.

## Observations

*Morphology of the Neurosecretory System.* The area of the ventral hypothalamus, where the neurons show a "Gomori-positive" reaction, is particularly
broad in the mouse-eared bat and extends up to 1.2 mm in the antero-posterior
axis and 2.8 mm in the lateral plane. The anterior end of the NSO reaches the
optic chiasma occupying a lateral position in relation to it. The posterior border
of the nucleus appears at the most rostral region of the pars tuberalis. Although
the NSO is paired, some cells wedged between the fibres of the optic tract and the
ventral surface of the hypothalamus bring the two parts together. The distribution
of cells in the NSO allows the distinction of three regions, one anterior (NSOa),
with neurons situated in front of the optic tract, the other, medialis (NSOm) with
neurons distributed within this tract, and lastly the posterior (NSOp), formed by

cells placed on the caudal side of the optic tract (Fig. 1). The anterior and posterior parts of the NSO are formed by numerous and compact cell groups, whereas the medial part is more scattered. Cells forming this part are arranged in a single layer or, in some places, in two layers.

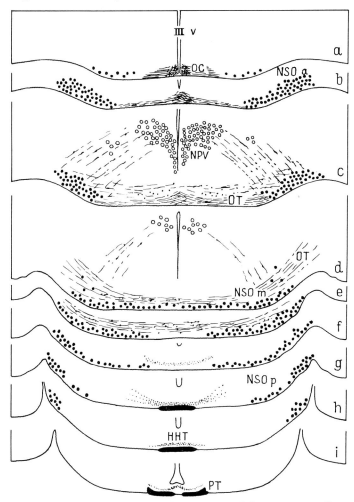

Fig. 1 a–i. Semischematic diagram showing distribution of "Gomori-positive" neurons in the hypothalamus of the mouse-eared bat. The drawing was made with an Abbé apparatus from transverse serial sections of the hypothalamus. The distances between individual sections differ. The true distance between sections a and i is 1 mm. *HHT* hypothalamo-hypophysial tract, *NPV* nucleus paraventricularis, *NSO a, m, p* nucleus supraopticus pars anterior, medialis and posterior, *OC* optic chiasma, *PT* pars tuberalis, *III V* third ventricle. ×35

On both sides of the third ventricle there is the nucleus paraventricularis directly adjoining the ependymal lining of the ventricle. The cells of this nucleus are rather scattered and their largest concentration is visible only in the dorso-lateral part of the nucleus. Hence in contrast to the NSO, the spatial distribution of the NPV in the mouse-eared bat is typical of mammals. A small and scattered

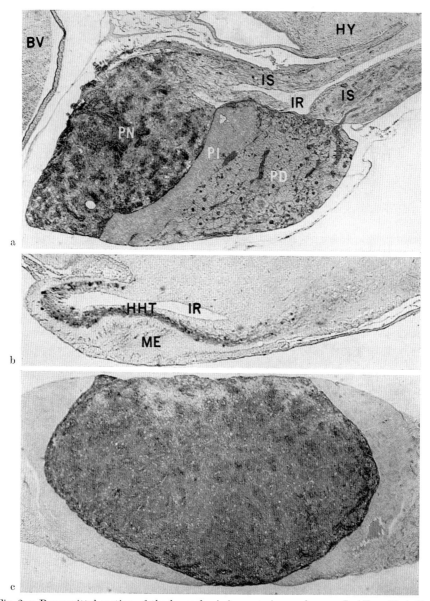

Fig. 2. a Parasagittal section of the hypophysis in a specimen of group I. AF. ×80. b Parasagittal section of the infundibular stem in a specimen of group I. AF. ×90. c Frontal section of the hypophysis in a specimen of group II. Note that laterally the pars nervosa is surrounded by pars intermedia and pars distalis. Also note quantity and distribution of AF-positive substance in pars nervosa in Fig. a and c, as well as lack of this substance in the median eminence in Fig. b. *BV* blood vessel, *IS* infundibular stem, *ME* median eminence, *PD* pars distalis, *PI* pars intermedia, *PN* pars nervosa. AF. ×80

group of AF- and CHP-positive neurons, situated laterally to the NPV, corresponds to the accessory paraventricular nucleus described by TROYER (1965) in *Myotis lucifugus lucifugus* (Fig. 1 c).

Relatively numerous axons derived from the cells of NSO-pars anterior run towards the opposite side of the hypothalamus. Due to this fact the axons from the right and left nucleus are thoroughly mixed prior to the formation of a compact, common tract. The majority of axons leaving the NPV run by the shortest way to the NSO cells in the more lateral position. Hence the formation of the hypothalamo-hypophysial tract (HHT), containing fibres from both nuclei, NSO and NPV, takes place already at the pars anterior of the NSO, while at the level of the pars caudalis of the NSO it appears as a compact tract well separated from other structures of the hypothalamus. A certain number of fibres leaving the NPV runs directly backwards joining the HHT in the infundibular stem. There the HHT fibres are distributed directly under the ependymal layer lining the infundibular recess. The majority of axons of this tract is situated in the ventral wall of the infundibulum, which is much thicker than the dorsal wall.

The ventral wall of the infundibular stem forms the median eminence (ME), clearly separated owing to several characteristic features: (1) The infundibular wall reaches here the greatest thickness and is delimited on both sides by deep fissures filled with connective tissue, and/or the cells of the pars tuberalis. (2) The broad infundibular recess, appearing on cross section as a dorso-ventrally flattened cavity, forms in the centre of the ME a narrow, vertical fissure. (3) Capillaries of the ME penetrate the whole depth of the palisade layer, whereas in other areas of the infundibular stem they are situated just under the surface. (4) The infundibular stem is surrounded by the pars tuberalis except for the region corresponding to the median eminence.

The hypothalamo-hypophysial tract ends in the neurohypophysis where the familiar accumulation of neurosecretory terminals around the vascular network is seen. Single neurosecretory axons were also found in the pars intermedia; the pars distalis is devoid of neurosecretory fibers.

*Group I: Hibernating Animals.* The quantity of "Gomori-positive" substance in the cytoplasm of NSO cells is small. Fine granules of this substance are in general evenly distributed in the cell body. Numerous cells are partially or completely devoid of neurosecretory substance, while exceptional cells are heavily loaded with granules (Fig. 3a). The average volume of cell nuclei in the pars anterior, medialis and posterior of the NSO amounts to 348.60, 325.66 and 386.25 $\mu^3$, respectively. The differences among these values are not significant, and this criterion has no functional meaning. The mean nuclear volume for the whole NSO amounts to 353.54 $\mu^3$ in the first group.

The NPV cells are smaller than the NSO cells. Their cytoplasm contains moderate amounts of neurosecretory substance, evenly distributed. The mean nuclear volume in nine specimens studied is 282.18 $\mu^3$ (range from 226.24 to 334.88 $\mu^3$).

The proximal portions of the HHT axons are in some places slightly thickened. In the infundibular stem the whole hypothalamo-hypophysial tract is strongly "Gomori-positive", and the bead-like varicosities of axons reach the size of large spheres, deeply stained with AF or CHP. The median eminence does not contain neurosecretory substance outside of the HHT, whereas the pars nervosa is full of it. It is mainly located around blood vessels and directly under the surface of the pars nervosa (Fig. 2a, b).

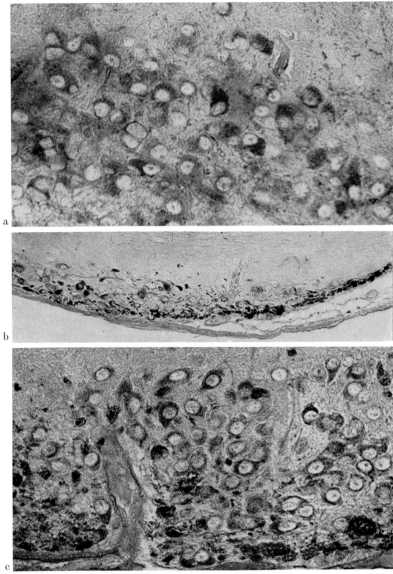

Fig. 3. a Part of n. supraopticus in a specimen of group I. The cytoplasm in some cells is heavily loaded with AF-positive substance, but in the majority of cells it appears in smaller amounts, and selectively stained granules are scattered evenly in the perikarya. Frontal section. AF. ×500. b Lower magnification of ventral part of the hypothalamus containing NSO cells. Numerous Herring bodies and fragments of axons strongly stained with aldehyde fuchsine are visible. Group II. Frontal section. ×180. c Fragment of n. supraopticus in a specimen of group II. Many cells are totally, or almost totally, devoid of fuchsinophilic granules. In other cells such granules occupy a juxtanuclear position. Large amounts of AF-positive substance situated beyond the perikarya are visible. Cross-section. ×500

*Group II: Active Animals.* The quantity of neurosecretion is markedly reduced in the cells of both neurosecretory nuclei, especially in the NSO. The "Gomori-positive" granules are irregularly distributed in the cytoplasm and accumulate mainly in a juxtanuclear position. Many cells are completely devoid of these granules. The volume of cell nuclei does not differ significantly. In the NPV cells it amounts to 271.72 $\mu^3$ on the average, varying from 210.34 to 328.82 $\mu^3$, whereas in the NSO it equals 345.04 $\mu^3$ with the following values corresponding to the pars anterior, medialis and posterior, respectively: 342.52, 351.12 and 341.49 $\mu^3$. The area of the nucleus supraopticus is rich in neurosecretory substance localized extracellularly, and gives a strong "Gomori-positive" reaction (Fig. 3 b, c). On the other hand, the hypothalamo-hypophysial tract in the region of the infundibular stem contains only negligible amounts of neurosecretion. The pars nervosa, on the contrary, is rich in this substance being distributed there almost evenly and only slightly condensed in the vicinity of blood vessels (Fig. 2 c). Emphasis should also be placed on the accumulation of AF- and CHP-positive granules around capillaries in the palisade layer of the median eminence.

## Discussion

A characteristic feature of the neurosecretory system of *Myotis myotis* is the wide distribution of NSO cells in the ventral hypothalamus. A similarly widespread nucleus supraopticus was described in other species of bats (BARRY, 1958; AZZALI, 1953, 1954; TROYER, 1965). Although some cells of the NSO-pars posterior occupy sites corresponding to those of other nuclei of the hypothalamus (see: TROYER, 1965), they are typical secretory neurons, both in *Myotis myotis* and other species of bats. Hence it is difficult to decide whether the characteristic appearance of the NSO in bats results from the territorial expansion of its cells, or from modulations of cells of other nuclei of the hypothalamus. The distinction of three regions of the NSO is quite arbitrary, since no morphological or functional differences have been demonstrated.

The majority of HHT fibres reach the pars nervosa where the axons end in the proximity of blood vessels. The presence of neurosecretory granules in the vascular area of the median eminence in specimens captured in June indicates, however, that some HHT fibres have their endings there, and that the "Gomori-positive" substance may be released into the hypophyseal portal system. Similar observations indirectly indicating a participation of "Gomori-positive" neurosecretion in the control of pars distalis activity were made in amphibians, reptiles and birds (FARNER and OKSCHE, 1962; KOBAYASHI, 1964; KOBAYASHI *et al.*, 1965; JASIŃSKI and GORBMAN, 1967; ZAMBRANO and DE ROBERTIS, 1968a). The possibility of a functional association between the "Gomori-positive" neurosecretory system and sexual activity in mammals is postulated among others by HAGEDOORN (1966) and ZAMBRANO and DE ROBERTIS (1968b).

Differences in the amount and distribution of neurosecretory substance in the mouse-eared bat in the final stage of hibernation and during summer activity are small, with the exception of the HHT. Still they indicate a conspicuous correlation between the activity rhythm of the neurosecretory system and the actual level of metabolism. Moderate amounts of neurosecretory granules present in the NSO or NPV cells, strong "Gomori-positive" reaction of HHT fibres, and accumulation of neurosecretion in the perivascular portions of axons indicate a relatively high activity of the whole system in the final period of hibernation.

In connection with the requirement for water retention in hibernating bats several suggestions emerge:

1. Biological adaptations of the hibernation period (see: Introduction) reduce the loss of water and in consequence probably inhibit the release of neurosecretion.

2. Even though the neurosecretory system abounds in Gomori-positive substance during hibernation (Azzali, 1955; Barry, 1954; Troyer, 1965; Shapiro et al., 1966), this does not amount to total inhibition of its synthesis and release. It only seems that a radical slowdown of metabolic processes is accompanied by a reduction of the impulses leading to the release of neurosecretion.

3. Lack of fundamental differences in the quantity of neurosecretion in the pars nervosa from hibernating and active specimens suggests that bats might acquire the ability of water retention under the influence of small amounts of ADH. A refractory reaction of the neurosecretory system to osmotic stress is known to occur in some vertebrates (Howe and Jewell, 1959; Uemura, 1964; Jasiński and Gorbman, 1967), but only among those inhabiting hot and dry regions.

4. The pars intermedia in bats is large (Green, 1951; Herlant, 1956). The relationship between the development of the pars intermedia and tolerance to desiccation shown by Legait and associates (Legait and Legait, 1962; Legait et al., 1963) is valid probably also in bats.

## Summary

The morphology of the hypothalamo-hypophysial neurosecretory system of the mouse-eared bat, Myotis myotis Borkhausen, in the final stage of hibernation (March) and during summer activity (June) is described. The neurosecretory substance in the supraoptic and paraventricular nuclei, and especially in the hypothalamo-hypophysial tract, appears in larger quantities in hibernating bats than in active specimens. The pars nervosa of the hypophysis abounds in this substance in both groups of bats, although in hibernating animals it is markedly accumulated in close vicinity to blood vessels. Determinations of the nuclear volume in cells of the NSO and NPV showed no significant differences between the two groups of bats.

It seems that during hibernation the synthesis and release of neurosecretory material are markedly slowed down but not entirely inhibited. This and other suggestions concerning water retention during hibernation are briefly discussed.

### References

Allen, G. M., Bats. New York: Dover Publications, Inc. 1962.
Azzali, G.: Ricerche sulla neurosecrezione ipotalamica nei chirotteri. Riv. Biol. 45, 131–149 (1953).
— L'apparato neurosecretorio diencefalo-ipofisario negli animali ibernanti (chiroptera e Myoxus glis). Arch. ital. Anat. Embriol. 59, 142–158 (1954).
— Il comportamento dell'apparato neurosecretorio ipotalamo-ipofisario nell'ibernazione e nell'ipotermia artificiale. Acta neuroveg. (Wien) 11, 72–89 (1955).
Bargmann, W., Scharrer, E.: The site of origin of the hormones of the posterior pituitary. Amer. Scientist 39, 255–259 (1951).
Barry, J.: De l'existence de voies neurosécrétoires hypothalamotélencéphaliques chez la chauve souris (Rhinolophus ferrum equinum) en état d'hibernation. Bull. Soc. Scient. Nancy 13, 126–136 (1954).
— Des voies neurosécrétoires extrahypophysaires et le problème de l'action nerveus e centrale des hormones posthypophysaires. J. Méd. Lyon 20, 1065–1074 (1958).

BROSSET, A.: La biologie des Chiroptères. Paris: Masson & Cie. 1966.

FARNER, D. S., OKSCHE, A.: Neurosecretion in Birds. Gen. comp. Endocr. **2**, 113–147 (1962).

GAISLER, J.: The winter activity of coulour-marked bats in the cavities of Květnice. Probl. Spel. Res. **2**, 207–229 (1966).

GREEN, J. D.: The comparative anatomy of the hypophysis, with special reference to its blood supply and innervation. Amer. J. Anat. **88**, 225–311 (1951).

HAGEDOORN, J. P.: Hypothalamic neurosecretory activity in relation to the reproductive cycle in the common striped skunk (*Mephitis mephitis nigra*; order Carnivora). Z. Zellforsch. **75**, 1–10 (1966).

HARMATA, W.: The thermopreferendum of some species of bats (Chiroptera). Acta theriol. **14**, 49–62 (1969).

HERLANT, M.: Corrélations hypophyse-génitales chez la femelle de la Chauve-Souris, *Myotis myotis*. Arch. Biol. (Liège) **68**, 89–280 (1956).

HOWE, A., JEWELL, P. A.: Effects of water deprivation upon the neurosecretory material of the desert rat *(Meriones meriones)* compared with the laboratory rat. J. Endocr. **18**, 118–124 (1959).

JASIŃSKI, A., GORBMAN, A.: Hypothalamic neurosecretion in the Spadefoot Toad, *Scaphiopus hammondi*, under different environmental conditions. Copeia **2**, 271–279 (1967).

— — HARA, T.: Activation of the preoptico-hypophysial neurosecretory system through olfactory afferents in fishes. In: Neurosecretion (F. STUTINSKY, ed.), p. 106–123. Berlin-Heidelberg-New York: Springer 1967.

KOBAYASHI, H.: Histochemical, electron microscopic and pharmacologic studies on the median eminence. Excerpta med. Intern. Congr. **83**, 570–576 (1964).

— HIRANO, T., OOTA, Y.: Electron microscopic and pharmacological studies on the median eminence and pars nervosa. Arch. Anat. micr. **54**, 277–294 (1965).

KOWALSKI, K.: Cave dwelling bats in Poland and their protection [in Polish with English summary]. Ochrona Przyrody **21**, 58–77 (1953).

KRZANOWSKI, A.: Some major aspects of population turnover in wintering bats in the cave at Puławy (Poland). Acta theriol. **3**, 27–42 (1959).

— Weight dynamics of bats wintering in the cave at Puławy (Poland). Acta theriol. **4**, 249–264 (1961).

LEGAIT, E., LEGAIT, H., CHARNOT, Y.: Etude histophysiologique de la «pars intermedia» de l'hypophyse de quelques ongulés. Ann. Endocr. (Paris) **70**–79 (1963).

LEGAIT, H., LEGAIT, E.: Relationships between the hypothalamus and pars intermedia in some mammals and amphibians. Mem. Soc. Endocr. **12**, 165–173 (1962).

RAPOLA, J., HEINONEN, E.-L., HELPINEN, A., HENRIQUES, U.: Metamorphosis and neurosecretion of *Xenopus laevis*. Acta endocr. (Kbh.). **49**, 305–311 (1965).

SHAPIRO, B. I., IVANIAN, A. K., NOMONOKOVA, L. M.: Seasonal changes in nuclei of anterior hypothalamus, subcommissural organ and epiphysis in some bats (Chiroptera). Arch. Anat. Gistol. Embryol. [in Russian] **51**, 7, 42–48 (1966).

SUOMALAINEN, P.: Stress and neurosecretion in the hibernating hedgehog. Bull. Mus. Comp. Zool. **124**, 271–284 (1960).

TINKLE, D. W., PATTERSON, I. S.: A study of hibernating populations of *Myotis velifer* in Northwestern Texas. J. Mammalogy **46**, 612–633 (1965).

TROYER, J. R.: Neurosecretion in the hibernating bat. The morphology of the hypothalamo-hypophyseal system. Anat. Rec. **151**, 77–92 (1965).

— Neurosecretory material in the supraoptico-hypophyseal tract of the bat throughout the hibernating and summer periods. Anat. Rec. **162**, 407–424 (1968).

UEMURA, H.: Effects of water deprivation on the hypothalamo-hypophysial neurosecretory system of the grass parakeet, *Melopsittacus undulatus*. Gen. comp. Endocr. **4**, 193–198 (1964).

ZAMBRANO, D., DE ROBERTIS, E.: Ultrastructure of the peptidergic and monoaminergic neurons in the hypothalamic neurosecretory system of Anuran Batracians. Z. Zellforsch. **90**, 230–244 (1968a).

— — The effect of castration upon the ultrastructure of the rat hypothalamus. I. Supraoptic and paraventricular nuclei. Z. Zellforsch. **86**, 487–498 (1968b).

# Contribution à l'étude du système hypothalamo-neurohypophysaire au cours de l'hibernation

E. Legait, C. Burlet* et J. Marchetti**

**Key words:** Hypothalamo-neurohypophysial system — *Eliomys quercinus* — Hibernation — Histophysiology.

*Summary.* During the winter, the temperature of the environment plays an important role in the modifications of the hypothalamo-neurohypophyseal system of the garden doormouse.

At $4°C$, the first phase of hibernation shows periods of hypoactivity separated by phases of hormone release and important hormonal synthesis. At the end of hibernation, hypoactivity is observed. The contents of the neurohypophysis in A.D.H. are as follows: 1.54 UI before hibernation; 6.35 UI in the middle of the winter; 4.19 shortly before awakening; 2.10 UI one hour after awakening.

At $22°C$, the periods of varying activity are reversed.

Acid phosphatase activity does not seem to intervene in the liberation of anti-diuretic hormone but is increased in the neurohypophysis during phases of release and decreased in the supraoptic nuclei during phases of inactivity.

The hypothalamo-neurohypophyseal system plays an important role during the alternating periods of awakening and sleep in the winter and spring. Adrenalectomy, which suppresses hibernation, determines hyperactivity of this system. Absence of dormancy may be due to increased sensitivity to stress of the hypothalamic nuclei and increased hormone release.

The successive periods of discharge of the posthypophyseal hormones at the beginning of hibernation influence the physiological evolution of the other endocrine glands that are hypoactive at the beginning of hibernation but present histological signs of activation before awakening.

## Introduction

Les modifications endocrinologiques provoquées par l'hibernation sont le plus souvent interprétées comme la conséquence d'une phase de repos induite par la léthargie; la plupart des glandes endocrines présentent, au moins dans la première partie du sommeil, des signes histophysiologiques d'hypoactivité; cependant quelques auteurs ont déjà signalé l'évolution tout à fait particulière des éléments intervenant dans l'homéostasie électrolytique, c'est-à-dire la zone glomérulée du cortex surrénal (Engel, Raths et Schultze, 1957; Gabe, Agid, Martoja, M. C. Saint-Girons et H. Saint-Girons, 1964; Bloch et Canguilhem, 1966) et le système

---

* Laboratoire d'Histologie, Faculté de Médecine, Nancy (Directeur: Professeur E. Legait).
** Laboratoire de Physiologie, Faculté de Médecine, Nancy (Directeur: Professeur P. Arnould). — Section du Métabolisme hydrominéral (Directeur: Professeur M. Boulange).

hypothalamo-neurohypophysaire (Azzali, 1953; Suomalainen, 1956; Gabe et coll., 1964). Ces auteurs observent, au cours de l'hiver, une charge neurosécrétoire accrue dans la neurohypophyse puis une disparition rapide du neurosécrétat au cours du réveil printannier. Cette accumulation pendant le sommeil est attribuée par certains à un hyperfonctionnement des centres neurosécrétoires, par d'autres à un arrêt de l'excrétion hormonale à partir de la neurohypophyse.

C'est pour tenter d'apporter des preuves à l'une ou à l'autre de ces hypothèses que nous avons entrepris ce travail.

## Matériel et méthodes

Cette étude porte sur 350 lérots (*Eliomys quercinus* L.) adultes mâles ou femelles; 250 sont placés dans des conditions de température et d'éclairement proches de l'environnement naturel, 80 sont conservés durant toute l'année à une température de 20 à 22°C; sur les animaux restants, nous avons recherché les influences de certaines conditions expérimentales sur le système neurosécrétoire supra-optique: la surrénalectomie bilatérale, l'anesthésie à l'éther ou à l'alcool, le stress au bruit, des injections intrapéritonéales de dexaméthasone[1] (500 μg/100 g de poids corporel) et de L8 Vasopressine[1] (3 mU/100 g de poids corporel, 3 fois par semaine durant 5 semaines).

L'étude histophysiologique du système hypothalamo-neurohypophysaire est effectuée par les techniques suivantes:

Les recherches volumétriques et caryométriques sont effectuées sur coupes à la paraffine de l'hypophyse et des régions hypothalamiques fixées au Bouin Hollande sublimé et colorées à l'hématoxyline chromique phloxine ou au P.A.S. bleu alcian (pH 0,2) orange G.

Les détections histoenzymologiques se font sur coupes à la congélation de 10 à 15 μ d'épaisseur pour les hypophyses, de 20 à 25 μ pour l'hypothalamus après fixation de 1 à 3 heures dans du formol neutre froid à 10%.

Les acétylcholinestérases sont mises en évidence par la méthode de Koelle et Geesey (1961) après incubation dans le D.F.P. ($10^{-4}$ M) pour inhiber les cholinestérases non spécifiques.

Les phosphatases alcalines, pH 9, par la méthode de Gomori.

Les phosphatases acides par la méthode de Burstone (1961) utilisant le naphtol-As-Mx-phosphate et le Fast-Red-Violet-Salt. Le dosage colorimétrique de ces activités est effectué à l'aide d'une semi-micro-méthode utilisant le P-nitrophénylphosphate à ($2.10^{-3}$ M) sur broyat total de la neurohypophyse ou des régions disséquées du Noyau Supra Optique (N.S.O.) dans un milieu tamponné par un mélange acétate-acétique sans adjonction d'ions activateurs. L'activité, mesurée à l'aide du spectrophotomètre Eppendorf à la longueur d'onde de 405 mμ, est exprimée en μg de p-nitrophénol libéré par mg de tissu en 40 minutes d'incubation à 37°C.

L'hormone antidiurétique neurohypophysaire est dosée par la méthode de l'inhibition de la diurèse du rat éthanolisé en surcharge hydrique (méthode de Berde et Cerletti, 1961). Nos solutions sont préparées à partir d'extrait acide de neurohypophyse isolée, déshydratée pendant 24 heures dans l'acétone froid puis sous vide en présence d'anhydride phosphorique pendant 3 heures. Chaque fragment est pesé à 0,5 μg près, à l'aide de l'électrobalance Cahn-Gram. L'activité hormonale est exprimée en unité d'hormone antidiurétique contenue dans chaque neurohypophyse ou rapportée à 0,1 mg de poids sec.

## Resultats

### A. Le système hypothalamo-neurohypophysaire du lérot

#### a) Les noyaux supra-optiques (N.S.O.)

Au cours de la vie active, l'aspect histologique des N.S.O. est peu différent de celui des autres Rongeurs; le peu d'abondance du neurosécrétat à l'intérieur des corps cellulaires et le long des fibres est assez caractéristique. Les noyaux hypo-

1 Nous remercions très vivement les Laboratoires Roussel qui ont aimablement fourni la dexaméthasone et les Laboratoires Sandoz qui nous ont procuré la L8 Vasopressine.

thalamiques se distinguent électivement du reste du tissu nerveux par une importante activité acétylcholinestérasique qui se trouve concentrée à la surface des corps cellulaires. Peu riches en phosphatases alcalines, ils présentent une très forte activité phosphatasique acide ; des dosages colorimétriques de ces activités à l'aide du p-nitrophénylphosphate et du naphtol-As-Mx-phosphate font apparaître deux pH optimaux l'un à $4,4 \pm 0,2$, l'autre à $5,4 \pm 0,2$ ; le fluorure de sodium (0,01 M) provoque une baisse de 45% de ces activités, le tartrate de sodium (0,01 M) les diminue également de 25%, le citrate de sodium (0,01 M) ne détermine pas d'activation. Les caractéristiques de ces activités enzymatiques sont assez proches de celles observées par d'autres auteurs sur des types cellulaires différents : prostate, Fadl Man et King (1949) — cellules hépatiques, Goodlad et Mills (1957), Schuel et Anderson (1964) — cellules sanguines, Seeman et Palade (1967). Les hydrolases sont concentrées dans des granules cytoplasmiques plus nombreux dans le péricaryon que dans le cytoplasme périphérique ; la plus grande partie de ces granules sont les lysosomes décrits en nombre important dans toutes cellules nerveuses et plus particulièrement dans les cellules neurosécrétoires (Zambrano et de Robertis, 1966 ; Cotte et Picard, 1968). Cependant un certain nombre de ces formations peuvent être les granules neurosécrétoires, en cours de maturation, observés par Osinchak (1964) chez le rat. Les localisations de ces hydrolases sont identiques aux deux pH optimaux.

### b) La neurohypophyse

Des travaux antérieurs, effectués dans ce laboratoire (Legait et Roux, 1961 ; Legait, 1963 ; Contet, 1968), ont déjà souligné l'importance relative de la neurohypophyse des hibernants par rapport aux autres Rongeurs : loir 39,3%, lérot en activité 29,8%, lérot en hibernation 35,9%, muscardin : en été 27,3% en hiver 43,8%, souris albinos 10,9%, rat 7%.

Bien qu'au cours de la période d'activité des mois de mars et d'avril, la substance chromohématoxynophile de la neurohypophyse ne soit pas abondante, le contenu en hormone antidiurétique reste appréciable ; $3,31 \pm 1,72$ UI.

L'activité acétylcholinestérasique très discrète est le plus souvent diffuse autour des capillaires ; quelques rares fibres nerveuses, incluses dans le tractus neurosécrétoire ou se terminant au contact des capillaires sont révélées par cette activité enzymatique.

Les phosphatases alcalines neurohypophysaires sont exclusivement vasculaires comme chez la plupart des espèces déjà étudiées (Arvy, 1966). Nous retrouvons dans le parenchyme neurohypophysaire les deux pH optimaux des activités phosphatasiques acides, avec, cependant, des localisations différentes (Fig. 1) ; au pH le plus acide, elles sont diffuses dans le parenchyme et peuvent se trouver en plus forte quantité dans des amas ovoïdes de taille et de localisation identiques au corps de Herring. Au pH le moins acide, elles sont concentrées dans les parois capillaires et dans quelques rares corps de Herring. Lors d'une étude de ces mêmes activités enzymatiques dans la neurohypophyse d'autres Rongeurs et Batraciens (Burlet et Burlet, 1967), nous avons constaté que seuls les hibernants et les Batraciens possèdent des capillaires neurohypophysaires riches en hydrolases acides ; chez le rat, la souris, le mérion, ce sont les pituicytes et leurs prolongements qui présentent cette activité. L'équipement enzymatique particulier de ces capillaires nous a conduit comme d'autres auteurs (KAYSER, 1967) à établir une relation fonctionnelle entre le système neurosécrétoire des Batraciens qui sont des poïkilothermes et celui des Rongeurs hibernants qui le deviennent en hiver.

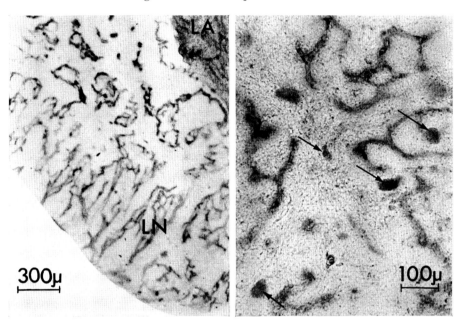

Fig. 1. Activité phosphatasique acide de la neurohypophyse; les capillaires présentent cette activité ainsi que des éléments de taille et de localisation identiques aux corps de Herring (flèche)

## B. Modifications du système hypothalamo-neurohypophysaire au cours de l'hibernation

Nous avons étudié les variations histophysiologiques de l'appareil neurosécrétoire au cours de l'hibernation sur deux lots d'animaux: le premier est maintenu à la température du laboratoire (20 à 22°C); les animaux, dans ce cas, ne présentent jamais de périodes de sommeil au sens strict, mais uniquement des phases de repos le plus souvent diurnes; ils se nourrissent normalement, leur poids augmente régulièrement au cours de l'hiver. Au printemps le pannicule adipeux est très développé, chez les mâles les testicules sont petits; des plages conjonctives envahissent la zone intermédiaire entre glomérulé et fasciculé de la corticosurrénale, ces images rappelant les signes de dégénérescence observés dans les surrénales de souris âgées.

Le second lot d'animaux est placé à la température constante de 4°C. Ces animaux s'endorment dans les 24 ou 48 heures qui suivent et présentent dans la première moitié de l'hibernation (40 à 50 jours) des phases de sommeil entrecoupées de courtes périodes de réveil nocturnes, la léthargie est plus profonde au cours de la seconde partie de l'hiver. Les animaux maigrissent progressivement, bien qu'ils puissent absorber de la nourriture lors des réveils. A la fin de chaque période de sommeil ils ont une vessie remplie d'urine qui se vide à l'occasion du réveil spontané. Au printemps le tractus et les glandes génitales sont développés, les cellules de la corticosurrénale histologiquement actives présentent de nombreuses figures de mitoses.

Les variations du système hypothalamo-neurohypophysaire pour chaque lot expérimental sont résumées dans les Fig. 2 et 3.

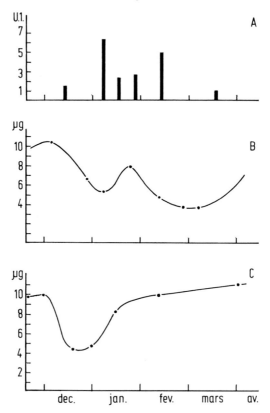

Fig. 2A–C. Evolution de l'appareil neurosécrétoire d'animaux maintenus à 22°C. A Contenu neurohypophysaire d'A.D.H. B Activités phosphatasiques neurohypophysaires à pH 4,4. C à pH 5,4

Nour constatons d'emblée que les évolutions sont inverses suivant les conditions de température.

A 22°C les premiers mois de l'hiver correspondent à une phase d'hypoactivité alors qu'une période d'hyperactivité se déroule ensuite. Les cellules neurosécrétoires sont peu importantes, très chromophiles, un certain nombre d'entre elles se picnosent. La neurohypophyse très volumineuse au début de l'hiver (0,460 mm³) contenant une quantité appréciable d'A.D.H. (6,49 UI) est moins développée en mars (0,280 mm³) et pauvre en A.D.H. (1,00 UI); le neurosécrétat est peu abondant.

A 4°C par contre, la période d'hyperactivité du système hypothalamo-neurohypophysaire se déroule au cours de la première moitié de l'hibernation, la fin de l'hibernation se traduisant par une phase d'hypoactivité; les cellules neurosécrétoires conservent de gros noyaux (9,4 μ de diamètre, 9,1 μ pour les animaux placés à 22°C). Dans cette première période les activités acétylcholinestérasiques restent très importantes. Dans la neurohypophyse on observe trois pics d'activité phosphatasique vasculaire. Au cours du premier pic d'activité qui se situe dans les 16 premières heures de l'hibernation, le contenu neurohypophysaire d'A.D.H.

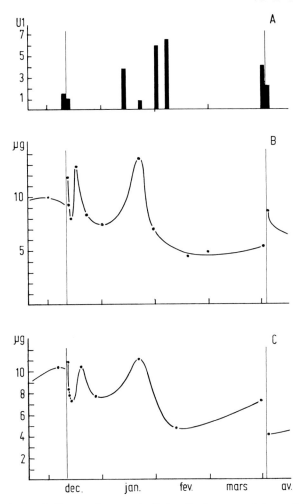

Fig. 3 A–C. Evolution de l'appareil neurosécrétoire d'animaux maintenus à 4°C. A Contenu neurohypophysaire d'A.D.H. B Activités phosphatasiques neurohypophysaires à pH 5,4. C à pH 4,4

passe de 1,54 UI à 1,09 UI. Au niveau du troisième pic, 40 à 43 jours après le début de l'hibernation, l'A.D.H. passe de 3,97 UI à 0,99 UI. Ces périodes de libération d'A.D.H. accompagnées des modifications histoenzymologiques de la neurohypophyse déclencheraient les phénomènes physiologiques entrainant les réveils; effectivement BENETATO (1966–1967) à provoqué le réveil et ses modifications physiologiques en injectant de la vasopressine à des spermophiles en hibernation.

C'est au milieu de l'hiver que le volume de la neurohypophyse est le plus important (0,447 mm³) et la quantité d'A.D.H. maximale (6,35 UI). Les pituicytes se vacuolisent et leurs noyaux s'hypertrophient.

La fin de l'hibernation se traduit par une chute d'activité des hydrolases acides à la fois du N.S.O. et de la neurohypophyse, le contenu d'A.D.H. neurohypophysaire diminue légèrement et passe de 6,35 UI à 4,19 UI en 50 jours; de nombreux corps de Herring riches en phosphatases acides sont identifiables.

Le réveil expérimental se traduit par une décharge brutale d'A.D.H.; dans les 20 premières minutes, le contenu hormonal de la neurohypophyse passe de 4,19 UI à 2,10 UI, puis 60 minutes après à 2,44 UI, le volume neurohypophysaire diminue brusquement de 0,431 à 0,319 mm³.

Comme de nombreux auteurs, nous pouvons donc conclure que la température de l'environnement en tant que facteur exogène, a une influence déterminante sur le déclenchement et l'évolution du sommeil hibernal; nous pouvons préciser que les modifications physiologiques du système hypothalamo-neurohypophysaire sont étroitement liées à l'abaissement de la température.

Lorsque les animaux sont placés dans des conditions proches de la nature, les activités phosphatasiques des noyaux supra-optiques restent importantes et en quantité relativement constante; dans la neurohypophyse l'évolution ne semble plus comparable, elles présentent des variations plus rapides et plus amples.

Habituellement rencontrées dans les cellules à métabolisme très actif; la présence de ces enzymes sur la membrane des granules neurosécrétoires immatures (Osinchak, 1964), dans les parois des capillaires neurohypophysaires et parfois dans les corps de Herring, nous a conduit à rechercher leur participation éventuelle aux processus de synthèse et de libération de l'hormone antidiurétique (A.D.H.).

## C. Modifications des activités phosphatasiques acides au cours de l'élaboration et de la libération de l'hormone antidiurétique

Au cours des mois d'octobre et de novembre, nous avons appliqué à certains animaux des stress: agressions systémiques ou anesthésie à l'éther, qui provoquent une augmentation de l'A.D.H. circulante (Lutz, Koch et Miahle-Voloss, 1967); d'autres lérots sont placés dans des conditions qui augmentent de façon appréciable la diurèse: anesthésie à l'alcool ou injection intrapéritonéale de dexaméthasone (Miahle-Voloss, Lutz et Koch).

Les variations des activités phosphatasiques acides sont indiquées dans les tableaux 1 et 2.

Nous constatons que les deux types d'activités enzymatiques évoluent dans le même sens au cours des phases de libération hormonale, consécutives à des agressions de courte durée (4 à 5 minutes pour le stress au son, 2 minutes pour l'anesthésie à l'éther); seules les activités neurohypophysaires se modifient. Par contre lorsque l'on place les animaux dans des conditions qui augmentent la diurèse, on constate que seules les activités enzymatiques hypothalamiques diminuent de 35% alors que celles de la neurohypophyse ne varient pas.

Il est donc possible de penser que ces enzymes n'interviennent pas directement dans le processus de libération puisque leurs modifications dans la neurohypophyse ne suivent pas toutes les variations d'excrétions hormonales; leur augmentation

Tableau 1. *Activités phosphatasiques acides à pH 4,4*

| Conditions expérimentales | Noyaux supraoptiques | | Neurohypophyse | |
|---|---|---|---|---|
| Animaux témoins lot No 1 | 6,16 | 0 | 6,29 | 0 |
| Animaux stressés par le son | 5,74 | −7% | 11,31 | +79% |
| Animaux anesthésiés à l'ether | 6,24 | 0% | 9,02 | +43% |
| Animaux soumis à la dexaméthasone (1 h) | 5,24 | −14% | 5,78 | −8% |
| Animaux témoins lot No 2 | 6,00 | 0 | 8,71 | 0 |
| Animaux anesthésiés à l'alcool | 4,95 | −17% | 9,26 | +6% |
| Animaux soumis à la dexaméthasone (16 h) | 3,92 | −35% | 9,36 | +7% |

Tableau 2. *Activités phosphatasiques acides à pH 5,4*

| Conditions expérimentales | Noyaux supraoptiques | | Neurohypophyse | |
|---|---|---|---|---|
| Animaux témoins lot No 1 | 6,69 | 0 | 8,03 | 0 |
| Animaux stressés par le son | 5,23 | −22% | 12,73 | +59% |
| Animaux anesthésiés à l'éther | 7,93 | +19% | 11,16 | +39% |
| Animaux soumis à la dexaméthasone (1 h) | 7,68 | +15% | 8,65 | +8% |
| Animaux témoins lot No 2 | 6,33 | 0 | 9,74 | 0 |
| Animaux anesthésiés à l'alcool | 6,35 | 0% | 9,06 | −7% |
| Animaux soumis à la dexaméthasone (16 h) | 3,96 | −37% | 9,69 | 0% |

lors de la libération de l'A.D.H. pourrait être plutôt envisagée comme une con-séquence des modifications métaboliques qui suivent l'excrétion (DOUGLAS, ISHIDA et POISNER, 1965; SACHS, SHARE, OSINCHAK et CARPI, 1967). Dans les éléments semblables aux corps de Herring, nous avons mis en évidence outre la présence d'hydrolases acides, du glycogène, des activités phosphorylasiques et glucose-6-phosphatasiques (LEGAIT et coll., 1967); ces formations pourraient peut-être, être envisagées comme des corps de Herring ne possèdant plus d'activité hormonale et en voie de résorption. Lors des arrêts de l'excrétion hormonale, la chute des activités phosphatasiques des corps cellulaires pourrait refléter la dimi-nution des activités métaboliques modifiant vraisemblablement elles-mêmes, l'ex-citabilité des cellules neurosécrétoires.

## Discussion

Le système hypothalamo-neurohypophysaire présente donc une évolution tout à fait particulière au cours de l'hibernation; les noyaux hypothalamiques con-servent des signes histophysiologiques et enzymologiques d'activité; des décharges neurohypophysaires d'A.D.H. correspondent à des périodes de réveil spontané plus nombreuses au début de l'hiver.

L'importance de l'action de ce système sur les alternances «éveil-sommeil» peut également être mise en évidence par l'étude des hibernants surrénalectomisés au cours des mois de novembre et décembre. KAYSER et PETROVIC (1958) avaient déjà remarqué que de tels animaux n'hibernent pas. Nous avons pour notre part effectué des constatations identiques, l'étude du système hypothalamo-neurohypo-physaire d'animaux surrénalectomisés nous montre que les noyaux hypothalami-ques possèdent de très gros noyaux (11,31 µ de diamètre, 9,40 chez les hibernants normaux), le neurosécrétat granulaire intracytoplasmique est peu abondant, les activités acétylcholinestérasiques et phosphatasiques acides sont plus importantes chez les opérés que chez les témoins, ce qui suggère un métabolisme plus actif et une excitabilité plus grande (Fig. 4). Dans la neurohypophyse, de nombreux corps de Herring sont identifiables et se présentent partiellement remplis de substance colorable par l'hématoxyline chromique ou le bleu alcian. La neurohypophyse d'un animal très peu actif, 14 jours après l'opération est criblée de lacunes et n'est pas

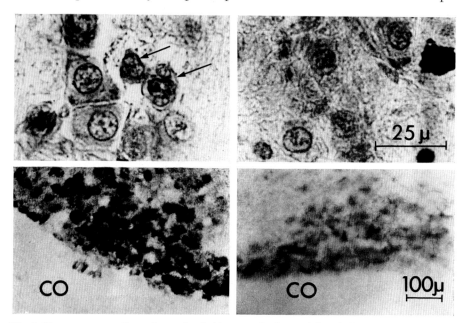

Fig. 4. Noyau supra-optique, à gauche de lérot surrénalectomisé et à droite de lérot témoin. Les photographies supérieures montrent les cellules neurosécrétoires colorées à l'hématoxyline chromique phloxine; après surrénalectomie on peut remarquer un début de pycnose (flèches). Les photographies inférieures montrent l'activité acétylcholinestérasique

sans rappeler une image que nous avions observé dans la neurohypophyse d'un animal normal sacrifié en septembre.

L'absence de sommeil de l'animal opéré serait donc la conséquence d'une hyperactivité soutenue du système hypothalamo-neurohypophysaire, c'est à dire, une plus grande sensibilité au stress et des décharges accrues d'hormone anti-diurétique.

Enfin, les quelques investigations que nous avons faites sur d'autres glandes endocrines: adénohypophyse, corticosurrénale, glandes génitales montrent que seuls les animaux ayant hiberné à basse température possèdent un peu avant le réveil et dès le printemps un système endocrine parfaitement fonctionnel. Chez le hérisson, Dubois et Girod (1967) ont constaté que dès février, les types cellulaires de l'adénohypophyse présentent des signes d'activité.

Nous avons voulu savoir si les décharges d'hormones neurohypophysaires peuvent intervenir dans l'évolution des glandes endocrines au cours de l'hibernation. Au cours des mois de décembre et janvier, nous avons donc fait des injections intrapéritonéales de 3 mU d'hormone antidiurétique 3 fois par semaine, pendant 5 semaines; un certain nombre de témoins reçoivent du sérum physiologique. Nous ne possédons actuellement que des résultats fragmentaires, mais il est intéressant de noter qu'à la suite des injections d'A.D.H., les animaux obèses perdent jusqu'à $^1/_4$ de leur poids. D'autre part, alors que l'adénohypophyse des animaux maintenus à 22°C est plus petite que celle des animaux qui hibernent (1,294 et 1,589 mg), l'adénohypophyse des animaux traités à l'A.D.H. est plus grosse que celle des animaux réveillés et ayant hiberné (1,919 et 1,830 mg).

En conclusion, nous pensons que le système hypothalamo-neurohypophysaire, très bien développé chez les hibernants, possède une signification physiologique particulière. Le début de l'hibernation se traduit par une série de décharges d'hormone post-hypophysaire accompagnées de réveils spontanés; la neurohypophyse possèdant à tout moment une charge importante en hormone antidiurétique, des stimulations extérieures accidentelles ou naturelles comme le réchauffement printannier peuvent provoquer une libération massive d'A.D.H., déclenchant le processus physiologique du réveil. Ces excrétions hormonales ne sont peut-être pas sans rapport avec l'évolution d'un certain nombre de glandes endocrines qui sont en phase de repos au début de l'hibernation et en état d'activité quelques temps avant le réveil.

## Résumé

Au cours de l'hiver, la température de l'environnement joue un rôle important sur les modifications du système hypothalamo-neurohypophysaire:

— à 4°C, la première partie de l'hibernation se traduit par des périodes d'hypoactivité séparées par des phases d'excrétion et de synthèse hormonales intenses; la fin de l'hibernation se caractérise par une hypoactivité; le contenu neurohypophysaire d'A.D.H. est de 1,54 UI avant l'hibernation; 6,35 UI au milieu de l'hiver; 4,19 un peu avant le réveil; 2,10 UI, 60 minutes après le réveil.

— à 22°C les évolutions sont inverses.

Les activités phosphatasiques acides ne semblent pas intervenir dans le déclenchement de la libération de l'hormone antidiurétique mais sont néanmoins augmentées au niveau de la neurohypophyse lors des phases d'excrétion et diminuées au niveau des noyaux supra-optiques lors des phases d'inhibition.

Ainsi le système hypothalamo-neurohypophysaire joue un rôle important sur les alternances réveil-sommeil au cours de l'hiver et au réveil printannier; la surrénalectomie, qui supprime chez les hibernants la léthargie hivernale, déclenche une hyperactivité de ce système; la plus grande sensibilité au stress des noyaux hypothalamiques et par conséquent l'excrétion hormonale accrue serait la cause de l'absence de sommeil.

Enfin les excrétions successives d'hormones posthypophysaires au début de l'hibernation participeraient peut-être à l'évolution physiologique des autres glandes endocrines, qui sont au repos au début du sommeil, mais présentent des signes histologiques d'activation avant le réveil.

# Bibliographie

Abul-Fadl, M. A. M., King, E. G.: Properties of the acid phosphatases of erythrocytes and of the human prostate gland. Biochem. J. **45**, 51–60 (1949).

Arvy, L.: Histo-enzymologie des glandes endocrines. Paris: Gauthier-Villars 1963.

— Les phosphatases du tissu nerveux. Paris: Hermann 1966.

Azzali, G.: Ricerche sulla neurosecrezione ipotalamica nei chirotteri. Riv. Biol. **45**, 131–139 (1953).

Benetato, Gr.: L'action des hormones neurohypophysaires sur le système nerveux central. Probl. act. Endocr. et Nutr. No 10, 291–322 (1966).

— Danieluc, E., Nestianu, V., Gabrielescu, G.: Concerning the effect of adeno- and neurohypophysial hormones on animals under hibernation conditions. Rev. roum. Physiol. **2**, 199–209 (1965).

Berde, B., Cerletti, A.: Über die diuretische Wirkung von synthetischem Lysin-Vasopressin. Helv. physiol. Acta **19**, 135–150 (1961).

Bloch, R., Canguilhem, B.: Cycle saisonnier d'élimination urinaire de l'aldostérone chez un hibernant *Cricetus cricetus*. Influence de la température. C. R. Soc. Biol. (Paris) **160**, 1500–1502 (1966).

Burlet, C., Burlet, A.: Mise en évidence de plusieurs activités phosphatasiques acides au niveau du système hypothalamo-hypophysaire. C. R. Soc. Biol. (Paris) **161**, 11, 2236–2240 (1967).

Burstone, M. S.: Histochemical demonstration of phosphatases in frozen section with Naphtol-As-phosphate. J. Histochem. Cytochem. **9**, 146–150 (1961).

Contet, J. L.: Recherches histophysiologiques sur le système hypothalamo-hypophysaire du muscardin (*Muscardinus avellanarius*). C. R. Ass. Anat. **141**, 719–727 (1968).

Cotte, G., Picard, D.: Etude ultrastructurale des neurones du noyau supra-optique du rat. Bull. Ass. Anat. (Nancy) **141**, 738–747 (1968).

Douglas, W. M., Ishida, A., Poisner, A. M.: The effect of metabolic inhibitors on the release of vasopressin from the isolated neurohypophysis. J. Physiol. (Lond.) **181**, 753–759 (1965).

Dubois, P., Girod, C.: Observations préliminaires sur l'ultrastructure des cellules antéhypophysaires chez le hérisson (*Erinaceus europaeus* L.) durant la période hivernale. C. R. Soc. Biol. (Paris) **161**, 813–816 (1967).

Engel, R., Raths, P., Schultze, W.: Die Aktivität der Zona glomerulosa beim Hamster und Goldhamster in Wachzustand, Winterschlaf und nach Belastungen. Z. Biol. **109**, 381–386 (1957).

Gabe, M., Agid, R., Martoja, M., Saint-Girons, M. C., Saint-Girons, H.: Données histophysiologiques et biochimiques sur l'hibernation et le cycle annuel chez *Eliomys quercinus* L. Arch. Biol. **75**, 1–187 (1964).

Goodlad, G. A. J., Mills, G. T.: The acid phosphatase of the rat liver. Biochem. J. **66**, 346–354 (1957).

Kayser, C.: Evolution de l'homéothermie incomplète. Les concepts de Claude Bernard sur le milieu intérieur, colloque international organisé pour la célébration du centenaire de la publication de l'introduction à l'étude de la médecine expérimentale de Claude Bernard (1965), p. 285–323. Foundation Singer-Polignac. Paris: Masson & Cie. 1967.

— Petrovic, A.: Rôle du cortex surrénalien dans le mécanisme du sommeil hivernal. C. R. Soc. Biol. (Paris) **152**, 519–522 (1958).

Koelle, G. B., Geesey, C. N.: Localization of acetylcholinesterase in the neurohypophysis and its functional implications. Proc. Soc. exp. Biol. (N.Y.) **106**, 625–628 (1961).

Legait, E., Legait, H., Burlet, C., Burlet, A.: Modifications de la charge glycogénique, des activités phosphorylasiques et glucose-6-phosphatasique au niveau du lobe nerveux de l'hypophyse. C. R. Soc. Biol. (Paris) **160**, 1659–1661 (1966).

Legait, H.: Recherches histophysiologiques sur le lobe intermédiaire de l'hypophyse. Nancy: Société d'impressions typographiques 1964.

— Roux, M.: Données morphologiques sur la pars intermedia de l'hypophyse des rongeurs. Bull. Ass. (Nancy) **113**, 462–468 (1961).

Lutz, B., Koch, B., Mialhe-Voloss, C.: Libération de l'Hormone antidiurétique au cours d'agressions systémique et neurotrope chez le rat. C. R. Acad. Sci. (Paris), Sér. D **266**, 1166–1168 (1968).

MIAHLE-VOLOSS, C., LUTZ, B., KOCH, B.: Effet inhibiteur de la dexaméthasone sur la sécrétion de la vasopressine et dosage de l'hormone antidiurétique. C. R. Acad. Sci. (Paris), Sér. D **264**, 2145–2147 (1967)

OSINCHAK, J: Electron microscopic localization of acid phosphatase and thiamine pyrophosphatase activity in hypothalamic neurosecretory cells of the rat. J. Cell Biol. **21**, 35–47 (1964).

SACHS, H., SHARE, L., OSINCHAK, J., CARPI, A.: Capacity of neurohypophysis to release vasopressin. Endocrinology **81**, 755–770 (1967).

SCHUEL, H., ANDERSON, N.: The distribution of acid phenyl-phosphatase activities in rat liver bei fractionated in the zonal ultracentrifuge. J. Cell Biol. **21**, 309–323 (1964).

SEEMAN, P. M., PALADE, G. E.: Acid phosphatase localization in rabbit eosinophils. J. Cell Biol. **34**, 745–756 (1967).

SUOMALAINEN, P.: Stress and neurosecretion in the hibernating hedgehog. Bull. Mus. Comp. Zool. **124**, 271–282 (1960).

ZAMBRANO, D., DE ROBERTIS, E.: The secretory cycle of supraoptic neurons in the rat. A structural functional correlation. Z. Zellforsch. **73**, 414–431 (1966).

# Weitere Befunde zum enzymhistochemischen Verhalten von Infundibulum und Hypophysenhinterlappen der Ratte nach beidseitiger Adrenalektomie

H. G. Goslar und R. Bock

Anatomisches Institut der Universität Bonn (Germany)

**Key words:** Infundibulum — Neural lobe — Rat — Adrenalectomy — Enzymes — Histochemistry.

Am Infundibulum der Rattenhypophyse lassen sich 3 Zonen unterscheiden: Das Ependym, die Zona interna und die Zona externa. Der in der Zona interna verlaufende Tractus supraoptico-hypophyseos kann aufgrund seines Neurosekretgehaltes nach dem Prinzip der Gomori-Methode (Gomori, 1941) elektiv dargestellt werden (Bargmann, 1949, u.a.). In der Zona externa, in der sich normalerweise nur wenige „Gomori-positive" Granula finden, verlaufen und endigen die Nervenfasern des tubero-hypophysären Systems.

Nach bilateraler Adrenalektomie ist eine in der 2. Woche p. o. einsetzende Vermehrung „Gomori-positiver" Granula im Bereich der Zona externa nachzuweisen (Arko, Kivalo und Rinne, 1963; Stöhr, 1969). Die Menge der auftretenden Granula kann durch Gaben von Corticoiden beeinflußt werden (Bock, v. Forstner, aus der Mühlen und Stöhr, 1969). Diese Befunde lassen annehmen, daß die besagten Granula als morphologisches Äquivalent eines Corticotropin-releasing factors oder seines Trägerproteins interpretiert werden können. Eine morphologische Zuordnung der Granula zu Nerven- oder Ependymfasern war aufgrund der lichtmikroskopischen Untersuchungen bisher noch nicht möglich.

Enzymhistochemische Untersuchungen an der Neurohypophyse bilateral adrenalektomierter Ratten ergaben neben einer Zunahme der Aminopeptidasen-Aktivität in der Zona externa infundibuli eine Abnahme der Esterasen-Aktivität in Ependym und Gliazellen (Pituicyten) von Infundibulum und Hypophysenhinterlappen (Bock und Goslar, 1969). Letzterer Befund führte zu der Vermutung, daß die betreffenden Zellen in den Regelkreis Nebenniere — Zwischenhirn — Hypophysenvorderlappen eingeschaltet sein und die in ihnen beobachteten Enzymveränderungen in unmittelbarem oder mittelbarem Zusammenhang zur Vermehrung der „Gomori-positiven" Granula in der Zona externa stehen könnten. Um einer Klärung dieses Problems näherzukommen, versuchten wir, die Esterasen im Tanycytenependym des 3. Ventrikels und in den Pituicyten des Hypophysenhinterlappens zu charakterisieren. Aus vorausgegangenen Blockierungsexperimenten hatte sich ergeben, daß die Enzyme Organophosphat-empfindlich und PCMB (p-Chlormercuribenzoat)-resistent sind, also der Gruppe der Aliesterasen angehören. Weitere Untersuchungen galten der Frage der Substratspezifität, vor allem in bezug auf die Länge der Fettsäurekette. Wir verwendeten hierfür relativ junge, männliche Wistarratten (Gewicht: 120–150 g) mit noch niedriger α-Naph-

thylacetatesterasen-Aktivität in Tanycyten und Pituicyten, um eine Substrat-
bedingte Steigerung der Reaktionsintensität besser erkennen zu können.

An Zwischenhirnschnitten dieser Tiere wurde die Spaltbarkeit der folgenden
Ester geprüft: α-Naphthylacetat, -propionat, -butyrat, -valerat, -capronat,
-caprylat, -nonanoat, -laurat und -myristat; Naphthol-AS-acetat, -ASMX-acetat,
-AS-D-acetat, -AS-D-Chlor-acetat.

Eine vergleichende Beurteilung der Reaktionsstärke bei Verwendung verschiedener Ester erfolgte immer nur an aufeinanderfolgenden Serienschnitten
*eines* Tieres. Die Untersuchungen ergaben ein Optimum der Spaltbarkeit bei
α-Naphthylbutyrat. Die im Vergleich zu α-Naphthylacetat oder -propionat zu
beobachtende Zunahme der Reaktionsintensität betraf Perikaryen und Fortsätze
der Tanycyten im Infundibulum und in der Wand des 3. Ventrikels. Ein gleiches
Verhalten zeigten die Pituicyten des Hypophysenhinterlappens. Bei steigender
Kettenlänge der Fettsäure wurde die Reaktion wieder schwächer, und zwar zunächst in den Perikaryen, dann auch in den Fortsätzen der Tanycyten und Pituicyten. Mit α-Naphthyllaurat oder -myristat ergab sich keine Reaktion mehr.
Letzterer Befund widerspricht in gewisser Weise früheren Ergebnissen, nach denen
im Bereich des Tanycytenependyms Tween 20 und Tween 60 (jedoch nicht
Tween 80) gespalten werden. Beide Beobachtungen sind jedoch miteinander zu
vereinbaren, wenn man einen störenden Einfluß der Naphtholkomponente an-
nimmt. Hierfür spricht, daß Ringsubstitution die Spaltbarkeit von α-Naphthylacetat verschlechtert.

Die untersuchten Esterasen lassen sich demnach wie folgt charakterisieren:
Es handelt sich weder um echte Lipasen (keine Reaktion mit Tween 80) noch
um Cathepsin-artige Enzyme (keine PCMB-Empfindlichkeit). Da ihre optimale
Aktivität das Buttersäure-Substrat betrifft, liegt es nahe, auch ihr physiologisches
Substrat in einem Ester dieser Fettsäure zu sehen. Hierfür käme z. B. ein Ester der
γ-Aminobuttersäure in Betracht, einer Substanz, die eine Rolle bei der Erregungs-
übertragung im Zentralnervensystem spielen soll. Von dieser Überlegung ausgehend
ist die Möglichkeit in Erwägung zu ziehen, daß die Glia- und Ependymelemente
der Neurohypophyse im Sinne einer Informationsübermittlung in den Regelkreis
Nebenniere — Zwischenhirn — Hypophysenvorderlappen eingeschaltet sind.

## Literatur

ARKO, H., KIVALO, E., RINNE, U. K.: Hypothalamo-neurohypophysial neurosecretion after
    the extirpation of various endocrine glands. Acta endocr. (Kbh.) **42**, 293–299 (1963).
BARGMANN, W.: Über die neurosekretorische Verknüpfung von Hypothalamus und Neuro-
    hypophyse. Z. Zellforsch. **34**, 610–634 (1949).
BOCK, R., FORSTNER, R. v., AUS DER MÜHLEN, K., STÖHR, PH. A.: Beiträge zur funktionellen
    Morphologie der Neurohypophyse. III. Über die Wirkung einer Corticoid- oder ACTH-
    Behandlung auf das Auftreten „gomoripositiver" Granula in der Zona externa infundibuli
    von Ratten und Mäusen nach beidseitiger Adrenalektomie oder Hypophysektomie. Z. Zell-
    forsch. **96**, 142–150 (1969).
— GOSLAR, H. G.: Enzymhistochemische Untersuchungen an Infundibulum und Hypo-
    physenhinterlappen der normalen und beidseitig adrenalektomierten Ratte. Z. Zellforsch.
    **95**, 415–428 (1969).
GOMORI, G.: Observations with differential stains on human islets of Langerhans. Amer. J.
    Path. **17**, 395–406 (1941).
STÖHR, PH. A.: Über quantitative Veränderungen „gomoripositiver" Substanzen in Infun-
    dibulum und Hypophysenhinterlappen der Ratte nach beidseitiger Adrenalektomie.
    Z. Zellforsch. **94**, 425–433 (1969).

# Elektronenmikroskopische Untersuchungen lichtmikroskopisch „gomoripositiver" Granula in Infundibulum und Hypophysenhinterlappen bilateral adrenalektomierter Ratten*

W. Wittkowski, R. Bock und C. Franken

Anatomisches Institut der Universität Bonn (West-Germany)

**Key words:** Infundibulum — Neural lobe — Rat — Adrenalectomy — Granules — Ultrastructure.

Bei der Ratte ist die Zona externa infundibuli lichtmikroskopisch so gut wie frei von gomoripositivem Material. Elektronenmikroskopisch enthalten die Nervenfasern der Zona externa normalerweise zahlreiche granuläre und agranuläre Vesikel verschiedener Größenordnung. Nach bilateraler Adrenalektomie kommt es lichtmikroskopisch zu einer erheblichen Vermehrung gomoripositiver Substanzen in der Zona externa. Unsere Bemühungen, ein ultrastrukturelles Äquivalent dieser Veränderung zu finden, blieben bei Anwendung herkömmlicher, in der Elektronenmikroskopie gebräuchlicher Fixierungs- und Kontrastierungsmethoden ohne Erfolg. Wir versuchten daher, die bei den lichtmikroskopischen Untersuchungen angewandte histologische Technik auf die Elektronenmikroskopie zu übertragen. Ein geeignetes Verfahren fand sich in der Chromalaun-Gallocyaninfärbung nach Bock (1966), die an Pikrinsäure-Formol-fixierten Schnitten ausgeführt wurde. Die Schnitte werden nach Abschluß des Färbeprozesses und Entwässerung mit Zyklonlack überzogen und getrocknet, anschließend vom Objektträger abgelöst und nach nochmaliger Trocknung mit Phosphorpentoxyd in Vestopal W eingebettet.

Nach der Einbettung sind mittels Stereomikroskop lichtmikroskopisch gomoripositiv erscheinende Strukturen wie neurosekretorische Ganglienzellen oder Herring-Körper noch deutlich erkennbar. Sie können mit dem Ultrotom gezielt geschnitten und im Elektronenmikroskop auf ihre Feinstruktur untersucht werden. Gomoripositive Substanzen stellen sich dann elektiv als Ansammlungen elektronendichter Granula dar (Abb. 1a, 2, 3). Mit Ausnahme der Zellkerne, die sich gut gegen das umgebende Cytoplasma abgrenzen lassen, sind andere Zellstrukturen kaum sichtbar (Abb. 2). An einem Herring-Körper der Zona interna ist das Ergebnis der Methode genauer zu studieren (Abb. 1a). Er besteht aus einer Anhäufung feingekörnter, wechselnd elektronendichter Elementargranula und bietet somit ein Bild, das bisherigen elektronenmikroskopischen Darstellungen des Herring-Körpers sehr ähnlich ist. Der Unterschied besteht lediglich darin, daß bei Glutaraldehydfixierung und Osmium-Bleikontrastierung der Kern der Granula

---

* Mit dankenswerter Unterstützung durch das Landesamt für Forschung NRW.

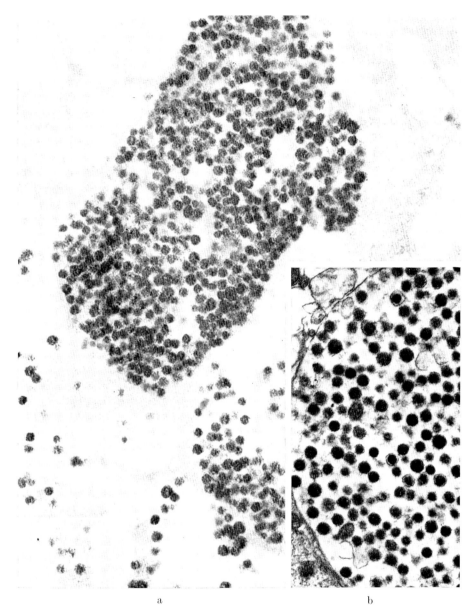

a                                    b

Abb. 1. a Herring-Körper in der Zona interna infundibuli einer adrenalektomierten Ratte nach Färbung mit Chromalaun-Gallocyanin. Endvergr. 18900×. b Ausschnitt aus einem Herring-Körper der Zona interna einer normalen Ratte bei Fixierung mit Glutaraldehyd und Osmium-Bleikontrastierung. Endvergr. 18900×

von einem Hof und einer Membran umgeben ist (Abb. 1b), während die angewandte Technik lediglich den Kern der Granula erfaßt.

Bei der elektronenmikroskopischen Untersuchung der gomoripositiven Strukturen in der Zona externa bilateral adrenalektomierter Ratten zeigte sich, daß

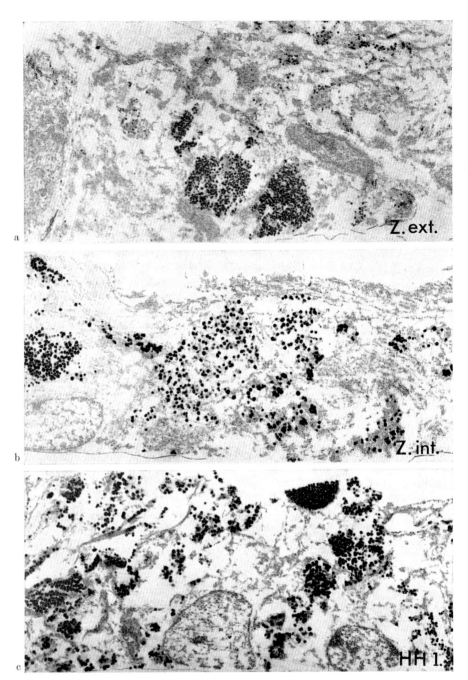

Abb. 2a—c. Übersichtsfotographien aus Zona externa, Zona interna und Hypophysenhinterlappen einer adrenalektomierten Ratte; Färbung mit Chromalaun-Gallocyanin; die Breite der
Bildstreifen entspricht der Dicke des lichtmikroskopischen Schnittes (10 μ). Die Grenzen
zwischen Gewebe und Vestopal sind zum Teil deutlich markiert. Die drei verschiedenen Ge-
webspartien enthalten in unterschiedlicher Ausdehnung und Dichte Ansammlungen von
Elementargranula. Klar erkennbar sind auch die Kerne der Pituicyten. Endvergr. a—c:
6290×

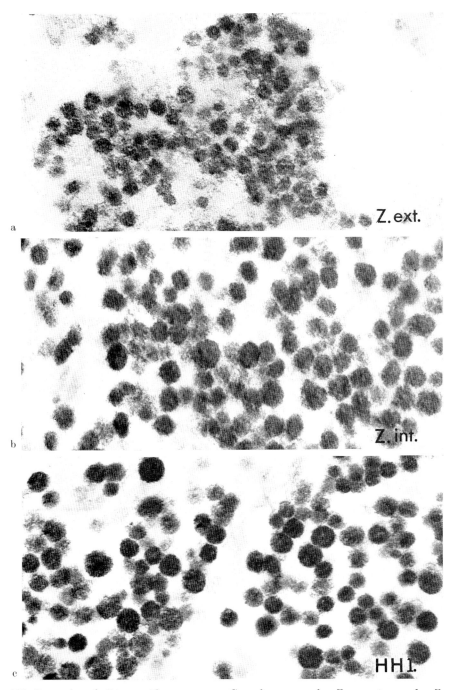

Abb. 3a—c. Ausschnittsvergrößerungen von Granulagruppen der Zona externa, der Zona interna und des Hypophysenhinterlappens. Die Granula in der Zona externa erscheinen deutlich kleiner als die in den beiden anderen Gewebsbezirken. Färbung mit Chromalaun-Gallocyanin. Endvergr. a—c: 48 600 ×

auch diese aus Elementargranula bestehen (Abb. 2a, 3a). Die Granula bilden meist kleinere Gruppen, ausnahmsweise treten sie auch in Form größerer Ansammlungen auf. Nach ersten vergleichenden Messungen scheinen sie mit einem Durchmesser von 700–1100 Å kleiner zu sein als die Elementargranula im Bereich der Zona interna und des Hypophysenhinterlappens, die Durchmesser zwischen 1000 und 1500 Å aufweisen (Abb. 3a, b, c). Dieser Befund würde darauf hinweisen, daß es sich bei den gomoripositiven Substanzen der Zona externa und der Zona interna um zwei verschiedene disulfidgruppenhaltige Peptide handelt.

## Literatur

Bock, R.: Über die Darstellbarkeit neurosekretorischer Substanz mit Chromalaun-Gallocyanin im supraoptico-hypophysären System beim Hund. Histochemie 6, 362–369 (1966).

# Structure and Function of the Liquor Contacting Neurosecretory System

I. Vigh-Teichmann and B. Vigh

Department of Histology and Embryology, Medical University (Head: I. Törö), Budapest (Hungary)

**Key words:** Neurosecretory nuclei — Vertebrates — Liquor contacting neurons.

The term *"liquor contacting neuronal system"* is used by us for elements of the central nervous system that are directly contacting the cerebrospinal fluid by their special, ventricular nerve endings (VIGH, TEICHMANN and AROS, 1968; VIGH, 1968a, b, 1969b; VIGH-TEICHMANN, 1968, 1970).

The *paraventricular organ* (Fig. 1a) was the first area where we could demonstrate liquor contacting neurons (VIGH, 1966). The paraventricular organ (or organon vasculosum hypothalami) (KAPPERS, 1920/21) is one of the ependymal organs of the third ventricle. The organ consists of a special ependyma and of a group of monoamine-containing neurons which was named nucleus organi paraventricularis (VIGH, 1966, 1967a, b, 1968a, 1969a; VIGH and TEICHMANN, 1966; VIGH, TEICHMANN and AROS, 1967; VIGH-TEICHMANN, VIGH and AROS, 1968; TEICHMANN, VIGH and AROS, 1968). The dendrites of these neurons protrude into the 3rd ventricle where they form bulb-like, ciliated nerve endings (RÖHLICH and VIGH, 1967; VIGH, 1968a, 1969b; BRAAK, 1968; PEUTE, 1968).

The second liquor contacting area we detected in the central nervous system, is the so-called *preoptic recess organ* (TEICHMANN and VIGH, 1968; VIGH-TEICHMANN, 1968; VIGH-TEICHMANN, RÖHLICH and VIGH, 1969; VIGH-TEICHMANN, VIGH and AROS, 1969). Its structure (Fig. 1b) resembles that of the paraventricular organ in so far as the ventricular dendrites of their nerve cells form also bulb-like, ciliated terminals in the lumen of the preoptic recess. Contrary to the paraventricular organ where a primary catecholamine and tryptamine can be observed with fluorescence histochemistry in the neurons, those of the preoptic recess organ are characterized by a content of noradrenaline.

On the basis of the morphological similarity of the liquor contacting neurons with receptor cells (*i.e.* regio olfactoria, taste buds, sensory cells of the skin of lower invertebrates, etc.), we think these liquor contacting neurons to be receptors.

Finally, we concluded that also the classic, Gomori-positive neurosecretory *preoptic nucleus* belongs to the liquor contacting neuronal system (TEICHMANN and VIGH, 1968; VIGH-TEICHMANN, 1968, 1970; VIGH-TEICHMANN and VIGH, 1968/69) as the neurosecretory cells build up bulb-like, ciliated liquor terminals (Fig. 1c). This relation to the cerebrospinal fluid casts new light on our knowledge of the neurosecretory system. Therefore, we tried to investigate the connection of the

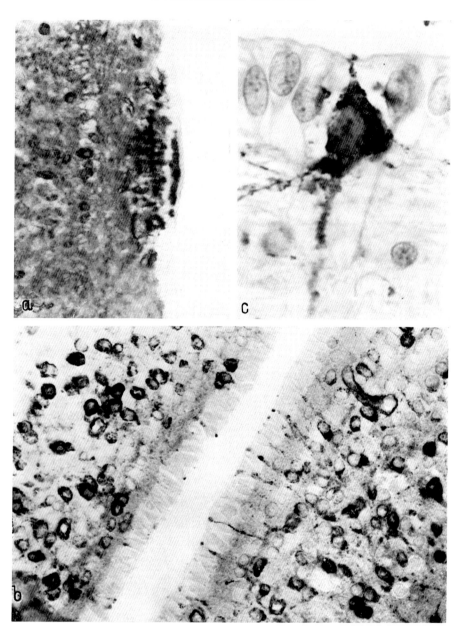

Fig. 1. a Paraventricular organ of *Lacerta viridis*. AChE reaction, incubation 90 min. Note distal neurons of the organ, their ventricular dendrites and liquor terminals showing a considerable activity for AChE. ×280. b Preoptic recess organ of *Rana esculenta*. AChE reaction, incubation 60 min. Nerve cells situated mostly farther away from the ventricle are AChE-positive. Note their ventricular dendrites forming bulb-like, AChE-positive liquor-terminals in the preoptic recess. ×280. c This hypendymal, neurosecretory cell of the preoptic nucleus of the frog, *Rana esculenta*, forms a bulb-like terminal in the lumen of the 3rd ventricle. Chrome alum gallocyanine according to Bock. ×1,120

other neurosecretory territories with the ventricular system. The following structures were studied in different vertebrates: 1. the Gomori-positive paraventricular
nucleus, 2. the nucleus lateralis tuberis, 3. the caudal neurosecretory system, and
4. the infundibular (arcuate) nucleus.

## Material and Methods

Brains of 80 fishes, amphibians, reptiles, birds and mammals (*Cyprinus carpio, Anguilla
vulgaris, Ameiurus nebulosus*; *Ambystoma mexicanum, Triturus cristatus, Rana esculenta*;
*Lacerta viridis, Lacerta agilis, Anguis fragilis, Natrix natrix, Emys orbicularis*; *Gallus domesticus*; *Erinaceus roumanicus, Cavia cobaya, Felis domestica, Rattus norvegicus*), furthermore
8 urophyses of the fishes mentioned above, and pieces of different parts of the spinal cord
(of *Anguilla vulgaris, Cyprinus carpio, Ambystoma mexicanum, Rana esculenta, Lacerta viridis,
Emys orbicularis, Gallus domesticus, Erinaceus roumanicus, Rattus norvegicus*) have been
studied enzyme-histochemically (see also VIGH-TEICHMANN, VIGH and AROS, 1970) and with
routine staining methods.

Acetylcholinesterase reaction (AChE) (KARNOVSKY and ROOTS, 1964) was performed on
cryostat sections (10 μ thick) of materials fixed in 4% formol-Calcium for 2.5 h at 4°C. Iso-
OMPA (final concentration $10^{-5}$ M) served as an inhibitor of unspecific cholinesterase in the
presence of acetylthiocholiniodide. Time of incubation: 60 and 90 min respectively.

For control, materials were fixed in Bouin's fixative and embedded in paraffin. The serial
sections (5 μ thick) were stained with haematoxylin eosin, aldehyde fuchsin according to
GABE (1953) and chrome alum gallocyanine (BOCK, 1966). Furthermore, semithin sections of
materials embedded in araldite, were stained with toluidine blue-azur II. For data concerning our
electron microscopic material see VIGH-TEICHMANN, VIGH and KORITSÁNSZKY (1970).

## Results

### 1. Neurosecretory Paraventricular Nucleus

In our material, the most demonstrative picture of the paraventricular
nucleus was obtained in reptiles (Fig. 2a). The neurons of this nucleus are localized
in several rows parallel to the ependyma. The cells situated near the ventricle
are mostly bipolar and lie closely side by side. Their ventricular processes protrude
into the lumen of the 3rd ventricle where they form bulb-like, ciliated endings
(Fig. 2b). The basal bodies of the cilia give rise to long rootlet fibers (VIGH-TEICH-
MANN, VIGH and KORITSÁNSZKY, 1970). The neurons situated farther away from
the ventricle seem to send also ventricular processes into the cerebrospinal fluid. Electron microscopically, we observed two kinds of bulb-like terminals: a) nerve endings
containing neurosecretory elementary granules and b) nerve endings with relatively numerous mitochondria. On the ventricular dendrites, synapses were found
in a fibrous zone between the hypendymal neurosecretory cells and the ependyma.
The rows of neurons of the paraventricular nucleus are separated from each other
by synaptic zones where the collaterals of the processes of neighbouring rows of
neurons form connections. Not only the perikarya, but also the nerve processes
and ventricular terminals show a remarkable AChE activity.

### 2. Nucleus lateralis tuberis

In the fishes we studied, the nucleus lateralis tuberis consists of large neurons
situated farther away from the ventricle, and of smaller nerve cells arranged near
the ependyma. We observed that the hypendymal neurons possess a ventricular

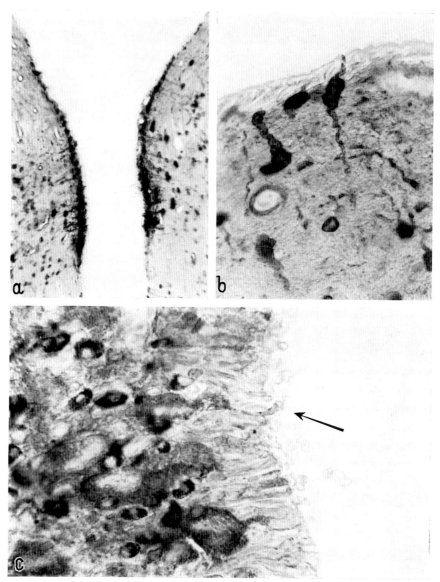

Fig. 2. a Paraventricular nucleus of *Emys orbicularis*. AChE reaction after blocking of unspecific cholinesterase with Iso-OMPA 10$^{-5}$ M, incubation 90 min. Ca. ×88. b The ventricular
dendrite of this bipolar, hypendymal neurosecretory cell passes by the ependyma and builds
up a small terminal in the 3rd ventricle. AChE reaction with Iso-OMPA, incubation 90 min.
×448. c Liquor contacting neuron (arrow) of the nucleus lateralis tuberis of *Cyprinus carpio*,
dehydrated for 20 hrs. The rather small, strikingly AChE-positive nerve cells belong to the
neighbouring anterior, periventricular nucleus. AChE reaction with Iso-OMPA, incubation
90 min. Ca. ×550

process which enters the ventricle and forms a rather large, club-like terminal
(Fig. 2c). The perikarya, nerve processes and liquor-terminals show only a moderate reaction for AChE.

## 3. Caudal Neurosecretory System

Around the *central canal* in the territory of the urophysis of fishes, we found small, bipolar neurons displaying a strong acetylcholinesterase activity in dehydrated animals (Fig. 3a). These nerve cells are localized mostly in one ventral and two lateral groups. All these cells, too, send a process into the lumen of the central canal where it builds up a bulb-like liquor-terminal. The processes and their ventricular endings show AChE positivity. Such small, bipolar, liquor contacting neurons could be demonstrated not only in the territory of the urophysis but also in other segments of the central canal of the spinal cord. This spinal liquor contacting system is present also in amphibians, reptiles, birds and mammals.

## 4. Nucleus infundibularis

In *Lacertilian* and *Testudo* species, the infundibular nucleus—the arcuate nucleus of mammals—is composed mainly of bipolar neurons (Fig. 3b). Two types of neurons can be distinguished already in semithin sections: a) cells with a light cytoplasm, and b) cells with a more dense cytoplasm. The dendrites of the nerve cells pass by the ependymal cells, and enter the 3rd ventricle where they form bulb-like terminals.

With the electron microscope (VIGH-TEICHMANN, VIGH, KORITSÁNSZKY and AROS 1970), we observed that the liquor-terminals bear cilia, and the basal bodies of the latter give rise to long rootlet fibers. There are two kinds of ventricular nerve processes and bulb-like endings: one type is filled with numerous mitochondria and some dense-core vesicles, the other contains ergastoplasm, numerous microtubuli and some large granulated vesicles. The neck of the nerve ending is attached to the neighbouring ependymal cells by desmosome-like structures.

The nerve cells of the infundibular nucleus which are situated ventrally, in the territory of the median eminence, likewise build up liquor-terminals (Fig. 3c). The neurites of the nucleus run arched to the outer surface of the median eminence and infundibulum and to the tuberal part of the adenohypophysis lying in the tissue of the hypothalamus.

Part of the cells of the infundibular nucleus shows a strong acetylcholinesterase activity. This enzyme reaction can be demonstrated in the perikarya, in their ventricular dendrites and nerve terminals, and in their neurites. The latter can be traced into the median eminence and to the tuberal part of the adenohypophysis. It is interesting to note that AChE activity could be observed at the surface of the tissue of the pars tuberalis lying in the hypothalamus.

The ependyma covering the infundibular nucleus has a special, stratified structure. As the morphological picture of the special ependyma and of the neuronal components of the infundibular nucleus is analogous to the structure of the paraventricular organ and to similar liquor contacting territories, we consider it as a link of the liquor contacting neuronal system and call it "tuberal organ".

## Discussion

We found that not only the neurosecretory preoptic nucleus but also the paraventricular nucleus of higher vertebrates contains liquor contacting neurons, and so this nucleus, too, belongs to the liquor contacting neuronal system (Fig. 4). For

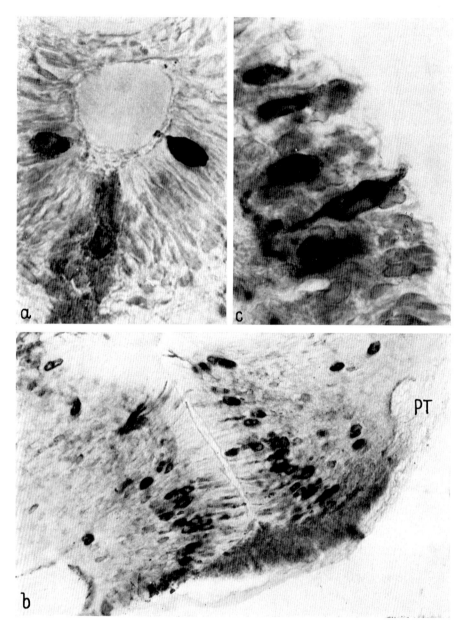

Fig. 3. a Central canal in the territory of the urophysis of the carp, *Cyprinus carpio*, dehydrated for 20 hrs. Note two strongly AChE-positive, bipolar neurons forming liquor contacting terminals. AChE reaction with Iso-OMPA, incubation 90 min. ×806. b Infundibular nucleus of *Lacerta viridis*. Part of the neurons are strongly AChE-positive. Their ventricular dendrites pass by the stratified ependyma and enter the ventricular lumen. PT: tuberal part of the adenohypophysis limited by an AChE-positive structure. AChE reaction with Iso-OMPA, incubation 90 min. ×280. c A strongly AChE-positive, bipolar neuron of the infundibular nucleus of *Emys orbicularis*. Its ventricular dendrite forms a bulb-like terminal in the ventricular lumen. AChE reaction with Iso-OMPA, incubation 90 min. ×806

distinguishing these areas from other liquor contacting territories, we use the term *liquor contacting neurosecretory system*. It is interesting that not only the classic Gomori-positive, neurosecretory nuclei form liquor terminals, but also the Gomori-negative nucleus lateralis tuberis. At present, it is not yet elucidated whether the neurons we observed on the level of the urophysis in the central canal, belong to the caudal neurosecretory system, or whether they form a general spinal network in the whole spinal cord.

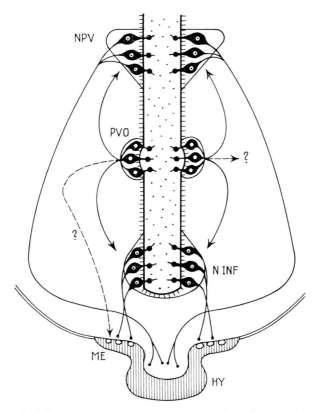

Fig. 4. Scheme of the liquor contacting neurosecretory system. *NPV* nucleus paraventricularis, *PVO* paraventricular organ, *N INF* nucleus infundibularis, *ME* median eminence, *HY* hypophysis. The 3rd ventricle dotted

The most interesting fact is that the infundibular nucleus, too, belongs to the liquor contacting neuronal system. This nucleus is well known to send neurites to the median eminence and to be an important component of the hypothalamic control of the adenohypophysis (SZENTÁGOTHAI, FLERKÓ, MESS and HALÁSZ, 1968). The liquor contacting neuronal system was considered by us as representing the morphological basis of a direct informative connection between central nervous system and cerebrospinal fluid. Since the paraventricular and infundibular nuclei and other neurosecretory cell groups form liquor contacting cells we can suppose that they are also in close informative connection with the cerebrospinal fluid. It is presumable that neurosecretory material or releasing factors may be secreted into the ventricle from these areas. Considering the structure of these nerve endings, however, we think them to be receptors, and so the neurosecretory hypothalamo-neurohypophyseal and hypothalamo-adenohypophyseal systems must directly get information from the cerebrospinal fluid (Fig. 4). These neurosecretory nuclei play an important role in the hormonal regulation of the organism. Now, we can suppose also a function in the regulation of the cerebrospinal fluid.

## Summary

The paraventricular nucleus, the infundibular nucleus, the nucleus lateralis tuberis and nerve cells in the urophysis of different vertebrates were studied with histological and histochemical methods. These neurosecretory cell groups project bulb-like nerve terminals into the cerebrospinal fluid. Therefore, they are considered to represent a special part of the liquor contacting neuronal system, called by us "liquor contacting neurosecretory system". Part of the neurons of this system is characterized by acetylcholinesterase activity. The existence of these nerve endings proves that there is a direct informative link between the hypothalamo-neurohypophyseal and hypothalamo-adenohypophyseal systems and the cerebrospinal fluid. The possible physiological significance of these findings is discussed.

## References

Bock, R.: Über die Darstellbarkeit neurosekretorischer Substanz mit Chromalaun-Gallo-cyanin im supraoptico-hypophysären System beim Hund. Histochemie 6, 362–369 (1966).
Braak, H.: Zur Ultrastruktur des Organon vasculosum hypothalami der Smaragdeidechse (Lacerta viridis). Z. Zellforsch. 84, 285–303 (1968).
Gabe, M.: Sur quelques applications de la coloration par la fuchsine-paraldéhyde. Bull. Micr. appl., Ser. II, 3, 153–162 (1953).
Kappers, C. U. A.: Die vergleichende Anatomie des Nervensystems der Wirbeltiere und des Menschen, Bd. I u. II. Haarlem: De Erven F. Bohn 1920/21.
Karnovsky, M. J., Roots, L.: A direct "coloring" thiocholin method for cholinesterases. J. Histochem. Cytochem. 12, 219–221 (1964).
Peute, J.: Fine structure of the paraventricular organ of Xenopus laevis tadpoles. Z. Zellforsch. 97, 564–575 (1968).
Röhlich, P., Vigh, B.: Electron microscopy of the paraventricular organ in the sparrow (Passer domesticus). Z. Zellforsch. 80, 229–245 (1967).
Szentágothai, J., Flerkó, B., Mess, B., Halász, B.: Hypothalamic control of the anterior pituitary, 3rd ed. Budapest: Akadémiai Kiadó 1968.
Teichmann, I., Vigh, B.: Histochemical investigation of the monoamine-containing neurons of the paraventricular organ and the preoptic recess of amphibians (Rana esculenta, Ambystoma mexicanum). Acta biol. Acad. Sci. hung. 19, 505 (1968).
— — Aros, B.: Histochemical studies on Gomori-positive substances. IV. The Gomori-positive material of the paraventricular organ in various vertebrates. Acta biol. Acad. Sci. hung. 19, 163–180 (1968).
Vigh, B.: Das Paraventrikularorgan und das periventrikuläre System des Zentralnerven-systems. VII. Unionskongr. der Anatomen, Histologen und Embryologen der SU, Tbilissi 1966.
— The paraventricular ependymal organ, a hypothalamic receptor? Gen. comp. Endocr. 9, 503 (1967a).
— A double innervation of the paraventricular organ in various vertebrates. IVth Symp. on Neurosecretion, Strasbourg 1966. In: Neurosecretion, ed. F. Stutinsky, p. 89–91. Berlin-Heidelberg-New York: Springer 1967.
— Examination on structure and function of the paraventricular organ. Thesis, Budapest 1968a.

VIGH, B.: The paraventricular organ, its structure and function. Symp. on circumventricular organs and cerebrospinal fluid, Reinhardsbrunn 1968. Jena: VEB Fischer 1969.
— Does the paraventricular organ have a receptor function? Ann. Endocr. (Paris) (1969a), in press.
— Das Paraventrikularorgan und das zirkumventrikuläre System. Budapest: Akadémiai Kiadó 1969b (in press).
— TEICHMANN, I.: Histologic and histochemical examination of the paraventricular organ in various vertebrates. Acta morph. Acad. Sci. hung. **14**, 350 (1966).
— — AROS, B.: The "nucleus organi paraventricularis" as a neuronal part of the paraventricular ependymal organ of the hypothalamus. A comparative morphological study in various vertebrates. Acta biol. Acad. Sci. hung. **18**, 271–284 (1967).
— — — Das Paraventrikularorgan und das Liquorkontakt-Neuronensystem. 63. Verslg Anat. Ges. Leipzig 1968. Erg.-H. Anat. Anz. **125**, 683–688 (1969).
VIGH-TEICHMANN, I.: Hydrencephalocriny of neurosecretory material in amphibia. Symp. on circumventricular organs and cerebrospinal fluid, Reinhardsbrunn 1968. Jena: VEB Fischer 1969.
— Morphologische Untersuchung über die Beziehung zwischen periventrikulärer grauer Substanz und Liquor cerebrospinalis. (In Hungarian.) Thesis, Budapest 1970.
— RÖHLICH, P., VIGH, B.: Licht- und elektronenmikroskopische Untersuchungen am Recessus praeopticus-Organ von Amphibien. Z. Zellforsch. **98**, 217–232 (1969).
— VIGH, B.: The neurosecretory preoptic nucleus as a member of the liquor contacting neuronal system. Acta morph. Acad. Sci. hung **17**, 338 (1969).
— — AROS, B.: Phylogeny and ontogeny of the paraventricular organ. Symp. on circumventricular organs and cerebrospinal fluid, Reinhardsbrunn 1968. Jena: VEB Fischer 1969.
— — — Fluorescence histochemical studies on the preoptic recess organ in various vertebrates. Acta biol. Acad. Sci. hung. **20**, 425–438 (1969).
— — — Enzymhistochemische Studien am Nervensystem. IV. Acetylcholinesteraseaktivität im Liquorkontakt-Neuronensystem verschiedener Vertebraten. Histochemie **21**, 322–337 (1970).
— — KORITSÁNSZKY, S.: Liquorkontaktneurone im Nucleus paraventricularis. Z. Zellforsch. **103**, 483–501 (1970a).
— — — Liquorkontaktneurone im Nucleus lateralis tuberis von Fischen. Z. Zellforsch. **105**, 325–338 (1970b).
— — — AROS, B.: Liquorkontaktneurone im Nucleus infundibularis. Z. Zellforsch. **108**, 17–34 (1970).

# Zur Frage der ventriculären „gomoripositiven" Neurosekretion*

H. Leonhardt

I. Anatomisches Institut der Universität des Saarlandes, Homburg, Saar (Germany)

**Key words:** Neurosecretion — Ventricles — Cerebrospinal fluid.

In dem Maße, in dem die Kenntnisse über Neurosekretion zunehmen, mehren sich auch die Beobachtungen, die darauf hindeuten, daß Sekrete aus dem Gehirn in den Ventrikelliquor übertreten können. (Zusammenfassende Berichte und Lit. s. Sterba, 1969.)

Soweit die Mitteilungen auf fluorescenzmikroskopische und elektronenmikroskopische Untersuchungen zurückgehen (Sterba, 1961; Sterba und Weiss, 1967; Takeichi, 1967; Öztan, 1967; Röhlich und Vigh, 1967; Braak, 1968; Wittkowski, 1968, u.a.), wird an der „ventriculären Sekretion" schwerlich zu zweifeln sein. Allerdings sind darunter keine Beobachtungen von gomoripositivem, peptidergem Neurosekret, das sich elektronenmikroskopisch in Form der 1200 bis 3000 Å großen Elementargranula darstellt; ausgenommen die Beobachtung von Wittkowski (1968), bei der es sich um eine „degenerative Form" von Neurosekret handelt. Den zahlreichen Mitteilungen über ventriculäre Neurosekretion sog. gomoripositiven Materials liegen lichtmikroskopische Untersuchungen am chromalaunhämatoxylin- oder aldehydfuchsingefärbten Schnitt zugrunde (Bargmann, 1949, 1953, 1955; Bargmann, Hild, Ortmann und Schiebler, 1950; Stutinsky, 1953; Noda, Sano und Nakamoto, 1955; Legait, 1955; Okamoto, 1957; Fleischhauer, 1960; Eichner, 1963; Srebro, 1965; Dorst, 1968, u.a.). Der Übertritt von gomoripositivem Neurosekret ist trotz der zahlreichen Beobachtungen strittig und wird aufgrund der lichtmikroskopischen Befunde eher vermutet als bewiesen (Bargmann, 1953). Der Nachweis der Elementargranula (Bargmann und Knoop, 1967, u.a.) macht es möglich, die submikroskopischen Einzelheiten der gomoripositiven intraventriculären Neurosekretion elektronenmikroskopisch zu untersuchen und einer besseren Beurteilung zuzuführen.

Zunächst darf festgestellt werden, daß Axone mit Elementargranula in den perivasculären Spalten der portalen Gefäße nahe dem Ependym der Eminentia mediana bei mehreren Tierarten elektronenmikroskopisch beobachtet worden sind (Nishioka, Bern und Mewaldt, 1964; Röhlich, Vigh, Teichmann und Aros, 1965; Takeichi, 1965; Kobayashi, Oota, Uemura und Hirano, 1966; Rinne, 1966; Holmes, 1968; Wittkowski, 1968, u.a.). An dieser Stelle ist ein Übertritt von Neurosekret in den Ventrikelliquor zu erwarten, um so eher, als nahezu alle einschlägigen lichtmikroskopischen Beobachtungen im Infundibulum gemacht

---

* Die Untersuchung wurde mit dankenswerter Unterstützung durch die Deutsche Forschungsgemeinschaft durchgeführt.

wurden. Aus der Eminentia mediana des Kaninchens stammen die hier vorgetragenen Befunde. Es wurden Trichterfortsätze von 11 Tieren beiderlei Ge-
schlechts in den Monaten März bis November untersucht. Teils wurden lückenlose
Schnittserien, teils Auswahlserien in der Frontal-, Horizontal- und Sagittalebene
ausgewertet.

## Methode

Die Tiere wurden in Thiogenal-Narkose (Fa. Merck, Darmstadt) 120 bis maximal 240 sec
nach Eröffnung des Brustkorbes (Atemstillstand) mit körperwarmem Macrodex [10% salzfrei,
Fa. Knoll, Ludwigshafen; durch Veronalpuffer nach SJÖSTRAND (1956) auf pH 7,5 eingestellt]
unter 110 mm Hg Druck 60 sec durchspült und anschließend 10 min mit veronalgepufferter
6%iger Glutaraldehydlösung perfundiert. Präparation des Gehirns nach weiteren 20 min,
Nachfixierung in 4% OsO$_4$, verdünnt mit Veronalpuffer auf 2%. Entwässern und Einbetten
in Araldit (LUFT, 1961). Die Schnitte wurden mit Glasmesser auf dem Reichert-Mikrotom
(Sitte) hergestellt und mit Uranylacetat und Bleicitrat kontrastiert. Elektronenmikroskop:
Zeiss EM 9. Frl. HELGA WITZSCH danke ich für bewährt sorgfältige technische Assistenz.

Die folgenden Beobachtungen konnten in keinem Fall in der Wand des
III. Ventrikels oberhalb des Infundibulums gemacht werden, sondern *nur in der
Wand des Recessus infundibularis*.

## Lichtmikroskopische Übersicht

(Abb. 1a—g)

In der Wand des Trichters können eine Zona interna und externa unterschieden werden (vgl. DIEPEN, 1962; BARGMANN, 1968). Die Zona interna führt
ventrikelnah die sinusoiden portalen Gefäße, daran schließen sich longitudinal
verlaufende Fasern an, die z.T. Neurosekret führen (Tractus supraoptico-hypo-
physeus und tubero-hypophysiale Fasern). Die Zona externa hat Berührung mit
dem Trichterlappen der Adenohypophyse und mit den Gefäßen des „Mantel-
plexus", Anschnitte von „Spezialgefäßen" kommen in beiden Schichten vor. Bei
erweiterten perivasculären Spalten wird die streckenweise nur einfache Lage von
Ependymzellen stark gedehnt und verdünnt. Einige neurosekrethaltige Axone mit
beträchtlichem Kaliber gelangen offensichtlich in die perivasculären Spalten,
einige erscheinen aber auch innerhalb der dünnen Ependymlage, die den Liquor
des Recessus infundibuli von den perivasculären Spalten trennt (Abb. 2a). In
vielen Fällen ist nicht sicher zu entscheiden, ob das Neurosekret noch von Ependymcytoplasma bedeckt wird oder unbedeckt in den Ventrikel eintritt (Abb. 1d, e).
Vereinzelt treten faltenförmige oder fingerförmige Ausstülpungen der Ventrikelwand mit sinusoiden Gefäßen oder Neurosekretansammlungen auf. Diese Bil-
dungen sind mehr zirkulär orientiert, man sieht sie auf Sagittalschnitten besonders
deutlich (Abb. 1b). Derartige Protrusionen erwecken den Eindruck, daß Neurosekret abgeschnürt wird. Im Zusammenhang mit dem Auftreten solcher Gewebs-
leisten im Trichtergrund liegt Neurosekret ohne erkennbare Verbindung zur Ventrikelwand im Recessus (Abb. 1f). Ferner finden sich in solchen Fällen immer
einige intraventriculäre Zellen mit großen Cytosomen, die für Mastzellengranula
oder Phagolysosomen gehalten werden können (Abb. 1f, g). Im Rahmen derartiger
Befunde liegen etwa die zitierten lichtmikroskopischen Beobachtungen ventri-
culärer gomoripositiver Neurosekretion.

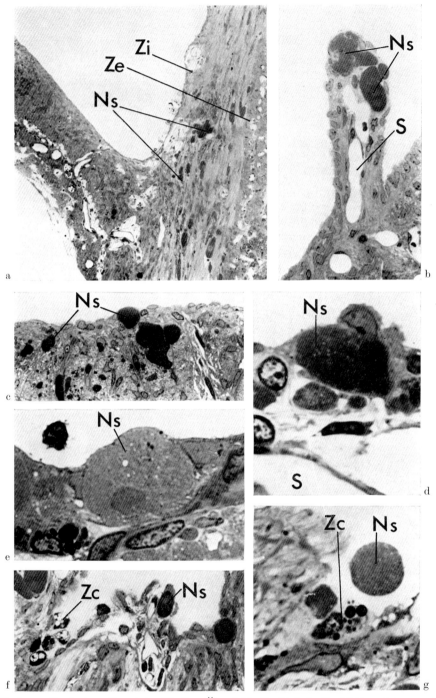

Abb. 1a–g. Kaninchen, Rec. infundibuli. a Übersicht, Sagittalschnitt; *Zi* Zona interna mit sinusoiden Portalgefäßen; *Ns* Neurosekretführende Bahn; *Ze* Zona externa. b Ausstülpung der Trichterwand; *Ns* Neurosekret; *S* sinusoides Portalgefäß. c *Ns* Neurosekret unter und im

## Elektronenmikroskopische Untersuchung

Die weiten perivasculären Spalten der sinusoiden Gefäße sind sowohl auf der Endothel- als auch auf der Gehirnseite von einer Basalmembran begrenzt. Die Spalten können stark erweitert oder zu verästelten Basalmembranlabyrinthen kollabiert sein, die dann Duplikaturen bilden. Innerhalb dieser Spalten liegen neurosekretführende Axone; die Eminentia mediana des Kaninchens ist, wie auch bei anderen Tierarten schon wiederholt festgestellt, eine neurohämale Region (OOTA und KOBAYASHI, 1963; RÖHLICH, VIGH, TEICHMANN und AROS, 1965; RINNE, 1966; MONROE, 1967; OKSCHE, 1967; HOLMES, 1968, u.a.). Wirkstoffe, die hier freigesetzt werden, gelangen in die sinusoiden Gefäße, die auch beim Kaninchen ein gefenstertes Endothel besitzen (Abb. 2 b–d).

Wo liegt aber das Sekret, von dem vermutet wird, es könnte in den Liquor gelangen?

1. In den Fällen, in denen noch ein geweblicher Zusammenhang zwischen Sekret und Ventrikelwand besteht, wird das neurosekretführende Axon regelmäßig von einer dünnen Ependymschicht bedeckt. Im äußersten Fall liegt die Neurosekretkugel innerhalb einer Ependymzelle apikal noch unter einer 840 Å dicken Cytoplasmakappe (Abb. 3a). Hier kann dann lichtmikroskopisch der Eindruck entstehen, das Neurosekret liege auf dem Ependym. Die verformbare Ependymzelle kann dabei stark gedehnt, das Neurosekret ins Ventrikellumen vorgetrieben werden (vgl. auch NISHIOKA, BERN und MEWALDT, 1964).

Stärkere Auflösung zeigt, daß die Größe der Elementargranula zwischen 1100 und 2400 Å variiert, ihre Substanzdichte wechselt; leere Bläschen dieser Größe kommen nur vereinzelt vor (Abb. 3a–c). Das Plasmalemm des Axons wird noch von einem weiteren Plasmalemm, das zur Ependymzelle gehört, umgeben. Beide Plasmalemmata halten einen konstanten Abstand von etwa 200 Å zueinander. Folgendes ist auffallend: a) An umschriebenen Stellen ist der intercelluläre Spalt zisternenartig erweitert. Das Ependymplasmalemm zeigt Einstülpungen ins Cytoplasma in Form einer unregelmäßigen Membranvesikulation. In räumlich enger Nachbarschaft liegen intracelluläre Vacuolen. b) Die Intercellularspalten zwischen Ependymzellen sind an zahlreichen Stellen spindelförmig stark erweitert. Die Erweiterungen reichen bis nahe an die apikale Oberfläche der Zellen, sind dort aber immer durch Zonulae adhaerentes und occludentes verschlossen (Abb. 3d).

2. In den anderen Fällen, in denen intraventriculäres Neurosekret ohne gewebliche Verbindung zur Ventrikelwand auftritt, kann es sich um nackte Axone handeln, die mit Elementargranula gefüllt sind. Auch Querschnitte von fingerförmigen neurosekretführenden Vorstülpungen der Wand können selbstverständlich bei entsprechender Schnittführung ohne Wandverbindung bleiben. Bei nackten neurosekretführenden Axonen umgibt nur das Axonplasmalemm das Neurosekret (Abb. 4). Die Elementargranula variieren im gleichen Maße, wie in den perivasculären und intraependymalen Axonen, doch findet man bei nackten intra-

Ependym. d *Ns* Neurosekret im einschichtigen Ependym über dem sinusoiden (*S*) Portalgefäß, fraglicher Austritt in Ventrikel. e *Ns* Neurosekret im Ependym, vermutlicher Austritt in Ventrikel. f Ns im Ependym, Austritt in Ventrikel; *Zc* Zelle mit Cytosomen. g Ns im Ventrikel; *Zc* Zelle mit Cytosomen. Vergr.: a Obj. 6 Ok. 10, b, c, f Obj. 25 Ok. 10, d, e, g Obj. 40 Ok. 10. Färbung nach RICHARDSON

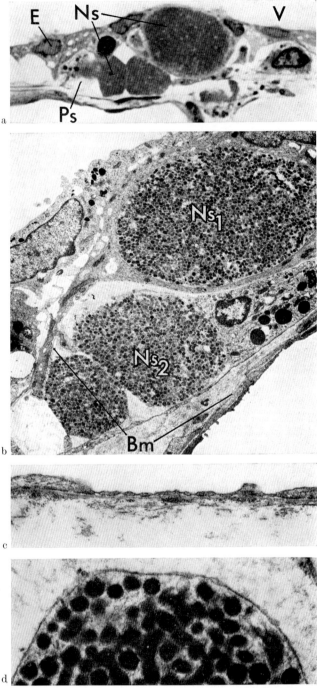

Abb. 2a–d. Kaninchen, Rec. infundibuli. a *Ns* Neurosekret in Gefäßnähe, lichtmikroskopisch Beziehung zu *V* Ventrikel, *E* Ependym und *pS* perivasculärem Spalt unklar; Färbung nach RICHARDSON. b Elektronenmikroskopisch; *Ns 1* in Ependymzelle; *Ns 2* im perivasculären Spalt; *Bm* Basalmembran. c Fenestriertes Endothel des sinusoiden Portalgefäßes. d Plasmalemm und Elementargranula des perivasculären Axons. Vergr.: a Obj. 40 Ok. 10, b 1700 × 3, c 6000 × 3, d 6000 × 5,5

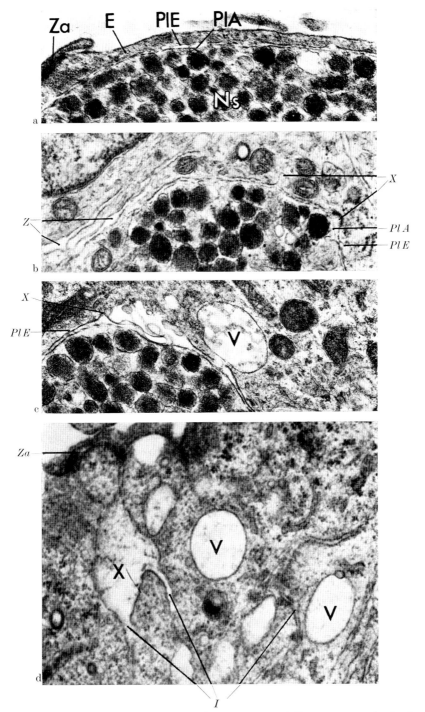

Abb. 3a–d. Kaninchen, Rec. infundibuli. a Plasmalemm und Elementargranula des intraependymalen Axons; *E* Ependymkappe über neurosekretführendem Axon Ns; *PlE* Ependymplasmalemm; *PlA* Axonplasmalemm; *Za* Zonula adhaerens. b *PlA* Axonplasmalemm; *PlE*
Ependymplasmalemm mit Membranvesikulation x; *Z* Zisternen. c *PlE* Ependymplasmalemm
mit Membranvesikulation x; *V* Vacuole. d *I* Intercellularspalt zwischen Ependymzellen;
*x* starke Erweiterung; *V* intracelluläre Vacuolen oder Anschnitte von x; *Za* Zonula adhaerens.
Vergr. a–d 6000×5,5

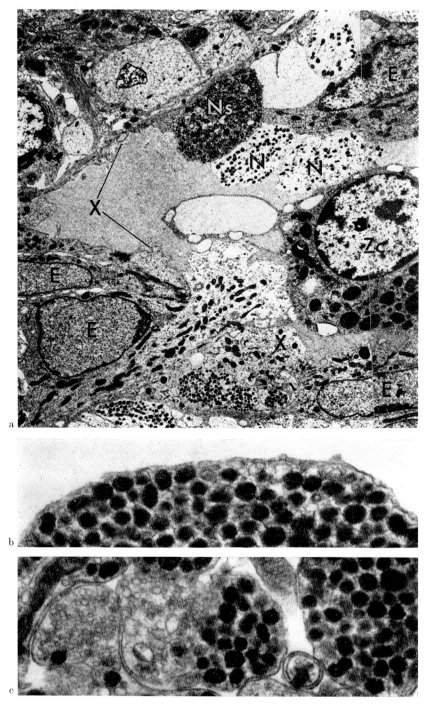

Abb. 4a–c. Kaninchen, Rec. infundibuli. a Boden des Recessus, Übersicht. Intraventriculäre Axone: *Ns* neurosekretführend; *N* ohne Neurosekret; *E* Ependymzellkern; *x* Ependymdefekte; *Zc* Zelle mit Cytosomen; *V* Ventrikel. b Plasmalemm und Elementargranula des intraventriculären Axons. c Intraventriculäre Axone mit Elementargranula und leeren Bläschen. Vergr. a 1700 × 3, b, c 6000 × 5,5

ventriculären Axonen immer eine größere Anzahl leerer Bläschen, häufig auch substanzdichte feinkörnige Massen in der Umgebung des neurosekretorischen Axons.

Wichtigste Begleiterscheinung dieser nackten intraventriculären Axone ist in unseren Präparaten immer ein Ependymdefekt. In keinem Fall tritt das nackte neurosekretführende Axon lediglich intracellulär, wie von den gewöhnlichen nackten Axonen bekannt (LEONHARDT und LINDNER, 1967; LEONHARDT und BACKHUS-ROTH, 1969) oder intercellulär, wie bei den Mitochondrienkugeln im Zentralkanal beobachtet (LEONHARDT, 1967), durch das Ependym. Jedesmal wird ein kleines Areal der Trichterwand von Ependym entblößt gefunden. Häufig erscheinen in dem betroffenen Areal Züge einer sehr faserreichen Glia, die sonst in der Eminentia mediana nur spärlich vorkommt. Bemerkenswert ist ferner, daß gleichzeitig mit nackten Axonen im Ventrikel große runde Zellen mit dichtem Kern auftreten, die zahlreiche substanzdichte, feingranulierte Körner, ähnlich denen von Mastzellen, und Vacuolen enthalten (Abb. 4a).

## Diskussion

Die Befunde geben Anlaß zu folgenden Fragen: 1. Kann in den Fällen, in denen die neurosekretführenden Axonanschwellungen noch von Ependym bedeckt sind, ein Substanztransport in den Liquor stattfinden? 2. Handelt es sich in den anderen Fällen, in denen die Axone intraventriculär liegen und ein Ependymdefekt besteht, um ein Artefakt, wodurch Axonen und Bindegewebszellen der Eintritt in den Recessus ermöglicht wird?

ad 1: Strukturen, die im Zusammenhang mit einem Substanztransport aus dem Axon über das Ependymcytoplasma in den Ventrikel stehen können, sind die umschriebenen intercellulären Erweiterungen zwischen Axonplasmalemm und Ependymplasmalemm, die Membranvesikulationen des Ependymplasmalemms, die Vacuolen im Ependym und die intercellulären Erweiterungen zwischen Ependymzellen. Wenn man es im Hinblick auf diese Strukturen für möglich hält, daß Stoffe aus dem Axon ins Ependym gelangen, wäre es vorstellbar, daß die Vergrößerung der Spalten zwischen den Ependymzellen einem Stofftransport dient. Die intercelluläre Erweiterung könnte analog zur Vergrößerung des Intercellulärspaltes von Darmepithelien bei transcellulärem Stofftransport gesehen werden. Hier wie dort trennen die Zonulae adhaerentes und occludentes Plasmalemmbezirke voneinander, die gegen unterschiedliches extracelluläres Milieu gerichtet sind, beim Ependym Ventrikelliquor und Intercellularflüssigkeit. Die Möglichkeit, daß das Ependym als Vermittler zwischen intramuralem Neurosekret und Liquor cerebrospinalis auftritt, wird diskutiert (vgl. KNOWLES, 1967; STERBA und BRÜCKNER, 1967). Daß am Axonplasmalemm selbst keine besonderen Erscheinungen im Zusammenhang mit Stoffdurchtritt auftreten, spricht so lange nicht gegen einen Stofftransport, wie auch die perivasculären Axone dabei keine besonderen Differenzierungen zeigen (Abb. 3a–d).

ad 2: Ein Artefakt ist auch bei sorgfältigster Präparation kaum mit Sicherheit auszuschließen (vgl. dazu auch E. u. B. SCHARRER, 1954). Allerdings müßte nach dem Aussehen der Strukturen erwartet werden, daß das Artefakt vor der Fixierung entstanden ist. Die mechanische Schädigung von Hirngewebe nach Fixierung führt zu Zellbruchstücken, nicht zu Verformungen dieser Art. Auch das Aussehen der cytosomenhaltigen Zellen im Liquor läßt eher auf intravitale oder supravitale als auf postmortale Vorgänge schließen. Es ist unbekannt, welche Faktoren intravital zur Entblößung der Ventrikelwand von Ependym führen und ob diese noch physiologisch genannt werden können. Sicher scheint allerdings, daß dabei der Inhalt neurosekretführender Axone in den Liquor gelangt. Man findet kernhaltige und leere Bläschen in Größe der Elementargranula und gleichzeitig feingranuläre Massen im Liquor, ähnlich denen im perivasculären Spalt. In einigen intraventriculären Axonen treten stellenweise kleine, etwa 300 Å messende, leere Bläschen nach Art der Synapsenbläschen in Plasmalemmnähe auf (Abb. 4a–c).

Es bleibt also zunächst beides unentschieden, einerseits, ob die, sicher nicht artefiziell veränderten, intraependymalen neurosekrethaltigen Axone Stoffe an den Liquor abgeben, und andererseits, ob die sicher Stoffe an den Liquor abgebenden neurosekrethaltigen Axone auf artefizielle Weise in den Ventrikel geraten sind. Eine Klärung beider Fragen wird experimentell versucht. Dagegen muß festgestellt werden, daß sich aus dem untersuchten Material eine weitere Möglichkeit für den Übertritt von Material aus neurosekretführenden Axonen dieser Art in den Ventrikel zunächst nicht ergibt.

## Summary

Investigation by light-microscopy shows that "Gomori positive" neurosecretory material is to be found on the surface of the ependyma of the median eminence as well as in the cavity of the recessus infundibuli. The exact localization of these neurosecretory bodies was clarified electronmicroscopically in the rabbit. The neurosecretory material is characterized by elementary granules of 1,200 to 2,400 Å in diameter. One type of the intraventricular neurosecretory fibres extends towards the ventricular cavity pushing in a thin lammellar portion of the apical cytoplasm of an ependymal cell. A second type, by contrast, is not covered by any cytoplasm. In these cases, the ependymal layer shows a circumscript lesion and some intraventricular cells are found containing granules like those of mast cells. Problems concerning the release of the neurosecretory material and the lesion of the ependymal layer are discussed.

## Zusammenfassung

Lichtmikroskopische Untersuchungen zeigen, daß „gomoripositives" neurosekretorisches Material sowohl auf der Oberfläche des Ependyms der Eminentia mediana als auch im Ventrikellumen vorkommt. Mit Hilfe des Elektronenmikroskops wurde die genaue Lage dieser Neurosekretballen geklärt. Das Neurosekret besteht aus 1200–2400 Å großen Elementargranula. Der eine Typ der intraventriculären neurosekretorischen Fasern erstreckt sich in den Ventrikel hinein, indem er eine dünne Lamelle des apikalen Cytoplasmas einer Ependymzelle vor sich herdrängt. Ein zweiter Typ wird im Gegensatz dazu von keinerlei Cytoplasma bedeckt. Dabei zeigt die Ependymschicht immer einen umschriebenen Defekt und es treten intraventriculäre Zellen auf, die Granula, ähnlich denen der Mastzellen, enthalten. Fragen der Neurosekretabgabe und des Ependymdefektes werden diskutiert.

# Literatur

BARGMANN, W.: Über die neurosekretorische Verknüpfung von Hypothalamus und Neurohypophyse. Z. Zellforsch. **34**, 610–634 (1949).
— Über das Zwischenhirn-Hypophysensystem von Fischen. Z. Zellforsch. **38**, 275–298 (1953).
— Weitere Untersuchungen am neurosekretorischen Zwischenhirn-Hypophysensystem. Z. Zellforsch. **42**, 247–272 (1955).
— Neurohypophysis. Structure and function. In: Handbuch der experimentellen Pharmakologie, vol. XXIII (ed. B. BERDE). Berlin-Heidelberg-New York: Springer 1968.
— HILD, W., ORTMANN, R., SCHIEBLER, TH. H.: Morphologische und experimentelle Untersuchungen über das hypothalamisch-hypophysäre System. Acta neuroveg. (Wien) **1**, 233–271 (1950).
— KNOOP, A.: Über die morphologischen Beziehungen des neurosekretorischen Zwischenhirnsystems zum Zwischenlappen der Hypophyse (licht- und elektronenmikroskopische Untersuchungen). Z. Zellforsch. **52**, 256–277 (1960).
BRAAK, H.: Zur Ultrastruktur des Organon vasculosum hypothalami der Smaragdeidechse (*Lacerta viridis*). Z. Zellforsch. **84**, 285–303 (1968).
DIEPEN, R.: Der Hypothalamus. In: Handbuch der mikroskopischen Anatomie des Menschen, Bd. IV, S. 7. Hrsg. von W. BARGMANN. Berlin-Göttingen-Heidelberg: Springer 1962.
DORST, J.: Zur mikroskopischen Anatomie der proximalen Hypophyse des Hausschweines *(Sus scrofa domestica)* unter besonderer Berücksichtigung ihrer Pars neurohypophyseos. Z. mikr. Anat. **80**, 100–142 (1969).
EICHNER, D.: Zur Frage des Neurosekretübertrittes in den III. Ventrikel beim Säuger. Z. mikr.-anat. Forsch. **69**, 388–394 (1963).
FLEISCHHAUER, K.: Fluoreszenzmikroskopische Untersuchungen an der Faserglia. I. Beobachtungen an den Wandungen der Hirnventrikel der Katze (Seitenventrikel, III. Ventrikel). Z. Zellforsch. **51**, 467–496 (1960).
HOLMES, R. L.: The infundibular process of the genus *Meriones*. Z. Zellforsch. **85**, 256–263 (1968).
KNOWLES, F.: Neuronal properties of neurosecretory cells. Neurosecretion. IV. Internat. Symposium on Neurosecretion (F. STUTINSKY, ed.), p. 8–19. Berlin-Heidelberg-New York: Springer 1967.
LEGAIT, H.: Variations indépendantes d'activité des noyaux paraventriculaires et supraoptiques au cours du cycle annuel et de la couvaison chez la Poule Rhode-Island. C. R. Soc. biol. (Paris) **149**, 175–177 (1955).
LEONHARDT, H.: Zur Frage einer intraventrikulären Neurosekretion. Eine bisher unbekannte nervöse Struktur im IV. Ventrikel des Kaninchens. Z. Zellforsch. **79**, 172–184 (1967).
— BACKHUS-ROTH, A.: Synapsenartige Kontakte zwischen intraventrikulären Axonendigungen und freien Oberflächen von Ependymzellen des Kaninchengehirns. Z. Zellforsch. **97**, 369–376 (1969).
— LINDNER, E.: Marklose Nervenfasern im III. und IV. Ventrikel des Kaninchen- und Katzengehirns. Z. Zellforsch. **78**, 1–18 (1967).
— PRIEN, H.: Eine weitere Art intraventrikulärer kolbenförmiger Axonendigungen aus dem IV. Ventrikel des Kaninchengehirns. Z. Zellforsch. **92**, 394–399 (1968).
LUFT, J. H.: Improvements in epoxy resin embedding methods. J. biophys. biochem. Cytol. **9**, 409–414 (1961).
MONROE, B. G.: A comparative study on the ultrastructure of the median eminence, infundibular stem and neural lobe of the hypophysis of the rat. Z. Zellforsch. **76**, 405–432 (1967).
NISHIOKA, R. S., BERN, H. A., MEWALDT, L. R.: Ultrastructural aspects of the neurohypophysis of the white-crowned sparrow, *Zonotrichia leucophrys gambelii*, with special reference to the relation to neurosecretory axons to ependyma in the pars nervosa. Gen. comp. Endocr. **4**, 304–313 (1964).
NODA, H., SANO, Y., NAKAMOTO, T.: Über den Eintritt des hypothalamischen Neurosekrets in den dritten Ventrikel. Arch. hist. jap. **8**, 355–360 (1955).
ÖZTAN, N.: Neurosecretory processes projecting from the preoptic nucleus into the third ventricle of *Zoarces viviparus* L. Z. Zellforsch. **80**, 458–460 (1967).

Okamoto, S.: Neurosecretory pathways in the hypothalamo-hypophyseal system. Arch. hist. jap. (Okayama) 11, 165–193 (1957).

Oksche, A.: Eine licht- und elektronenmikroskopische Analyse des neuro-endokrinen Zwischenhirn-Vorderlappen-Komplexes der Vögel. In: Neurosecretion (F. Stutinsky, ed.). Berlin-Heidelberg-New York: Springer 1967.

Oota, Y., Kobayashi, H.: Fine structure of the median eminence and the pars nervosa of the bullfrog (Rana catesbeiana). Z. Zellforsch. 60, 667–687 (1963).

Rinne, U. K.: Ultrastructure of the median eminence of the rat. Z. Zellforsch. 74, 98–122 (1966).

Röhlich, P., Vigh, B., Teichmann, I., Aros, B.: Electron microscopy of the median eminence of the rat. Acta biol. Acad. Sci. hung. 15, 431–457 (1965).

— Vigh, B.: Electron microscopy of the paraventricular organ in sparrow (Passer domesticus). Z. Zellforsch. 80, 229–245 (1967).

Scharrer, E., Scharrer, B.: Neurosekretion. In: Handbuch der mikroskopischen Anatomie des Menschen, Bd. VI, S. 5. Hrsg. von W. Bargmann. Berlin-Göttingen-Heidelberg: Springer 1954.

Sjöstrand, F. S.: Electron microscopy of cells and tissues. In: Physical techniques in biological research, Vol. III, ed. by G. Oster and A. Pollister. New York: Academic Press 1956.

Srebro, Z.: The effect of endbrain lesions on hypothalamic neurosecretion and the formation of cytoplasmic inclusions in the ependyma of Xenopus laevis. Fol. biol. (Kraków) 13, 397–407 (1965).

Sterba, G.: Fluoreszenzmikroskopische Untersuchungen über die Neurosekretion beim Bachneunauge (Lampetra planeri Bloch). Z. Zellforsch. 55, 763–789 (1961).

Sterba, G. (Hrsg.): Circumventriculäre Organe und Liquor. Vorträge, gehalten auf dem Internat. Symposion Schloß Reinhardsbrunn 1968. Jena: VEB Gustav Fischer 1969.

— Brückner, G.: Zur Funktion der ependymalen Glia in der Neurohypophyse. Z. Zellforsch. 81, 457–473 (1967).

— Weiss, J.: Beiträge zur Hydrencephalokrinie: I. Hypothalamische Hydrencephalokrinie der Bachforelle (Salmo trutta fario). J. Hirnforsch. 9, 359–371 (1967).

Stutinsky, F.: La neurosécrétion chez l'anguille normale et hypophysectomisée. Z. Zellforsch. 39, 276–297 (1954).

Takeichi, M.: The fine structure of ependymal cells. Part II: An electron microscopy study of the soft-shelled turtle paraventricular organ, with special reference to the fine structure of ependymal cells and so-called albuminous substance. Z. Zellforsch. 76, 471–485 (1967).

Wittkowski, W.: Elektronenmikroskopische Studien zur intraventrikulären Neurosekretion in den Recessus infundibularis der Maus. Z. Zellforsch. 92, 207–216 (1968).

# Function of Lysosomes in Neurosecretory Cells*

Ch. Pilgrim

Department of Anatomy, University of Würzburg (Germany)

**Key words:** Neurosecretion — Lysosomes — Secretory cycle.

Neurosecretory cells of the rat show a remarkably high content of lysosomes which usually occur as so-called dense bodies (Osinchak, 1964). It can be assumed, therefore, that these organelles play an important, but as yet unknown, role in the function of the neurosecretory cell (Pilgrim, 1967). To investigate this problem, paraventricular and supraoptic nuclei were examined in the electron microscope in rats under normal conditions, after withdrawal of water for 8–14 days, and in the following recovery period. Attention was focussed mainly on the formation of lysosomes which could be shown to develop in three ways.

1. Dilatations of the smooth endoplasmic reticulum gradually fill with granular, electron-dense material strongly resembling the matrix of "mature" dense bodies (Fig. 1). Parallel with this increase in density, the dilated parts bud off from the endoplasmic reticulum and, through intermediate stages exhibiting a variety of sizes and shapes, eventually reach the spheroid form typical of dense bodies.

2. The innermost cisterna on the concave, mature face of the Golgi field detaches from the stack, and frequently becomes horseshoe-shaped. Eventually both ends meet, thereby enclosing some of the Golgi vesicles (Fig. 2). Thus, a multivesicular body is formed. Multivesicular bodies again develop into dense bodies by accumulating the same dense matrix as mentioned above (Fig. 3).

3. Cytoplasmic material (mitochondria, membrane fragments, ribosomes, elementary granules) are wrapped by elements of the smooth or rough reticulum (Fig. 4). This process results in the formation of autophagosomes or autolysosomes, known to appear in many other cell types under certain experimental or pathological conditions (De Duve and Wattiaux, 1966).

A functional interpretation of these three different types of lysosomes has to be based on the following points. It is known from enzyme-histochemical and autoradiographic investigations that neurosecretory cells have a very active metabolism (for ref. see Pilgrim, 1967, 1969). Obviously, this is due not only to a high rate of secretion but also to a high turnover of cellular constituents. A high turnover, on the other hand, requires effective mechanisms of degradation which must be comparable to the rate of formation of new macromolecules. Since self-digestion is commonly regarded to be the assignment of autolysosomes (De Duve and Wattiaux, 1966) their occurrence in normal animals and their increase in number in thirsting rats is easily explained.

* Supported by a grant from the Deutsche Forschungsgemeinschaft.

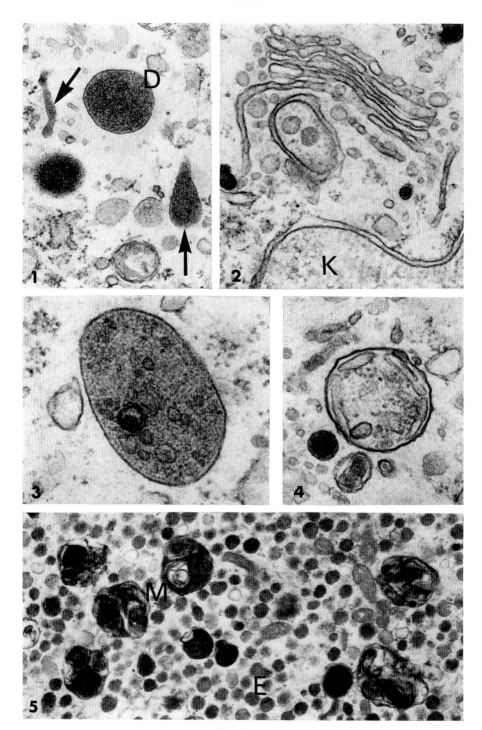

Fig. 1—5

With respect to the two other types of lysosomes described above (cf. par 1, 2), the hypothesis is set forth that these also represent certain forms of autolysosomes. In the course of the present investigation, a secretory cycle was detected in which the neurosecretory cell oscillates between phases of high secretory activity and restitution (PILGRIM, 1969). During this cycle, the perinuclear region which contains the Golgi apparatus, the smooth endoplasmic reticulum, and most of the lysosomes, is greatly expanded at the expense of the granular endoplasmic reticulum. This can be interpreted as being caused by a "flow" of membranes from the granular to the smooth compartment. The membranes are incorporated into the Golgi apparatus at its forming face, passed through it and segregated on its mature side. Eventually, they are digested in multivesicular bodies.

The third function of lysosomes is thought to be the degradation of intracisternal material which is transported towards the Golgi region along with the secretory products, but not meant for extrusion. It is suggested that this material does not reach the Golgi apparatus, but is digested inside the smooth endoplasmic reticulum, the digestion products accumulating in the dilatations described above. In both cases, the developing dense bodies should be considered as secondary lysosomes, their dense matrix representing a residue of lysosomal digestion.

The ultimate fate of most of the lysosomes seems to be that they are transformed into myelinated bodies. It is an interesting feature of the neurosecretory cell that during prolonged osmotic stress large amounts of myelinated bodies accumulate in the Herring bodies situated in the immediate vicinity of the hypothalamic nuclei (Fig. 5). They are regarded as local dilatations of dendrites which may serve as "garbage cans" for the waste products of lysosomal digestion the cell cannot afford to store in its cell body.

## References

DUVE, CH. DE, WATTIAUX, R.: Functions of lysosomes. Ann. Rev. Physiol. **28**, 435–492 (1966).

OSINCHAK, J.: Electron microscopic localization of acid phosphatase and thiamine pyrophosphatase activity in hypothalamic neurosecretory cells of the rat. J. Cell Biol. **21**, 35–47 (1964).

PILGRIM, CH.: Über die Entwicklung des Enzymmusters in den neurosekretorischen hypothalamischen Zentren der Ratte. Histochemie **10**, 44–65 (1967).

— Morphologische und funktionelle Untersuchungen zur Neurosekretbildung. Enzymhistochemische, autoradiographische und elektronenmikroskopische Beobachtungen an Ratten unter osmotischer Belastung. Ergebn. Anat. Entwickl.-Gesch. **41** (4), 1–79 (1969).

Fig. 1. Smooth endoplasmic reticulum containing dense, granular material (arrows). Its texture is similar to that of the matrix of a dense body (*D*). Supraoptic nucleus, normal rat. ×60,000

Fig. 2. Golgi cisterna enclosing Golgi vesicles, thus forming a multivesicular body. *K* nucleus. Supraoptic nucleus, 2 days after onset of rehydration. ×56,000

Fig. 3. Transformation of a multivesicular body into a dense body. Note the vesicles, partly obscured by the dense matrix. Supraoptic nucleus, normal rat. ×88,000

Fig. 4. Typical autophagosome containing membranes and ribosomes. Supraoptic nucleus, normal rat. ×56,000

Fig. 5. Herring body from the region of the supraoptic nucleus, containing elementary granules (*E*) and myelinated bodies (*M*). Water withdrawal for 14 days. ×25,000

# Morphological and Functional Relationships between the Hypothalamo-Neurohypophysial System and Cerebrospinal Fluid

E. M. Rodríguez*

Department of Pharmacology, University of Bristol (England)

**Key words:** Hypothalamus — Neurohypophysis — CSF — Morphology — Physiology.

## Morphological Relationships between the Hypothalamo-Neurohypophysial System and CSF

According to previous studies (RODRÍGUEZ *et al.*, 1970) the ventral group of neurons of the toad preoptic nucleus (VPO) gives origin to the Gomori-positive fibers that end in the neural lobe (Fig. 1). Many neurons of the VPO are bipolar with one process directed towards the hypophysial region ("hypophysial process") and the other one towards the ependymal lining of the preoptic recess ("ventricular process") (Fig. 2). The ventricular process is Gomori-positive in its initial portion more proximal to the perikaryon but is generally Gomori-negative in the vicinity of the ependyma (Fig. 2). Only occasionally the whole ventricular process, including its ventricular ending, is stained by the Gomori method (Fig. 3).

The ultrastructural study of these bipolar neurons shows that the "hypophysial process" is mainly loaded with neurosecretory granules, whereas the most proximal portion of the ventricular process contains numerous lysosome-like bodies and only a few neurosecretory granules (Fig. 4). The latter are practically lacking in the intraependymal and intraventricular portions of the process (Fig. 5). On the contrary, the lysosome-like bodies are generally present in the ventricular endings (Fig. 5), and sometimes are very large and numerous. Besides lysosome-like bodies, the ventricular endings contain numerous, large, elongated and dense mitochondria, one or two centrioles with one or more roots similar to the thin cilium-root, tubular formations resembling smooth endoplasmic reticulum, a variable number of vesicles of different sizes, a few pinocytotic vesicles, which are frequently seen to open into the ventricle, and a few multivesicular bodies (some of these formations are shown in Fig. 5).

It seems very possible that in the bipolar neurons of the VPO, the Gomori-positive reaction of the "hypophysial process" is due to the presence of neurosecretory granules, whereas in the most proximal portion of the ventricular process

* Fellow of the Consejo Nacional de Investigaciones Científicas y Técnicas de la República Argentina and partially supported by a Grant of the Wellcome Trust Foundation (England). The author wishes to thank Prof. H.-D. DELLMANN for providing certain facilities in his department.

Present address: Instituts de Histologia, Facultad de Ciencias Medicas, U.N.C., Mendoza, Argentina.

it appears to be mainly due to the presence of lysosome-like bodies. This would explain the discrepancy between the number of ventricular endings observed with the Gomori method and with the electron microscope, since the former would only reveal those endings containing a relatively high number of lysosome-like bodies. Lysosomes of some types of neurons have been shown to be Gomori-positive (STUTINSKY *et al.*, 1963; SANTOLAYA and RODRÍGUEZ, 1967). If some ventricular endings of the VPO neurons do contain numerous neurosecretory granules as have

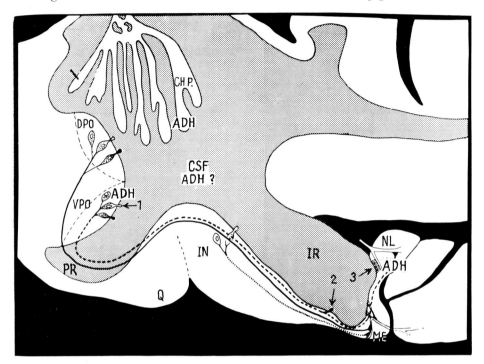

Fig. 1. Schematic representation of the hypothalamo-hypophysial systems. *DPO* dorsal group of neurons of the preoptic nucleus; *VPO* ventral group of neurons of the preoptic nucleus; *PR* preoptic recess; *Q* optic chiasma; *IN* infundibular neurons; *IR* infundibular recess; *ME* median eminence; *NL* neural lobe; *CSF* cerebrospinal fluid; *CH P* choroid plexus; *1* proximal ventricular process; *2* distal ventricular process; *3* ependyma connecting the CSF to a capillary of the neural lobe. The full and dotted lines represent the "hypothalamo-adenohypophysial system", and the broken line the "hypothalamo-neurohypophysial system". The antidiuretic hormone (*ADH*) is present in the preoptic nucleus, neural lobe, CSF and choroid plexus

been observed in the trout by MÜLLER (1969), they (the endings) must be very scarce in the toad, since among over 200 ventricular endings observed, none was loaded with neurosecretory granules.

In the infundibulum there are also Gomori-positive fibers which reach the infundibular recess of the third ventricle (Fig. 1). The electron microscope reveals that these ventricular endings do contain numerous neurosecretory granules of about 1,300–1,500 Å in diameter (Fig. 6). In addition, these endings contain a scarce number of mitochondria, neurotubules and neurofilaments. Because of their localization and their content, these ventricular processes are thought to be either lateral branches or actual endings of the "hypophysial processes" of the VPO neurons (Fig. 10). A similar type of process has been observed with the electron microscope in the infundibulum of the mouse (Wittkowski, 1968).

For discussion purposes, the short neuronal process which reaches the preoptic recess and which lacks neurosecretory granules will be called "proximal ventricular process", as opposed to the one which reaches the infundibular recess and which is loaded with neurosecretory granules, that will be called "distal ventricular process" (Fig. 10).

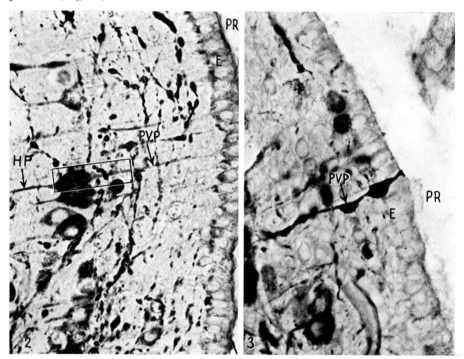

Fig. 2. Frontal section of the preoptic nucleus showing the bipolar neurons of the VPO. *HP* hypophysial process of a bipolar neuron; *PVP* proximal ventricular process; *E* ependyma; *PR* preoptic recess. The rectangle encloses an area similar to the one shown in Fig. 4. Aldehyde fuchsin. ×500

Fig. 3. Proximal ventricular process filled in its whole length with Gomori-positive material. *E* ependyma; *PR* preoptic recess. Aldehyde fuchsin. ×500

Most of the "hypophysial processes" of the VPO neurons reach the neural lobe and end on the perivascular basement membrane.

In summary, many neurons of the VPO are connected, through their ventricular processes, to the cerebrospinal fluid (CSF) and, through their "hypophysial processes", to the blood vessels of the neural lobe (Figs. 1, 10).

Fig. 4. Bipolar neurosecretory neuron of the VPO, showing the most proximal part of its proximal ventricular process (*PVP*) (similar to the area enclosed in rectangle of Fig. 2). *G* Golgi apparatus; *ER* rough endoplasmic reticulum; *L* lysosome-like bodies; *NG* neurosecretory granules; *N* nucleus. ×6,300

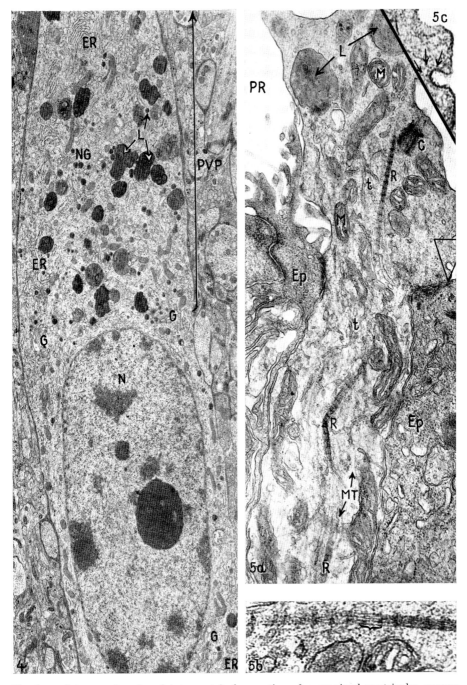

Fig. 5 a–c. Intraependymal and intraventricular portion of a proximal ventricular process. a *L* lysosome-like bodies; *M* mitochondria; *C* centriole; *R* root; *t* tubular formations; *MT* neurotubules; *Ep* ependyma; *PR* preoptic recess. ×26,000. b High magnification of a root shown in 5 a, revealing its fibrillar structure and periodical striations. ×65,000. c High magnification of the area framed in triangle of 5 a, showing the structure of the wall of a pinocytotic vesicle. The arrows point to short spines attached to the intracellular side of the vesicular wall. ×65,000

A few blood vessels of the neural lobe approach the ependymal layer, and at that point they are surrounded by the basal regions of the ependymal cells (Figs. 7, 8). The highly organized tubular system(s) and the presence of pinocytotic vesicles, which are seen in the cytoplasm and opening towards the ventricular lumen and towards the perivascular space, suggest that these ependymal cells transport some kind of material between blood vessels of the neural lobe and CSF. Therefore, it seems possible that the neural lobe blood, through a few subependymal capillaries, is linked to the CSF by way of a specialized transporting ependyma.

## Functional Relationships between the Hypothalamo-Neurohypophysial System and CSF

Antidiuretic hormone (ADH) has been shown to be present in the CSF of some mammals under certain experimental conditions (Heller et al., 1968; Vorherr et al., 1968). Preliminary studies support the possibility that ADH is also present in the amphibian CSF. Besides, it is certain that the toad choroid plexus does have an antidiuretic principle, which according to some pharmacological tests seems to be an antidiuretic hormone (Fig. 9) (see: Rodríguez and Heller, 1970). It has been shown by Heller et al. (1968) and Vorherr et al. (1968) that experimental conditions known to stimulate the release of neurohypophysial hormones into the blood (hemorrhage, electrical stimulus of the central end of a severed vagus nerve, ether anaesthesia), produce a rise of the antidiuretic activity of the CSF. Bearing this in mind, some experiments were carried out in order to further understand the probable relationships between the hypothalamo-neurohypophysial system and CSF. Dehydration by water deprivation, one of the most potent stimuli for the vascular release of the neurohypophysial hormones, when applied to toads during the winter, resulted in a decrease of the hormonal content of the neural lobe. Correlative histological studies showed a hypertrophy of the pituicytes *and* of the ependymal cells lining the neural lobe, whereas the ependyma of neighboring areas underwent no changes. The neurons of the VPO showed an increase in the amount of Gomori-positive material.

Dehydration also affected the choroid plexuses dramatically. Many choroidal cells were loaded with PAS-positive and Gomori-negative granules of about 2 μ in diameter. The granules were mainly localized at the base of the cell. The electron microscopical study showed that these granules have a limiting membrane which encloses a dense irregularly distributed material. The size of the granules ranges between 0.3 and 2 μ. Intercellular channels, normally seen in the choroid plexus, became shortened and dilated after dehydration. In a preliminary experiment, the antidiuretic activity of the choroid plexus of dehydrated toads was several folds that of the controls.

All the described observations give rise to an important question: *after potent stimuli, such as hemorrhage, dehydration, ether anaesthesia, etc., does all the amount of hormone which disappears from the hypothalamo-neurohypophysial tract, especially from the neural lobe, go to the blood stream, or is part of it released into the CSF?* The parallel rise in CSF and blood hormonal levels after a single stimulus (Heller et al., 1968; Vorherr et al., 1968) would be in favor of a positive answer to the

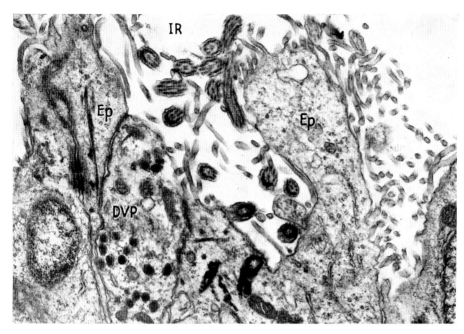

Fig. 6. Ependyma (*Ep*) of the infundibulum traversed by a distal ventricular process bearing neurosecretory granules (*DVP*). *IR* infundibular recess of the third ventricle. ×18,000

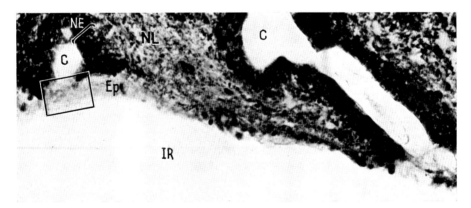

Fig. 7. Area of the neural lobe (*NL*) limiting the infundibular recess (*IR*) showing the presence of two capillaries (*c*) approaching the ependymal lining (*E*); *NE* neurosecretory endings of the palisade region. The rectangle indicates the approximate area where the electron micrograph of the next figure was taken. Aldehyde fuchsin. ×400

last possibility. Such a parallel rise in both compartments, blood and CSF, triggered by a single stimulus, may occur either because the whole neurosecretory neuron was stimulated and release occurred at *both*, the ventricular (the "distal ventricular ending") and the neurohypophysial endings, or because the elevation in the neural lobe blood levels of hormones stimulated the transport of ADH from the neural lobe blood to the CSF through the "transporting" ependyma. The

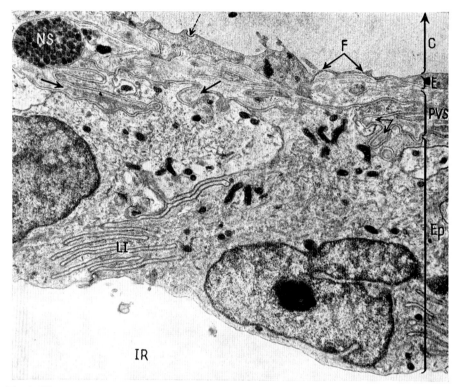

Fig. 8. Electron micrograph of an ependymal area similar to that enclosed in rectangle of Fig. 7, showing the numerous mitochondria and tubular formations of the ependymal cells. *C* capillary of the neural lobe; *E* endothelium; *PVS* perivascular space; *Ep* ependymal lining; *LI* lateral infoldings; *NS* neurosecretory fiber; *IR* infundibular recess; *F* fenestrations of the endothelium. The broken arrow indicates a pinocytotic vesicle in the endothelium. The full arrows point to processes of the perivascular space towards the ependyma. ×7,500

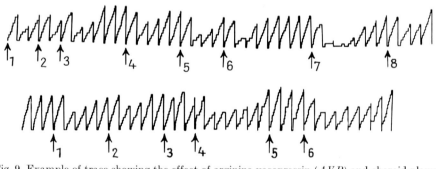

Fig. 9. Example of trace showing the effect of arginine vasopressin (*AVP*) and choroid plexus extracts (*CHP*) on the diuresis of water-loaded alcohol-anaesthetized rats. Top trace: 1→10 µU AVP; 2→5 µU AVP; 3→15 µU AVP; 4→0.1 ml CHP of the IVth ventricle (February); 5→30 µU AVP; 6→0.2 ml CHP of the IVth ventricle (February); 7→0.08 ml CHP of the IVth ventricle extracted in November and diluted ten times. 8→15 µU AVP. Bottom trace: 1→20 µU AVP; 2→10 µU AVP; 3→20 µU AVP treated with sodium thioglycollate; 4→0.05 ml CHP of IVth ventricle (December); 5→0.05 ml CHP of IVth ventricle (December) treated with sodium thioglycollate; 6→0.05 ml of CHP of IVth ventricle (December)

hypertrophy of this ependyma after dehydration would support the latter possibility. STERBA and BRÜCKNER (1967) have also suggested that the ependyma of
the lamprey neurohypophysis transports hormones from the nerve endings to the
CSF, and RODRÍGUEZ and LA POINTE (1969) have observed that in the lizard
neural lobe, the highly developed ependyma forms a link between the CSF, nerve
endings and blood vessels.

Under experimental conditions the blood levels of ADH are at least twice as
high as the CSF levels (HELLER *et al.*, 1968). Since the ratio between the blood
and CSF volumes varies between 100:1 and 200:1, this means that the amount
of ADH released into the CSF after a strong stimulus is at least 200–400 times
lower than the amount of ADH released into the blood stream. This ratio may
explain the relatively scarce neurosecretory fibers reaching the ventricle in comparison with those ending on the neural lobe capillaries, and also might explain
the relatively few capillaries of the neural lobe which contact the ependyma in
comparison with those which are entirely surrounded by neurosecretory endings.

Another possible explanation for the parallelism between the blood and CSF
levels of ADH may be the absence of a blood-CSF barrier to the neurohypophysial
hormones. HELLER *et al.* (1968) found that after the intravenous injection of ADH
in rabbits, the antidiuretic activity of the CSF rose quickly. This might have been
due either to a direct entrance of the exogenous hormone from the systemic blood
into the CSF (the presence of areas such as the lateral walls of the infundibular
recess, where very close contact between systemic blood vessels and ependyma
occurs, would support this possibility), or to the fact that the exogenous hormone
stimulated the release of endogenous hormone into the CSF. However, VORHERR
*et al.* (1968) did not find any entry of exogenous ADH into the CSF of dogs. Thus,
the important question whether the blood-CSF barrier is permeable to ADH or
not, remains to be answered. The answer is important because, if the barrier is
permeable to ADH, the parallel rise of blood and CSF ADH levels after stimulation,
may be explained simply by the *passage* of the hormone from the blood into the
CSF. But if the barrier is not permeable, a parallel rise can only be explained by
a parallel *release* of the hormone into the blood and into the CSF.

## Probable Functions of the Antidiuretic Hormone in the CSF

The role of the antidiuretic hormone in the CSF is entirely unknown. Based on
morphological, physiological and pharmacological observations, the following
*working* hypotheses are postulated.

### 1. Feed-Back Mechanism

KNOWLES and VOLLRATH (1966) have suggested that the neurosecretory fibers
ending on ependymal cells of the neuro-intermediate lobe stimulate them to release
a substance which, by travelling in the CSF, reaches the intraventricular dendrites
of the preoptic nucleus neurons, thus establishing a feed-back mechanism from
the distal to the proximal parts of the hypothalamo-hypophysial system. This
hypothesis could be widened by suggesting that the substances released into the
CSF are the neurohypophysial hormones themselves (Fig. 10). The capability of
the ependymal cells of the neurohypophysis to phagocytize neurosecretory ma-

terial (Sterba and Brückner, 1967), the ultrastructure of the "proximal ventricular endings", which points to the possibility that they have absorptive or
sensory properties rather than a secretory function, and the changes observed in
the neuronal perikarya after the intraventricular injection of a neural lobe extract,
are all facts in favor of this first hypothesis. However, it is difficult to visualize
how a feed-back mechanism may be mediated by the fed system's own secretory
product.

## 2. The CSF as a Second Pathway for the Release of the Neurohypophysial Hormones

The possibility that the CSF neurohypophysial hormones are absorbed by the
choroid plexus and then transferred into the blood stream has been suggested by
Tramezzani *et al.* (1956) and by Rodríguez (1964). Pharmacological studies
strongly suggest that the choroid plexus contains ADH, and there is good
evidence indicating that the antidiuretic principle of the choroid plexus is absorbed from the CSF (for references see: Rodríguez and Heller, 1970). Although
this hypothesis is attractive, the main objection would be, why there should be
two pathways of release of the same hormone. Vorherr *et al.* (1968) have postulated that the CSF might provide a reservoir for the *slow* release of *small* amounts
of ADH into the circulation via the arachnoid villi. Grinnell *et al.* (1968) have
found that the intravenous infusion of "sub-antidiuretic amounts of ADH"
(0.1 µU/kg/min) to anaesthetized and conscious dogs produced an increase of the
urine flow. The diuresis occurred principally when the urine flow before the infusion
started was low. It could then be possible that this second release pathway through
the choroid plexus provides the systemic circulation with "sub-antidiuretic
amounts of ADH" with subsequent diuretic effects.

## 3. ADH in CSF and Osmoreceptors

The different stimuli known to produce ADH release seem to act upon the
hypothalamic neurosecretory neurons through at least two different mechanisms.
Some stimuli like hemorrhage, positive and negative pressure respiration, pain,
etc. follow afferent pathways which are exclusively nervous (see reviews by:
Sawyer and Mills, 1966; Rothballer, 1966; Heller, 1966; Ginsburg, 1968).
On the other hand, there is a second group of stimuli (dehydration by water
deprivation or by injection of hypertonic saline) which seems to be exclusively or
principally humoral. It is a well established fact that hypertonicity of plasma

Fig. 10. Schematic representation of the morphological and functional relationships between
the preoptic-neurohypophysial system and CSF. Only one type of neurosecretory neuron
(bipolar) is shown. *PVP* proximal ventricular process; *HP* hypophysial process; *DVP* distal
ventricular process; *EpP* ependyma of the preoptic recess; *DE* differentiated ependyma of the
preoptic recess; *EpI* ependyma of the infundibulum; *EpNL* ependyma of the neural lobe.
Arrow A represents the group of stimuli which are mediated by nervous pathways whose
terminal neurons are cholinergic (*CE*) and/or aminergic (*AE*). Arrow B represents the group
of stimuli which are principally or exclusively humoral (osmotic stimuli) and which would
stimulate the PVP. After the neurosecretory neuron has been stimulated, it then propagates
the stimulus to its hypophysial process (arrows 1), what would then cause release of ADH
into both, the CSF, through the DVP, and the neural lobe capillaries, through the vascular

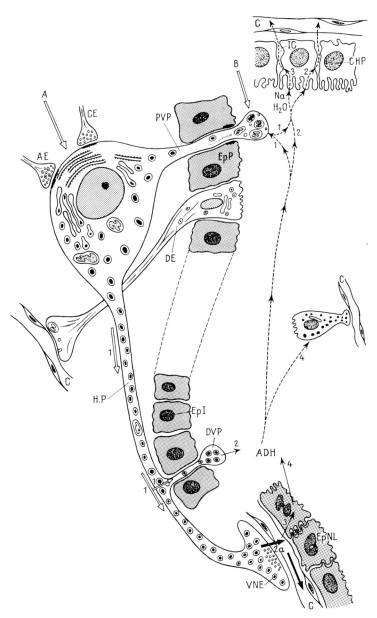

nerve ending (*VNE*). The different thickness of arrows 2 and 2a indicates that the amount of ADH released into the blood is much larger than that released into the CSF. It also seems possible that some of the hormone present in the neural lobe capillaries is, by way of a transporting ependyma (*EpNL*), released into the CSF (arrows 3 and 4). The dotted arrows indicate possible functions of the ADH present in the CSF: *1* feed-back mechanism from the distal to the proximal part of the hypothalamo-neurohypophysial system; *2* a second pathway of vascular release of ADH through the choroid plexus (*CHP*); *3* promotion of sodium (Na) and water ($H_2O$) transport from CSF into the blood, through the intercellular channels (*IC*) of the choroid plexus; *4* stimuli for the release of other biologically active principles. For explanation see text causes release of ADH from the neural lobe into the systemic circulation (Verney, 1947; Ames et al., 1950). By evidence from blood distribution, Jewell and Verney (1957) suggested the presence of osmoreceptors in a restricted area of the diencephalon. However, the nature and precise localization of the osmoreceptive elements still remains to be clarified.

That ADH release may be promoted by two completely different mechanisms has been further substantiated by the experiments of Saito et al. (1969) who found that the isolated diencephalon, without nervous connections with the adjacent nervous structures, could release ADH in response to an infusion of hypertonic saline, but on the contrary, nervous connections between diencephalon and mid-brain were indispensable to ADH release in response to hemorrhage. Another striking observation in favor of the presence of more than one mechanism for the release of ADH is the one reported by Moll and de Wied (1962), who found that the regenerated neural lobe following posterior lobectomy, released ADH in response to dehydration but release did not occur after hemorrhage.

It seems reasonable to assume that the cholinergic and aminergic nerve fibers which make synaptic contact with the neurosecretory neurons of the hypothalamus (Fig. 10A) represent the final neurons of the afferent nervous pathways followed by the first group of stimuli (see above). On the other hand, there are several observations supporting the possibility that the "proximal ventricular process" (PVP) of the neurosecretory cells is the structure sensitive to the osmotic stimuli (Fig. 10B), which then would be finally mediated via the CSF. The supporting observations are:

a) The PVP are localized in the area suggested by the experiments of Jewell and Verney (1957).

b) The blood and CSF levels of sodium are in equilibrium, since the ratio between the concentrations of sodium in blood and CSF is practically 1 (Davson, 1967). Intravenous injection of sodium is followed by a progressive rise in the CSF sodium until equilibrium is re-established (Fishman, 1959). In summary, after vascular infusion of hypertonic saline, not only the blood but also the CSF becomes hypertonic, although with some delay.

c) The perfusion of the cerebral ventricles with hypertonic saline produced anti-diuresis (Leusen and Lacroix, 1961). This antidiuretic effect of the intraventri-cular hypertonic saline disappeared after hypophysectomy, suggesting that the antidiuresis had been due to ADH release from the neurohypophysis (Anderson et al., 1969). These two experiments strongly suggest that some region of the ventricular walls must be sensitive to the CSF hypertonicity with a subsequent triggering of the systemic release of ADH.

d) The osmoreceptive function of the PVP would explain why the isolated diencephalon (diencephalic islands) releases ADH in response to osmotic stimuli, since according to the isolation technique used by Saito et al. (1969), the peri-ventricular structures of the hypothalamus were not damaged.

e) The ultrastructure of the PVP is very much in favor of a sensory function. The presence of cilia, numerous mitochondria and tubular formations is common to both the PVP and the free ends of the olfactory nerves, which are undoubtedly sensory (Graziadei and Bannister, 1967).

f) The presence of two types of neurosecretory neurons in the VPO (which is the part of the preoptic nucleus related to the neural lobe, see above), one with a ventricular process and the other without it (Fig. 1) could be due to the fact that the former are sensitive to osmotic stimuli and the latter to stimuli conducted through nervous afferents (see above).

If, as it seems to be well established, the hypertonicity of the CSF triggers the release of ADH, there must be some feed-back mechanism to inform the neurosecretory cells when to decrease or stop the release of hormones. The re-establishment of the plasma isosmolarity, and consequently that of the CSF, due to the peripheral effect of the released ADH may be the actual feed-back mechanism. However, it seems also possible that the osmosensitive neurons, through their "distal ventricular process" (Fig. 10) release into the CSF an amount of ADH proportional to the one released into the systemic blood (see above). The ADH released into the CSF could then promote the transport of sodium from the CSF to the blood, through the choroid plexus, until isosmolarity of the CSF is re-established, with a consequent disappearance of the osmotic stimulus. The choroidal epithelium would then be a target organ for ADH similar to the epithelium of the collecting tubules of the kidney or to that of the urinary bladder. In fact, these three structures share some ultrastructural characteristics, such as the presence of intercellular channels. It is known that ADH produces a dilatation of these channels in the collecting tubules (GANOTE et al., 1968), and similar expansions of the choroid plexus channels were observed after dehydration (see above). The gall bladder is another example in which sodium is pumped from epithelial cells into intercellular channels, which are distended when sodium transport is accelerated and collapsed when sodium transport is inhibited (TORNEY and DIAMOND, 1967).

LEUSEN and LACROIX (1961) found that the infusion into the CSF of hypotonic saline had a diuretic affect. This could have been due to the fact that the decrease of sodium concentration in the CSF reduced or stopped the release of ADH from the neural lobe. Following the same line of reasoning, it could be assumed that the diuretic effect of the intraventricularly injected ADH observed by NASHOLD et al. (1963) was due to a reduction of the CSF sodium level due to the trans-choroidal transport of sodium from the CSF to the blood promoted by the injected ADH.

The main objections to this third theory are: a) In mammals the neurons of the neurosecretory nuclei where ADH is synthetized apparently do not have an equivalent to the "proximal ventricular ending" observed in fishes and amphibians. However, the mammalian neurosecretory neurons do have Gomori-positive processes which reach the infundibular recess (BARGMANN, 1949; BARGMANN et al., 1950) and which may contain neurosecretory granules of about 1,300–1,500 Å (WITTKOWSKI, 1968). These processes very likely correspond to the "distal ventricular process" of the amphibians. LEONHARDT (1968) has described the presence of complicated nervous structures protruding into the hypothalamic region of the third ventricle of the rabbit. The simple PVP of lower species might very well be replaced, in more evolved species, by more complicated structures as that described by LEONHARDT. b) The CSF levels of ADH are increased after "non-osmotic" stimuli presumably mediated by nervous pathways (hemorrhage, VORHERR et al., 1968; vagal stimulation, HELLER et al., 1968).

## 4. The Neurohypophysial Hormones in the CSF as Stimuli for the Release of other Biologically Active Principles

NASHOLD et al. (1963) found that the intraventricular injection of 8-lysine vaso-pressin in the cat was associated with a significant rise of urine flow. The increased urine flow was accompanied by an increased osmolar clearance, which the authors regarded as due to an increased excretion of sodium. The intravascular admini-stration of the same dose of the hormone under similar conditions, produced the usual antidiuretic effect. CHAN and SAWYER (1968) found that the injection of 0.6 mU/oxytocin/kg into the third ventricle of the dog produced marked and prolonged "natriuresis". The same dose injected into a carotid artery occasionally produced a mild and short natriuresis, but was ineffective intravenously. The authors suggested that the intraventricular oxytocin may excite central structures to secrete a natriuretic hormone.

All these results clearly show that the neurohypophysial hormones produce different and sometimes, opposite results when they are injected into the blood or into the CSF. It could be assumed that the natriuretic property of the exogenous neurohypophysial hormones intraventricularly injected, is also a property of the endogenous neurohypophysial hormones which are released into the CSF after certain stimuli (Fig. 10).

## References

AMES, R. G., MOORE, D. H., DYKE, H. B. VAN: The excretion of posterior pituitary anti-diuretic hormone in the urine and its detection in the blood. Endocrinology **46**, 215–227 (1950).

ANDERSON, B., DALLMAN, M. F., OLSSON, F.: Observations on central control of drinking and of the release of antidiuretic hormone. Life Sci. **8**, 425–432 (1969).

BARGMANN, W.: Über die neurosekretorische Verknüpfung von Hypothalamus und Neuro-hypophyse. Z. Zellforsch. **34**, 610–634 (1949).

— HILD, W., ORTMANN, R., SCHIEBLER, TH. H.: Morphologische und experimentelle Unter-suchungen über das hypothalamisch-hypophysäre System. Acta neuroveg. (Wien) **1**, 233–271 (1950).

CHAN, W. Y., SAWYER, W. H.: Intracranial action of oxytocin on sodium excretion by conscious dogs. Proc. Soc. exp. Biol. (N.Y.) **127**, 267–270 (1968).

DAVSON, H.: Physiology of the cerebrospinal fluid. London: J. & A. Churchill Ltd. 1967.

FARNER, D. S., KOBAYASHI, H., OKSCHE, A., KAWASHIMA, S.: Proteinase and acid-phos-phatase activities in relation to the function of the hypothalamo-hypophysial neuro-secretory system of photostimulated and of dehydrated white-crowned sparrows. Progr. Brain Res. **5**, 147–156 (1964).

FISHMAN, R. A.: Factors influencing the exchange of sodium between plasma and cerebro-spinal fluid. J. clin. Invest. **38**, 1698–1708 (1959).

GANOTE, CH. E., GRANTHAM, J. J., MOSES, H. L., BURG, M. B., ORLOFF, J.: Ultrastructural studies of vasopressin effect on isolated perfused renal collecting tubules of the rabbit. J. Cell Biol. **36**, 355–367 (1968).

GINSBURG, M.: Production, release, transportation and elimination of the neurohypophysial hormones. In: Handbook of experimental pharmacology (ed. B. BERDE), vol. XXIII, p. 286–371. Berlin-Heidelberg-New York: Springer 1968.

GRAZIADEI, P., BANNISTER, L. H.: Some observations on the fine structure of the olfactory epithelium in the domestic duck. Z. Zellforsch. **80**, 220–228 (1967).

GRINNELL, E. H., KRAMAR, J. L., DUFF, W. M., LYDON, TH. E.: Further studies on the diuretic activity of antidiuretic hormone. Endocrinology **83**, 199–206 (1968).

HELLER, H.: Neural control of hormone secretion. J. Sci. Industr. Res. **25**, 298–302 (1966).

— HASAN, S. H., SAIFI, A. O.: Antidiuretic activity in the crebrospinal fluid. J. Endocr. **41**, 273–280 (1968).

JEWELL, P. A., VERNEY, E. B.: An experimental attempt to determine the site of the neuro-hypophysial osmoreceptors in the dog. Phil. Trans. B **240**, 197–234 (1957).

KNOWLES, F., VOLLRATH, L.: Neurosecretory innervation of the pituitary of the eels *Anguilla* and *Conger*. I. The structure and ultrastructure of the neurointermediate lobe under normal and experimental conditions. Phil. Trans. B **250**, 311–327 (1966).

LEONHARDT, H.: Bukettförmige Strukturen im Ependym der Regio hypothalamica des III. Ventrikels beim Kaninchen. Z. Zellforsch. **88**, 297–317 (1968).

LEUSEN, I., LACROIX, E.: Changes in osmolarity in the cerebral ventricles and diuresis. Endocrinology **68**, 719–721 (1961).

MOLL, J., WIED, D. DE: Observations on the hypothalamo-posthypophyseal system of the posterior lobectomized rat. Gen. comp. Endocr. **2**, 215–228 (1962).

MÜLLER, H.: In: Zirkumventrikuläre Organe und Liquor (ed. G. STERBA) Jena: VEB Gustav Fischer 1969

NASHOLD, B S., MANNARINO, E. M., ROBINSON, R. R.: Effect of posterior pituitary poly-peptides on the flow of the urine after injection in lateral ventricle of the brain of a cat. Nature (Lond.) **197**, 293 (1963).

RODRÍGUEZ, E. M.: Neurosecretory system of the toad *Bufo arenarum* Hensel and its changes during inanition. Gen. comp. Endocr. **4**, 684–695 (1964).

— LA POINTE, J.: Histology and ultrastructure of the neural lobe on the lizard, *Klauberina riversiana*. Z. Zellforsch. **95**, 37–57 (1969).

— HELLER, H.: Antidiuretic activity and ultrastructure of the toad choroid plexus. J. Endocr., **46**, 83–91 (1970).

— VEGA, J. A., LA MALFA, J. A.: The different origins of the neurosecretory hypothalamo-hypophysial tracts of the toad *Bufo arenarum* Hensel. Gen. comp. Endocr., in press (1970).

ROTHBALLER, A. B.: Pathways of secretion and regulation of posterior pituitary factors. Endocr. Centr. Nerv. Sys. **43**, 86–131 (1966).

SAITO, T., YOSHIDA, S., NAKAO, K.: Release of antidiuretic hormone from neurohypophysis in response to hemorrhage and infusion of hypertonic saline in dogs. Endocrinology **85**, 72–78 (1969).

SANTOLAYA, R. C., RODRÍGUEZ, E. M.: The reticular substance of the medulla oblongata of the albino rat. Histochemistry and ultrastructure of neurons and blood capillaries. Z. Zellforsch. **79**, 537–549 (1967).

SAWYER, W. H., MILLS, E.: In: Neuroendocrinology (eds. L. MARTINI and W. F. GANONG), vol. I, p. 187–216. New York-London: Academic Press 1966.

STERBA, G., BRÜCKNER, G.: Zur Funktion der ependymalen Glia in der Neurohypophyse. Z. Zellforsch. **81**, 457–473 (1967).

STUTINSKY, F., PORTE, F. A., TRANZER, J. D., TERMINN, Y.: Sur la signification des inclusions colorables par l'aldéhyde-fuchsine dans les neurones du système nerveux central du rat. C. R. Soc. Biol. (Paris) **157**, 2294–2296 (1963).

TORMEY, J. McD., DIAMOND, J. M.: The ultrastructural route of fluid transport in rabbit gall bladder. J. gen. Physiol. **50**, 2031–2060 (1967).

TRAMEZZANI, J. H., NEGREIROS DE PAIVA, C., SESSO, A.: Oxytocic activity of the toad's brain. Acta endocr. (Kbh.) **23**, 175–184 (1956).

VERNEY, E. B.: The antidiuretic hormone and the factors which determine its release. Proc. roy. Soc. B **135**, 25–105 (1947).

VORHERR, H., BRADBURY, M. W. B., HOGHOUGHI, M., KLEEMAN, C. R.: Antidiuretic hormone in cerebrospinal fluid during endogenous and exogenous changes in its blood level. Endocrinology **83**, 246–250 (1968).

WITTKOWSKI, W.: Elektronenmikroskopische Studien zur intraventrikulären Neurosekretion in den Recessus infundibularis der Maus. Z. Zellforsch. **92**, 207–216 (1968).

# Ultrastructure des granules neurosécrétoires du cobaye

St. Donev

Institut d'Histologie et d'Embryologie, Faculté de Médecine
(Chef de l'Institut: Prof. P. Em. Petkov), Sofia (Bulgaria)

**Key words:** Neurosecretory material — Elementary granules — Ultrastructure.

L'ultrastructure de la neurohypophyse du cobaye est relativement peu étudiée en comparaison avec celle des autres animaux de laboratoire (Barry, 1961; Barry et Cotte, 1961; Mazzuca, 1965; Wittkowski, 1967). Pour la première fois Barry et Cotte (1961) décrivent les granules neurosécrétoires du cobaye comme des granules denses, enveloppés d'une seule membrane et avec un halo périphérique clair. Le centre dense est le plus souvent rond, mais on rencontre des granules dans lesquels il a la forme d'un bâtonnet. Donev (1969) décrit deux types de granules neurosécrétoires chez le cobaye: type A et type B, ayant différente morphologie et dynamique d'apparition au cours de l'ontogénèse, ainsi que les changements dans l'activité fonctionnelle d'appareil hypothalamo-neurohypophysaire. Les granules neurosécrétoires du type A possèdent une structure interne caractéristique pareille à celle, décrite par Knowles (1960) chez *Squilla mantis* et par Bargmann et v. Gaudecker (1969) chez l'hérisson. Cette structure est différente de celle des granules neurosécrétoires chez la grenouille (Rodríguez, 1969), chez la souris (Bargmann et v. Gaudecker, 1969) et chez l'homme (Lederis, 1965). Ces descriptions de la structure interne des granules neurosécrétoires son faites uniquement à la base de la fixation osmique.

Le but de notre recherche était d'étudier la structure interne des granules neurosécrétoires du cobaye avec l'emploi de différents fixateurs et leurs changements dans de différents états fonctionnels de l'appareil hypothalamo-neurohypophysaire.

## Matériel et méthodes

24 cobayes en maturité sexuelle étaient examinés pendant différentes saisons de l'année: automne (novembre, décembre) et printemps (mars, avril).

Les animaux étaient sacrifiés par décapitation. Le cerveau était prélevé immédiatement après le sacrifice, on en séparait la région du nucleus supraopticus et la neurohypophyse. Fixateurs:

1. 2,5% de glutaraldéhyde dilué dans du tampon Millonig à 4°C pour 1 heure et fixé ensuite au 2% de tétroxyde d'osmium dilué dans du tampon Millonig pour 1 heure à 4°C suivant Sabatini et coll. (1964).

2. 2% de solution de tétroxyde d'osmium dans tu tampon Millonig pour 1 heure à 4°C (Palade, 1952).

3. $KMnO_4$ pour 2 heures à 0° (Sjöstrand, 1967).

Après déshydratation les prélèvements étaient inclus au Durcopan ACM. Le matériel était découpé à l'ultramicrotome OMU-2 (Reichert) en coupes grises. Les réseaux portant les coupes préparées étaient en plus contrastés à l'uranil acétate (WATSON, 1958), et au citrate de plomb (REYNOLDS, 1963). Les observations étaient faites au microscope électronique Hitachi HU-11A.

# Résultats

## 1. Fixation au glutaraldéhyde

Dans la neurohypophyse du cobaye on peut distinguer deux sortes de granules neurosécrétoires:

a) Type A-granules d'une taille de 1600–1800 Å environ. Elles possèdent un centre dense aux électrons, enveloppé d'une membrane unique. Entre le centre et la membrane on observe un «halo».

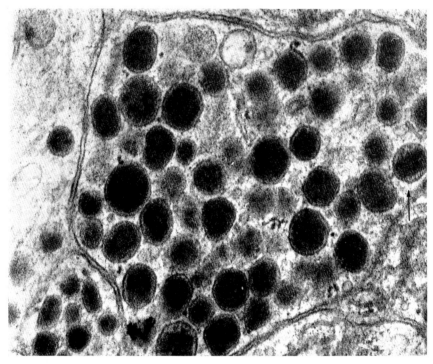

Fig. 1. Granules neurosécrétoires dans la neurohypophyse (automne). Dans le centre dense des granules on remarque la structure interne (flèche). Glutaraldéhyde, 52650×

Le centre dense a, le plus souvent, une forme ronde, mais on rencontre aussi des granules isolés dans lesquels le centre a la forme de bâtonnet ou de fuseau (Fig. 1). La densité du centre dans les granules isolés d'une terminaison nerveuse est assez différente. Dans certains des granules se fait voir un aspect filamenteux du centre dense. Celà ressort le mieux dans les granules de faible densité électronique. On peut y discerner une structure tubulaire caractéristique, qui, pourtant, n'est pas nettement exprimée dans la plupart des granules.

Dans les différents granules le halo périphérique varie de largeur. Il est le plus étroit dans les granules ayant un centre plus dense — 60 Å environ, mais peut atteindre jusqu'à 150–200 Å et même davantage. Bien qu'il semble plus clair que le centre du granule, il contient du matériel homogène sans structure déterminé d'une faible densité électronique (Fig. 1).

La membrane qui enveloppe le granule neurosécrétoire a des contours réguliers, arrondis. Dans les granules les plus denses elle est d'une épaisseur de 55–60 Å environ et paraît à une seule couche, mais dans les granules ayant un halo plus grand et une densité électronique plus faible on peut voir sa structure à trois couches: couche extérieure et intérieure osmiophile et couche extérieure et intérieure osmiophile et couche intérmédiaire claire.

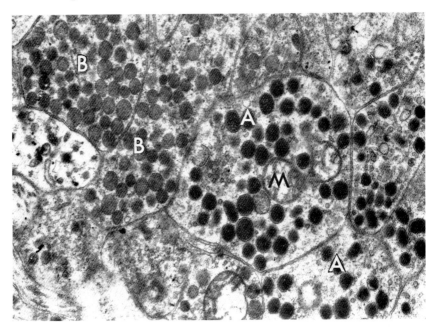

Fig. 2. Granules neurosécrétoires du type A et B dans la neurohypophyse (automne).
*M* mitochondries. Glutaraldéhyde, 20 800 ×

b) Type B-granules de dimensions pareilles à celles du type A (1600–1800 Å) mais d'une densité électronique plus faible, ne possèdent pas de halo périphérique et on ne peut pas voir la membrane périphérique qui les enveloppe (Fig. 2). Le centre du granule paraît complètement homogène et l'on ne voit pas de structure interne. Les granules du type A et du type B peuvent être observés dans différentes axones et terminaisons: on ne les rencontre jamais ensemble dans la même fibre nerveuse. Tous les granules du type B ont presque la même densité électronique.

## 2. Fixation au tétraoxyde d'osmium

La fixation au tétroxide d'osmium fait voir nettement certaines particularités de la structure interne des granules neurosécrétoires élémentaires.

Le centre dense des granules se présente sous la forme de trabécules dans certains des granules coupés en sens longitudinal, ou bien de tubules, si elles sont coupés transversalement. Mais le plus souvent on rencontre des formes coupées

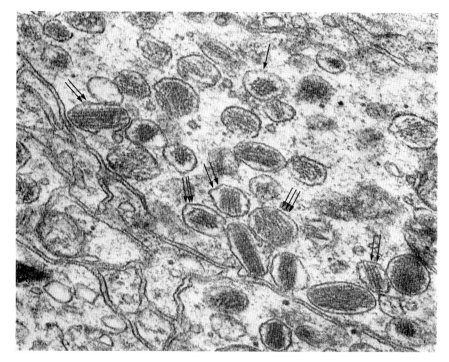

Fig. 3a. Granules neurosécrétoires à structure interne caractéristique. Tubules coupés transversalement (→), longitudinalement ($\overset{\longrightarrow}{\to}$), et obliquement ($\overset{\Rrightarrow}{\to}$). Tétroxyde d'osmium, 52 800 ×

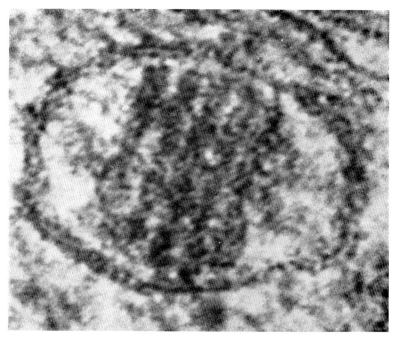

Fig. 3b. Granule neurosécrétoire à structure interne caractéristique. Tétroxyde d'osmium, 492 000 ×

obliquement (Fig. 3). Dans les coupes longitudinales elles se présentent comme des membranes parallèles à l'interieur du granule. Leur nombre varie de 3–4 jusqu'à plus de dix. Les dimensions et la structure des trabécules sont comme celle de la membrane élémentaire, qui enveloppe ce granule — de 70 à 90 Å, et lui ressemblent aussi par leur structure. Elles sont formés de deux couches extérieures foncées et d'une couche intermédiaire claire, ayant chaque une grosseur de 25–30 Å environ. Elles sont disposès trés régulièrement les unes à côté des autres à une

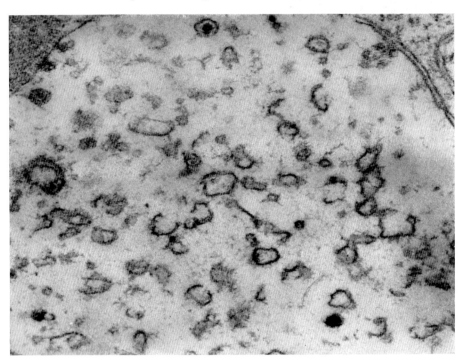

Fig. 4. Grandes vésicules membraneuses, restes des granules neurosécrétoires dans la neurohypophyse de cobaye sacrifié au printemps. On remarque la dissociation des couches de la membrane élémentaire. Tétroxyde d'osmium, 60000×

distance de 70–90 Å. Dans une coupe transversale elles représentent des canules disposées régulièrment avec un intèrieur clair, occupant le centre du granule. Dans certains granules on peut compter de centaines de canules coupées obliquement. Dans ces cas elles sont disposées assez serrées les unes à coté des autres et de cette manière le centre du granule paraît plus foncé.

Entre les canules qui forment le centre dense du granule et la membrane périphérique qui l'enveloppe se forme le halo périphérique. Il semble assez irrégulier à cause des contours irréguliers du centre du granule et il est complètement transparent.

La structure interne se rencontre dans tous les granules neurosécrétoires aussi bien dans la neurohypophyse que dans les péricarions du NSO.

La membrane qui enveloppe le granule neurosécrétoire a une structure à trois couches nettement exprimées et sa largeur varie suivant la densité électronique du granule de 60–95 Å environ. Dans beaucoup de cas l'épaisseur de la membrane n'est pas régulière dans toute sa longueur. Par endroits, dans des granules ayant une faible densité électronique, les deux couches périphériques foncées de la membrane forment des gonflements variqueux. A certains endroits on observe une interruption de la membrane. Pendant l'activité saisonnière de l'appareil hypothalamo-neurohypophysaire, au printemps, on observe dans la neurohypophyse presqu'exclusivement seulement des granules ayant perdu leur centre dense et présentés sous la forme de grandes vésicules membraneuses (Fig. 4). Celles-ci ont une forme irrégulière, elles sont fissurées et ridées, interrompues à plusieurs endroits. Leurs membranes élémentaires sont, dans certains cas, larges de plus de 100 Å et la structure à trois couches apparaît nettement. Aux endroits de l'interruption on voit la dissociation des trois couches et leur transformation en matière sans structure déterminée à faible densité électronique.

### 3. Fixation au permanganate de potassium

Ce fixateur ne nous a pas donné la possibilité de différencier les deux types de granules. Le centre des granules a une densité électronique très faible. Il est rempli de matière sans structure déterminée dans laquelle on observe par-ci par-là des structures semblables aux canules, avec un centre clair. La membrane périphérique est bien dessinée et on voit nettement sa structure à trois couches. Ce qui fait impression, c'est qu'on n'observe nulle part de halo périphérique.

## Discussion

Comme il fut indiqué par BARGMANN et KNOOP (1957), WEINSTEIN et coll. (1961), LA BELLA et SANWAL (1965), HELLER et LEDERIS (1962), les granules neurosécrétoires sont porteurs des neuro-hormones vasopressine et ocytocine. Il fut établi, qu'il y avait une activité directement proportionnelle entre leur densité électronique et leur activité hormonale (HARTMANN, 1958; HELLER et LEDERIS, 1962). En même temps la diminution de leur «osmiophilie» est considérée comme un signe de libération des hormones qu'ils portent.

En comparant les données obtenues par l'emploi de différents fixateurs dans l'examen de l'ultrastructure des granules neurosécrétoires du cobaye, nous trouvons que les granules se caractérisent par une plus grande densité électronique lors de la fixation au glutaraldéhyde. La densité est plus faible lors de la fixation au tétroxyde d'osmium et minime lors de la fixation au permanganate de potassium. En outre, les trois fixateurs décèlent dans les granules neurosécrétoires du type A une structure tubulaire caractéristique et qui est la plusnette lors de la fixation au tétroxyde d'osmium. Les deux types de granules neurosécrétoires ne peuvent pas être différenciés les uns des autres par la fixation au tétroxyde d'osmium et au permanganate de potassium.

Il est admis que le glutaraldéhyde, sans avoir une valeur histochimique, stabilise mieux les composants protidiques, alors que le tétroxyde d'osmium — les lipoprotides. Le permanganate de potassium détruit les composants purement protidiques, mais conserve bien les lipoprotides et particulièrement les structures membraneuses (PEASE, 1964; MILLONIG et MARINOZZI, 1968).

En se basant à la morphologie des trabécules et des tubules décrites à l'intérieur des granules neurosécrétoires et les possibilités de les faire ressortir par différents fixateurs, nous supposons qu'ils sont de nature lipoprotéique proche à celle de la membrane élémentaire du granule. Les protides conservés lors de la fixation au glutaraldéhyde masquent la structure de fond lipoprotéique que l'on peut voir dans la diminution du composant protidique au moment de laquelle le granule devient plus clair. Celà nous fait penser que la fixation au glutaraldéhyde conserve les composants protidiques du neurosécrétat Gomori-positif, appelé protéine de van Dyke. Ce dernier représente un complexe de la protéine d'Acher (neurophysine) et des nonapeptides de la vasopressine ou de l'ocytocine (van Dyke et coll., 1955; Acher et al., 1956; Polénov, 1968). De son côté la protéine de van Dyke est liée aux phospholipides (Handa et Kumamoto, 1958; Kurosumi et al., 1964) que Sloper (1966) lie à la membrane élémentaire du granule. Celà nous permet d'admettre que la structure interne des granules que nous décrivons participe en tant que structure de fond lipoprotéique à laquelle est liée la protéine biologiquement active de van Dyke.

En ce qui concerne le halo périphérique, nous l'examinons à la base de nos données comme un espace fonctionnel étroitement lié au «contenu hormonal» du granule, et au processus de libération de l'hormone du granule. La présence dans le halo de matériel à densité électronique faible lors de la fixation au glutaraldéhyde montre que c'est par là que passent les substances protidiques du centre dense du granule, avant leur sortie à travers la membrane élémentaire. Ses variations dans les différents fixateurs montrent qu'il n'a pas une structure stricte.

Nous attirons l'attention sur le fait, que la membrane élémentaire des granules neurosécrétoires avec ses trois couches, décrits par Bargmann et v. Gaudecker (1969) change de largeur suivant la densité électronique du granule. Dans les granules neurosécrétoires vidés elle atteint une largeur maximale, les trois couches étant considérablement dissociées et nettement exprimées. Nous estimons que c'est un signe de la participation active de la membrane élémentaire du granule neurosécrétoire aux processus de libération des neuro-hormones.

Nos observations montrent qu'à la fin de l'épuisement du «matériel osmiophile» du granule, sa membrane élémentaire se déchire précisément aux endroits où la dissociation de ses trois couches est la plus marquée. En même temps les membranes restantes des granules se désintègrent et se présentent sous forme sans structure déterminée. Il est possible q'une partie des produits de la désintégration sous un aspect moléculaire serait inclue de nouveau dans le métabolisme du neuron.

## Bibliographie

Acher, R., Chauvet, J., Olivry, G.: Sur l'existence éventuelle d'une hormone unique neurohypophysaire. I. Relations entre l'ocytocine, la vasopressine et la protéine de van Dyk- extraites de la neurohypophyse du boeuf. Biochim. biophys. Acta (Amst.) 22, 421–427 (1956).

Bargmann, W., Gaudecker, Br. v.: Über die Ultrastructur neurosekretorischer Elementar granula. Z. Zellforsch. 96, 495–504 (1969).

— Knoop, A.: Elektronenmikroskopische Beobachtungen an der Neurohypophyse. Z. Zellforsch. 46, 242–251 (1957).

BARRY, J.: Recherches morphologiques et expérimentales sur la glande diencéphalique de l'appareil hypothalamo-hypophysaire. Ann. sci. Univ. Besançon, 2ème sér. Zool et Physiol. **15**, 3–185 (1961).

— COTTE, G.: Etude préliminaire au microscope électronique de l'éminence médiane du cobaye. Z. Zellforsch. **53**, 714–724 (1961).

DONEV, ST.: Différenciation fonctionnelle de l'appareil hypothalamo-neurohypophysaire dans l'ontogénèse du cobaye et de certains mammifères. Thèse, 1969.

DYKE, H. VAN, ADAMSON, F., ENGEL, S.: Aspects of the biochemistry and physiology of the neurohypophysial hormones. Recent Progr. Hormone Res. **2**, 1–41 (1955).

HANDA, V., KUMAMOTO, T.: Studies on some properties of neurosecretory substance. Z. Zellforsch. **47**, 674–682 (1958).

HARTMANN, J. F.: Electron microscopy of the neurohypophysis in normal and histamine-treated rats. Z. Zellforsch. **48**, 291–308 (1958).

HELLER, H., LEDERIS, K.: Characteristics of isolated neurosecretory vesicles from mammalian neural lobes. Neurosecretion (H. HELLER and R. B. CLARK, eds.), p. 35–40. New York: Academic Press 1962.

KNOWLES, F. G. W.: A highly organized structure within a neurosecretory vesicle. Nature (Lond.) **185**, 710–711 (1960).

KUROSUMI, K., MATSUZAWA, T., KOBAYASHI, H., SATO, S.: On the relationship between the release of neurosecretory substance and lipid granules of pituicytes in the rat neurohypophysis. Gunma Symp. Endocrinol. **1**, 87–118 (1964).

LA BELLA, F., SANWAL, M.: Isolation of nerve endings from the posterior pituitary gland. J. Cell Biol. **25**, 179–193 (1965).

LEDERIS, K.: An electron microscopical study of the human neurohypophysis. Z. Zellforsch. **65**, 847–868 (1965).

MAZZUCA, M.: Structure fine de l'éminence médiane du Cobaye. J. Microscopie **4**, 225–238 (1965).

MILLONIG, G., MARINOZZI, V.: Fixation and embedding in electron microscopy. In: Advance in optical and electron microscopy, 2nd ed. by R. BARRER and V. P. COSSLETT, p. 251–341. London and New York: Academic Press 1968.

PALADE, G. E.: A study of fixation for electron microscop. J. exp. Med. **95**, 285 (1952).

PEASE, D. C.: Histological techniques for electron microscopy. New York and London: Academic Press 1964.

POLÉNOV, A. L.: Neurosécrétion hypothalamique. Léningrad: A. N. URSS, éd. «Nauka» 1968.

REYNOLDS, E. S.: The use of lead citrate at high pH as an electron-opaque stain in electron microscopy. J. Cell Biol. **17**, 208–212 (1963).

RODRIGUEZ, E. M.: Ultrastructure of the neurohaemal region of the toad mediane eminence. Z. Zellforsch. **93**, 182–212 (1969).

SABATINI, D. D., MILLER, F., BARRNETT, R. J.: Aldehyde fixation for morphological and enzyme histochemical studies with the electron microscope. J. Histochem. Cytochem. **12**, 57 (1964).

SJÖSTRAND, F. S.: Electron microscopy of cells and tissues, vol. I, Instrumentation and techniques. New York and London: Academic Press 1967.

SLOPER, J. C.: The experimental and cytopathological investigation of neurosecretion in the hypothalamus and pituitary. In: The pituitary gland, vol. I, p. 134–239. London 1968.

WATSON, M.: Staining of tissue sections for electron microscopy with heavy metals. J. biophys. biochem. Cytol. **4**, 475–478 (1968).

WEINSTEIN, H., MALAMED, S., SACHS, H.: Isolation of vasopressin containing granules from the neurohypophysis of the dog. Biochim. biophys. Acta (Amst.) **50**, 386–389 (1961).

WITTKOWSKI, W.: Synaptische Structuren und Elementargranula in der Neurohypophyse des Meerschweinchens. Z. Zellforsch. **82**, 434–458 (1967).

# Concluding Remarks

Howard A. Bern

Department of Zoology and its Cancer Research Genetics Laboratory
University of California, Berkeley (U.S.A.)

It would be pretentious to state that I have found it easy to satisfy Professor Bargmann's request to make some concluding remarks to this rich and extensive symposium. Indeed, I have found it a most formidable task, especially in view of the diversity and quantity of material presented. In seeking a point of departure which would universally be considered virtuous, I have settled on the virtue of brevity. I shall consider only a few points which I find particularly compelling as a consequence of the discussions we have had.

We have obviously not yet made the last discovery of new neurosecretory systems and of new parts of old systems. Among invertebrates, new neurohemal organs and new neurosecretory cell groups have been recently delineated in annelids, molluscs and arthopods. In most cases, their functional significance awaits future investigation. Regarding the vertebrate brain, we have been almost overwhelmed with new tracts and new cross-connections relative to the control of neurosecretory cells involved in adenohypophysial regulation, along with possible pathways to and from the ventricular system. Slide after slide has left us with a veritable aura of fluorescence. The hypothalamists have given us a picture of great complexity, with the indication that there may be species differences of importance, along with differences among classes of vertebrates. It is obvious from the discussions and the arguments that have ensued that many questions have yet to be answered, not the least of which concerns the cells of origin of many of the aminergic fiber tracts that have been described, as well as the cells actually producing the several hypothesized hypophysiotropic hormones. One is impressed with the abundance of evidence for axo-axonic contacts in the aminergic regulation of neurosecretory neurons in both cranial and caudal neurosecretory systems of vertebrates. Electrophysiologists will have to concern themselves in the future with the implication of these multiple inputs.

Concerning electrophysiology, we have had a paucity of the valuable information we seek presented at this symposium. Yet, in addition to the studies of hypothalamic units discussed here, recent data on the electrical properties of crustacean, insect and molluscan neurosecretory cells leave us with little doubt that the neurosecretory cell is truly neuronal, validating the essence of the original definition of the neurosecretory phenomenon. Its seems possible that these special neurons may still prove to possess consistently certain unique electrical properties, such as an action potential of prolonged duration, conceivably related to the temporal features discussed early in this symposium and to the release of mediators that do not operate as in classical impulse transmission.

One can raise a question at this point as to what are the "proper" (by this I mean profitable) relations between neurosecretionists and neurophysiologists. Certainly the adherents of our multidisciplinary, phenomenologically oriented field cannot afford to become submerged in the general areas of neurobiology, but we can well afford to become temporarily immersed in them. For example, two recent neurosciences "workshops" in the U.S.A. have concerned themselves with the Trophic Functions of Neurons and with Axoplasmic Transport, both topics of vital interest to students of neurosecretion. The purpose of this comment is to underline the important input to be obtained from other neurobiologists in the resolution of some critical questions faced by neurosecretionists, especially at the cellular and subcellular levels.

We have heard some reference to the distal flow of neurosecretory material. This is a subject of recurrent interest: at the first symposium this point was debated; at the last symposium Prof. BARGMANN raised the issue of axonal transport again. But what do *we* mean by axoplasmic flow? Which flow? The classical slow one of WEISS (1–3 mm/day)? Or the fast flow of 30–60 mm/day? Or the very fast flow of 350–400 mm/day? The existence of these several flows seems well established by now. In addition, one group of neurosecretionists has proposed a flow rate of 3,000 mm/day (3–10 times faster than the fastest flow of the ordinary neurobiologist) to explain the depletion of neurosecretory material observed by them. Retrograde flow has been mentioned as a possibility at our symposium. What is the evidence for this phenomenon, in ordinary as well as in neurosecretory nerve fibers?

Obviously we shall need to concern ourselves still more with the problem of transport. Nerve endings have to be supplied with the materials they are expected to release. This problem leads us to the allied question of local axonal synthesis of neurosecretory material. Can neurosecretory endings produce neurohormone locally and even package it? Can such peptidergic endings take up again their neurohormonal product, or one related to it (in analogy with this capacity of aminergic endings, referred to at this meeting) and store such materials by the reconstruction of granules in situ?

The release of neurosecretory products has been considered in detail. Much time has rightly been spent worrying about how the part we want—the neurohormone—gets out of the cell; much less concern has been raised with what the disposition may be of the parts we do not want: the carrier, the granule membranes (and probably some of the internum in view of the striking new information on the infrastructure of the granule itself), the little vesicles, the ends of microtubules, the stuff that arrives as a result of axoplasmic flow. The discussion of lysosomes represents a beginning of much-needed attention to the fate of materials other than the neurohormone itself. Similarly, there has been mention of the energetics of the release process, but little reference to the energetics of the transport process: essential to the continuous availability of material to be released. The evidence for basement membranes against which neurosecretory endings abut, has been impressed upon us, but often with the implication that they may serve as barriers rather than as facilitators of movement. Small matrixless gaps may in fact be physiologically harder to cross effectively than major thicknesses of basement membrane.

We have again faced the problem of the small vesicles in neurosecretory endings, and again felt that we now understood them, only to find that our fragmentation hypothesis was at best a fragmentary explanation. We can hardly afford to disregard these prominent features of neurosecretory endings, well recognizing that we may be dealing with several different populations of vesicles. As with the problem of axonal synthesis and uptake, one can suggest that application of the ultrastructural radioautographic techniques used by Droz will be needed in order finally to resolve the important issues still with us. And I think there is real cogency to Prof. Sloper's remark to me that the use of cytochemical methods at the electron-microscope level is essential to add meaning to the suggestive morphological images we have seen. The significance of lysosomes in neurosecretory cells obviously should not be underestimated, and one may ask how one can distinguish a typical elementary neurosecretory granule from a neighboring small lysosome. We have already seen numerous examples at this symposium of the admirable ingenuity of our fellow investigators in the application of a variety of techniques to the study of neurosecretory systems, including ultraradioautography.

We obviously are limited in our information as to the chemistry of neurosecretory hormones. We know our neurohypophysial octapeptides well, but we are thoroughly confused by our neurohypophysial hypophysiotropins. At the moment we seem to know more about the nature of the amines that control release of these hypophysiotropins. Some information is becoming available for crustacean neurohormones, but for the vast majority of neurosecretory systems, little or nothing is known of the chemistry of the active agents. Fortunately, the pharmacological approach is providing us with information vital to their isolation.

The discussion of the variety of mammalian neurophysins raises the question of carrier proteins in other neurosecretory systems, both vertebrate and invertebrate. If electron-dense granules mean anything by their appearance, they are presumably telling us that such hormone-protein complexes may not be unique to the vertebrate hypothalamic neurosecretory system.

This sketchy epilogue is indeed brief and indeed inadequate. The inadequacy of the summary, however, pays a compliment to the coverage of the symposium. It will be of interest to see which of the points I have felt compelled to make appear to be of significance at the next international symposium on neurosecretion, about which I would now like to make a few comments.

In 1953, a small group of biologists of great vigor met at the Stazione Zoologica di Napoli in an atmosphere of obvious *Gemütlichkeit* to conduct the first Convegno sulla Neurosecrezione. Of this group of pioneers, an important number have faithfully attended subsequent meetings and several are here at this symposium: Wolfgang Bargmann, Francis Knowles, Valdo Mazzi, Berta Scharrer, Fred Stutinsky, Ellen and Mathias Thomsen, Gerhard Zetler. Others also have remained true to the faith but regrettably could not attend this meeting. Some have dropped by the wayside; and some few, such as Bertil Hanström, whom we commemorate at this symposium, and Ernst Scharrer, to whom the last symposium was dedicated, are lost to us forever.

It is my pleasure to announce that in 1973, four years hence, *die neurosekretorische Bahn* will take us back to Naples, in celebration of the 20th anniversary of the first symposium. Prof. Francis Knowles has indicated his willingness to head the organization of this next—the sixth—symposium, and our grateful thanks and best wishes go with him in his efforts.

Und schließlich ist es eine angenehme Pflicht, Herrn Professor BARGMANN unseren herzlichsten Dank auszudrücken für seine Mühewaltung in der Organisation dieses erfolgreichen Symposiums. Ihm und dem ganzen Personal seines Anatomischen Instituts der Christian-Albrechts-Universität — der neuen Universität im alten Kiel — gilt unsere große Dankbarkeit für die warme Gastfreundschaft und für tatkräftige Hilfe in allen unseren Nöten und Wünschen.

Vielen Dank und auf Wiedersehen!

# Participants of the V<sup>th</sup> International Symposium on Neurosecretion

ABRAHAM, M., Dr., The Hebrew University of Jerusalem, Department of Zoology, Jerusalem/Israel

BARGMANN, W., Prof., Dr., Anatomisches Institut der Universität, D-2300 Kiel/Germany, F. R.

BARRY, J., Prof., Laboratoire d'Histologie Embryologie, Faculté de Médecine et Pharmacie, Lille/France

BAUMGARTEN, H. G., Dr., Anatomisches Institut, Abt. f. Neuroanatomie, D-2000 Hamburg/Germany, F. R.

BERN, HOWARD A., Prof., University of California, Department of Zoology, Berkeley, California/U.S.A.

BJÖRKLUND, ANDERS, Dr., Institute of Anatomy and Histology, Department of Histology, Lund/Sweden

BOCK, R., Dr., Anatomisches Institut, D-5300 Bonn/Germany, F. R.

BOER, H. H., Dr., Zoologisch Laboratorium, Vrije Universiteit, Amsterdam/Netherland

BONGA, S. E. WENDELAAR, Dr., Department of Zoology, Free University, Amsterdam/Netherlands

BRAAK, H., Dr., Anatomisches Institut der Universität, D-2300 Kiel/Germany, F. R.

BUDTZ, POVL E., Dr., Zoophysiological Laboratory A, The University of Copenhagen/Denmark

BURLET, C., Dr., Faculté de Médecine, Laboratoire d'Histologie, Nancy/France

DEKKER, RONALD A. F., Dr., Instituut voor Histologie en Microscopische Anatomie, Antwerpen/Belgium

DELLMANN, H.-D., Prof., Dr., University of Missouri, School of Veterinary Medicine, Columbia/U.S.A.

DONEV, ST., Dr., Institut d'Histologie et d'Embryologie, Sofia/Bulgaria

DOUGLAS, W. W., Prof., Department of Pharmacology, Yale University Medical School, New Haven, Connecticut/U.S.A.

DUVE, Dr., Copenhagen/Denmark

DYBALL, R. E. J., Dr., Department of Anatomy, The Medical School, Bristol/England

EGGENA, Dr., Copenhagen/Denmark

ETKIN, WILLIAM, Prof., Dr., Albert Einstein College of Medicine, Department of Anatomy, Bronx, N.Y./U.S.A.

FISCHER, ALBRECHT, Dr., Zoologisches Institut der Universität, D-5000 Köln/Germany, F. R.

FLAMENT-DURAND, JACQUELINE, Dr., Faculté de Médecine et de Pharmacie, Université Libre de Bruxelles/Belgium

FLEISCHHAUER, K., Prof., Dr., Anatomisches Institut, D-5300 Bonn/Germany, F. R.

FOLLENIUS, E., Prof., Faculté de Sciences, Laboratoire de Zoologie et d'Embryologie Expérimentale, Strasbourg/France

FUXE, KJELL, Prof., Karolinska Institutet, Department of Histology, Stockholm/Sweden

v. GAUDECKER, BRITA, Dr., Anatomisches Institut der Universität, D-2300 Kiel/Germany, F. R.

GOMARD, INGER MARIE, Dr., Institute of General Zoology, Copenhagen/Denmark

GOOS, H. J. T., Dr., Zoölogisch Laboratorium der Rijksuniversiteit, Utrecht/Netherlands

GOSLAR, H. G., Prof., Dr., Anatomisches Institut, D-5300 Bonn/Germany, F. R.

HAASE, EBERHARD, Dr., Institut für Haustierkunde, D-2300 Kiel/Germany, F. R.

HAUG, H., Prof., Dr., Anatomisches Institut der Universität, D-2300 Kiel/Germany, F. R.

v. HEHN, GERTRUD, Dr., Anatomisches Institut der Universität, D-2300 Kiel/Germany, F. R.

HELLER, H., Prof., Dr., Department of Pharmacology, The Medical School, Bristol/England

HÖKFELT, TOMAS, Dr., Karolinska Institutet, Department of Histology, Stockholm/Sweden

HØJAGER, BIRGITTE, Dr., Kopenhagen/Denmark

HOLMES, R. L., Prof., Department of Anatomy, The School of Medicine, Leeds/England

HOPE, DEREK B., Dr., University Department of Pharmacology, Oxford/England

JONGKIND, J. F., Dr., Netherlands Central Institute for Brain Research, Amsterdam/Netherlands

VAN DE KAMER, J. C., Prof., Dr., Zoölogisch Laboratorium der Rijksuniversiteit, Utrecht/Netherlands

KAPPERS, J. ARIËNS, Prof., Dr., Netherlands Central Institute for Brain Research, Amsterdam/Netherlands

KNOWLES, Sir FRANCIS, Prof., University of London King's College, Department of Anatomy, London/England

KORDON, CLAUDE, Dr., Collège de France, Laboratoire d'Histophysiologie, Paris/France

KRATZSCH, ERWIN, Dr., Frauenklinik der Freien Universität Berlin, Klinikum Steglitz, Hindenburgdamm 30, D-1000 Berlin 45/Germany

KRSULOVIC, JUAN, Dr., Zoologisches Institut der Karl Marx-Universität, Leipzig/Germany DDR

LEDERIS, KARL, Prof., Dr., Division of Pharmacology and Therapeutics, Faculty of Medicine, University of Calgary, Calgary 44, Alberta/Canada

LEONHARDT, HELMUT, Prof., Dr., I. Anatomisches Institut, D-6650 Homburg (Saar)/Germany, F. R.

LINDNER, E., Prof., Dr., Anatomisches Institut der Universität, D-2300 Kiel/Germany, F. R.

MARTINET, JACK, Dr., Laboratoire de Physiologie de la Lactation, Jouy-en-Josas/France

MAZZI, V., Prof., Istituto di Anatomia Comparata, Università di Torino, Torino/Italy

MEURLING, PATRICK, Dr., Zoological Institute, University of Lund, Lund/Sweden

MÜLLER, EUGENIO E., Dr., Department of Pharmacology School of Pharmacy, University of Pavia, Pavia/Italy

NOLTE, ANGELA, Prof., Dr., Zoologisches Institut, D-4400 Münster/Germany, F. R.

NORMANN, TOM CHRISTIAN, Dr., Institute of General Zoology, Copenhagen/Denmark

NOTENBOOM, C. D., Dr., Zoölogisch Laboratorium der Rijskuniversiteit, Utrecht/Netherlands

ÖZTAN, NEZIHE, Dr., Department of General Zoology, Faculty of Sciences, Istanbul/Turkey

OKSCHE, A., Prof., Dr., Anatomisches Institut, D-6300 Giessen/Germany, F. R.

OEHMKE, H. J., Dr., Anatomisches Institut, D-6300 Giessen/Germany, F. R.

OLIVEREAU, MADELEINE, Dr., Institut Océanographique, Paris/France

PAULSEN, FREDRIK, Dr., Ferring AB, Malmö/Sweden

PEHLEMANN, F.-W., Dr., Anatomisches Institut der Universität, D-2300 Kiel/Germany, F. R.

PETER, RICHARD E., Dr., University of Washington, Department of Zoology, Seattle, Washington/U.S.A.

PEUTE, J., Dr., Zoölogisch Laboratorium der Rijksuniversiteit, Utrecht/Netherlands

PFOCH, M., Dr., Anatomisches Institut der Universität, D-2300 Kiel/Germany, F. R.

PICARD, DOMINIQUE, Prof., Dr., Institut d'Histologie, Faculté de Médecine, Marseille/France

PILGRIM, CH., Dr., Anatomisches Institut, D-8700 Würzburg/Germany, F. R.

PRENTØ, POUL, Dr., Institute of General Zoology, Copenhagen/Denmark

RINNE, U. K., Prof., Dr., University of Turku, Department of Neurology, Turku/Finland

RODRÍGUEZ, E. M., Dr., Instituto de Histologia, Facultad de Ciencias Médicas, U.N.C., Casilla de Coneo 56, Mendoza, Argentinia.

SHARP, PETER J., Dr., Department of Zoology, Leeds/England

SLOPER, J. C., Prof., Dr., Charing Cross Hospital Med. School, Dept. of Experimental Pathology, London/England

SCHARRER, BERTA, Prof., Dr., Albert Einstein College of Medicine, Yeshiva University, Dept. of Anatomy, Bronx, N.Y./U.S.A.

SCHIEBLER, T. H., Prof., Dr., Anatomisches Institut, D-8700 Würzburg/Germany, F. R.

SCHNEIDER, H. P. G., Dr., Frauenklinik der Medizinisch-Naturwiss. Hochschule, D-7900 Ulm/Germany, F. R.

STAEMMLER, H.-J., Prof., Dr., Städtische Frauenklinik, D-6700 Ludwigshafen/Germany, F. R.

STENEVI, ULF, Dr., Institute of Anatomy and Histology, Lund/Sweden

STERBA, G., Prof., Dr., Zoologisches Institut der Karl Marx-Universität, Leipzig/Germany DDR

STUTINSKY, F., Prof., Dr., Institut de Physiologie et de Chimie Biologique, Laboratoire de Physiologie Générale, Strasbourg/France

THOMSEN, ELLEN, Prof., Dr., Institut for alm. Zoologi, v. Københavns Universitet, Universitetsparken 15, Copenhagen/Denmark

THOMSEN, M., Prof., Dr., Institut for alm. Zoologi, v. Københavns Universitet, Universitetsparken 15, Copenhagen/Denmark

THORN, NIELS A., Prof., Universitetets Medicinsk-Fysiologiske Institut C, Copenhagen/Denmark

UTTENTHAL, L. O., Dr., University Department of Pharmacology, Oxford/England

UHLMANN, K., Dr., Anatomisches Institut der Universität, D-2300 Kiel/Germany, F. R.

VIGH, B., Dr., Histologisch-Embryologisches Institut Medizinische Universität, Tüzoltó-u. 58, Budapest IX/Hungary

VIGH-TEICHMANN, INGEBORG, Dr., Histologisch-Embryologisches Institut/Medizinische Universität, Tüzoltó-u. 58, Budapest IX/Hungary

VILHARDT, HANS, Dr., Universitetets Medicinsk-Fysiologiske Institut C, Copenhagen/Denmark

VOLLRATH, LUTZ, Dr., Anatomisches Institut der Universität, D-8700 Würzburg/Germany, F. R.

VULLINGS, H. G. B., Dr., Zoölogisch Laboratorium der Rijskuniversiteit, Utrecht/Netherlands

WARBURG, M. R., Dr., Israel Institute for Biological Research, Ness-Ziona/Israel

WEATHERHEAD, BRIAN, Dr., University of London King's College, Department of Anatomy, London/England

WEITZMAN, MARY, Dr., Albert Einstein College of Medicine, Department of Anatomy, Bronx, N.Y./U.S.A.

WELSCH, U., Dr., Anatomisches Institut der Universität, D-2300 Kiel/Germany, F. R.

WILSON, FRED E., Prof., Dr., Kansas State University, Division of Biology, Manhattan, Kansas/U.S.A.

WITTKOWSKI, WERNER, Dr., Anatomisches Institut der Universität, D-5300 Bonn/Germany, F. R.

ZETLER, G., Prof., Dr., Institut für Pharmakologie, Medizinische Akademie, D-2400 Lübeck/Germany, F. R.

ZIMMERMANN, P., Dr., Anatomisches Institut, D-6300 Giessen/Germany, F. R.